INCREDIBLE YEARS

Helping Preschool Children
with Autism (2-5 years):
Parents and Teachers as Partners

Get Into Your Child's Attention Spotlight

- Face-to-Face Joint Activity
- Physical Prompts/Guiding Hands
- Partial Modeling, Prompt, & Wait
- Descriptive Commenting
- Intentional Communication
- Visual Prompts, Pictures
- Using Sensory Games & Songs
- Social Emotional Coaching
- Pretend & Puppet Play
- Getting in Child's Spotlight
- Ignore, Redirect, Distract
- Modeling & Repetition
- Persistence Coaching
- Nonverbal Gestures & Signs
- Child-Directed Play & Imitation

The Incredible Years

INCREDIBLE YEARS®

Helping Preschool Children with Autism (2-5 years): Parents and Teachers as Partners

CAROLYN WEBSTER-STRATTON, PH.D.

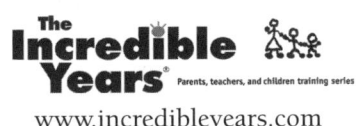

www.incredibleyears.com

Incredible Years
Helping Preschool Children with Autism (2-5 years):
Parents and Teachers as Partners

Copyright © 2021 by Carolyn Webster-Stratton. All rights reserved.

No part of this publication, as copyright herein, may be produced or used in any form or by any means including graphic, electronic or mechanical, including photocopying, recording, taping or information storage and retrieval systems, without the prior written permission of the publisher.

Book design by Janice St. Marie
Cover photos: www.istockphoto.com

Webster-Stratton, Carolyn
Incredible Years
Helping Preschool Children with Autism (2-5 years):
Parents and Teachers as Partners

Includes bibliographical references.
ISBN 978-1-892222-06-0

Publisher:
Incredible Years®, Inc.
1411 8th Avenue West
Seattle, WA 98119 USA
206-285-7565
www.incredibleyears.com

Printed in USA

*For Hudson, Amelia, Kalani, Charlie,
and all the other children,
parents, and teachers who have
taught me so much.*

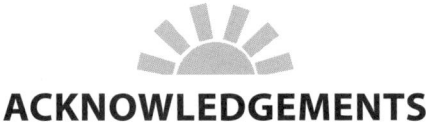

ACKNOWLEDGEMENTS

Thanks to Many Child Developmental Researchers

Many of the intervention principles, methods and ideas presented in the Incredible Years (IY) programs are the result of developmental and learning theory research that has been conducted over the past 50 years. While there are too many researchers to name everyone here, the IY interventions have a strong foundation in our understanding of the role played by early cognitive social learning theory, observational modeling, attachment, and child development theories. I am grateful for the opportunity to build on the theoretical and pioneering work by people such as Ainsworth, Bandura, Bowlby, Patterson, Piaget, and many others.

Moreover, in the past decade a great deal of research in neuroscience and autism has led to earlier recognition of children with signs of autism and the need to capitalize on brain neuroplasticity by providing intervention as soon as possible. We now understand more about how biological impairment or delays in children's social motivation, emotional sharing, joint attention, and their failure to spontaneously observe, imitate, model, or initiate behaviors with others results in a deficit of naturally occurring social learning and engagement opportunities in the social environment. These studies have resulted in more attention to the internal working of these children's minds, including cognitive and emotional dimensions. This has led to the development of more sophisticated, naturalistic, developmental and potentially more effective parenting interventions for young children on the autism spectrum. These interventions attempt to fill in children's brain deficits due to social withdrawal by helping parents and caregivers provide sensitive, responsive and scaffolded positive attention to children's internal motivations, intentional communication, and to cultivate or spotlight joint attention, beginning empathy for others, and self-initiated active learning.

These two IY video-based group-format autism parent and teacher programs build on and incorporate the empirically supported practices and core strategies I have learned from Applied Behavior Analysis (ABA) and the principles of operant conditioning (e.g, Skinner, Lovaas) as well as Pivotal Response Training (PRT) (e.g., Koegel, Schreibmann) and the Early Start Denver Model (ESDM) (e.g., Rogers, Dawson, Stern) with a focus on quality of caregiver relationships, positive affect, and responsivity. I am deeply grateful to many colleagues and autism researchers for expanding my understanding of how to help these children.

Special Thanks

Thanks to Dr. Jamila Reid, my friend and colleague, for her careful editorial review and thoughtful input regarding selection of scripts for this book. Special thanks to the Experimental Education Unit at the University of Washington, the teachers and the parents for making this program possible. Thanks to Ken Kortge for his amazing video skills capturing children's interactions with their parents and teachers which have made the program come to life. Thanks to Lisa Wallace Gloria for her help with illustrations and to Janice St. Marie for her book design. Finally, thanks to my husband John who continues to support my time and passion for this work.

CONTENTS

Acknowledgements 7
Introduction 17

CHAPTER ONE: Getting to Know Your Child   25

Signs and Characteristics of Children
  with autism spectrum Disorder   26
Getting to Know How Your Child is Incredible   28
      Understanding How and Why Your Child Communicates   28
      Understanding Your Child's Likes and Dislikes   32
      Knowing Your Child's Play Level   33
      Setting Realistic Goals   36
Helping Others Know How Your Child is Incredible   39
To Sum Up...   41

CHAPTER TWO: Getting in Your Child's Spotlight with Child-Directed Narrated Play   43

Introduction   43
Being Child-Directed & Getting in Your Child's Spotlight   45
      Imitation and Sound Exchange Games   48
Adding Interactive Interest to Play   49
Transition to a New Interactive Activity   51
Waiting for Your Child to Indicate Choice   53
      Pause to Wait for a Response from Child   54
Getting in Your Child's Spotlight by Following
  Your Child's Lead and Directions   56
      Face-to-Face Positioning   58
      Descriptive Commenting and Prompting   58
Imitation and Face-to-Face Play Interaction Games
  to Turn on Your Child's Voice   59
      Value of Imitation   62
Encouraging Verbal and Nonverbal Communication   62
      Wait and Direct Spotlight on Response   65
Prompt, Model, Gesture, and Imitate Language in Play   66
      Gentle Intrusions   69
      When not to Follow Your Child's Lead   70

Use Visual Prompts and Gestures As a Way for Less Verbal Children
to Indicate Choice or Request for Play Activity   71
    Teaching Children How to Use Picture Prompts   72
    How Many Objects or Pictures Can Be Put
      on a Choice Board?   74
    The "No" Visual Signal   75
    Helping Children to Say No   75
Using Sequenced Visual Prompts to Help Children
    Broaden their Play Activities   75
Spotlighting: Tips to Using Visual Prompts for Promoting
  Child-Directed Play Choices   79
Father Reflections about Being Child-Directed   81
Mother Reflections about Being Child-Directed   81
Teacher Reflections about Using Visual Prompts   81
To Sum Up...   82
Spotlighting: Getting in Your Child's Attention Spotlight
  During Play and Other Activities   83

CHAPTER THREE: Descriptive Commenting and Coaching Promotes Language Development   85

Introduction   85
Using Descriptive Commenting To Turn On Your Child's Voice   87
For Children with Less Language Model and Imitate
  Simple Sounds   88
Gesturing   89
Naming Objects and Actions When Using Request Gestures   90
Using the "One-Up" Rules for Expanding Language   90
Descriptive Commenting and Visual Prompts
  to Build Language   91
Spotlighting: Child-Directed Coached Play for Children
  with Limited Language   93
Pre-academic Coaching Promotes School Readiness Skills   94
Incorporating Pre-Academic Coaching into a Game   94
Teachers and Parents Checklist: Descriptive Commenting   95
Pre-academic Coaching Combined with
  Persistence Coaching   98

Spotlighting: Pre-Academic Coaching Promotes
   Children's Language Skills   100
E-Care Encourages Language and Reading Readiness   101
Spotlighting: Coaching Children's Reading Readiness
   with Extra-Care   107
Parent Reflections with Descriptive Commenting
and Pre-academic Coaching   108
Persistence Coaching   108
Persistence Coaching For a Child with More Language   109
Persistence Coaching for a Child with Less Language   111
Parent Reflections on Persistence Coaching   113
To Sum Up...   113
Spotlighting: Persistence Coaching Promotes
   Children's School Readiness Skills   114
Teachers and Parents Checklist: Preacademic
   and Persistence Coaching   115

**CHAPTER FOUR: Turing Up the Spotlight
on Your Child's Social Skills**   **117**

Introduction   117
Six Steps to Using the ABCs to Set Up Social
   Learning Opportunities   118
Getting in Your Child's Attention Spotlight with ABC   125
      Helping Your Child Learn to Make Requests   126
Engaging Your Child with Songs, Gestures,
   and Teaching Turn Taking   128
Making the Most of Music   131
Spotlighting: Connect with Your Child through Music   133
Coaching Turn Taking and Sharing   134
Spotlighting: One-on-One Parent-Child Coaching   136
Prompting Waiting, Asking, and Turn Taking   137
Encouraging Sharing and Noticing Others   140
Coaching Sibling Play   142
Spotlighting: Prompting Your Child's Social Awareness   144
Reading as a Joint Social Activity to Promote Social Skills   145

Using Sensory Physical Activities to Increase
  Social Interactions   148
Back and Forth Sensory Activities "I'm going to get you"   151
Mother Reflections about Sensory Routines   152
Spotlighting: Using Fun Sensory Physical Routines
  to Motivate Social Interactions   153
Face to Face and Joint Attention During Snack Time   154
Prompting Sharing, Helping, Verbal Responses, and Asking   156
Managing Children's Anxiety and Promoting Independence   160
Coaching to Foster Independence in Everyday Activities   162
Social Coaching During Mealtimes   164
Using Visual Prompts to Help Children Know How
  to Participate in Social Interactions   166
Parent Reflections about Social Coaching   168
To Sum Up...   169
Checklist: Teachers and Parents Social Skills Coaching   171

CHAPTER FIVE: Emotion Coaching Promotes Emotional Literacy—Spotlight Your Child's Feelings   173

Introduction   173
Modeling, Naming, and Prompting Emotion Language   174
Using Visual Prompts to Teach Your Child Emotion Words   177
Some Tips for Using and Making Feeling Pictures Prompts
  to Help Your Child Understand Feelings   179
Spotlight: Feeling Activities   180
Reading to Build Emotional Literacy   180
Combining Emotion Coaching with Physical
  Sensory Routines   184
Responding to Children's Unpleasant Emotions   186
Helping Children Learn that Unpleasant Emotions Change   188
Linking Helping Social Behavior to Feelings   189
Parent Reflections on Emotion Coaching   191
To Sum Up...   192
Spotlighting: Emotion Coaching   192
Checklist: Teachers and Parents Emotion Coaching   193

CHAPTER SIX: Using Pretend Play to Spotlight Empathy and Social Skills — 195

Introduction   195
Puppet Models and Prompts your Child's Social Skills   197
Puppet Models or Names Emotion and Prompts
  Beginning Empathy   199
Tailoring Your Puppet's Language   200
Parent Role   200
Using the Wally's Detective Books for Solving Problems
  at Home and at School   201
Using Pretend Play to Teach Helping Behavior   202
Using Pretend Play to Model and Teach Friendship Skills   204
Increasing Your Child's Symbolic Play Skills   205
Using Pretend Puppet Play to Promote Social Skills   208
Using Puppets to Promote Empathy   210
Using Puppets to Promote Empathy & Friendship Skills   214
Parent Self Reflections—Using Pretend Play   217
To Sum Up...   218
Spotlighting: Getting in Your Child's Spotlight with Pretend Play   219

Chapter Seven: Spotlighting Your Children's Emotion Self-Regulation Skills — 221

Introduction   221
Teaching Beginning Self-Regulation Skills—Breathing   222
Using the Calm Down Thermometer Visual Poster
  to Teach Calm Down Breathing   225
Visualizations: Using a Happy Thought or Memory Visualization
  to Calm Down   227
Using Puppets to Help Your Child Learn
  Self-Regulation Skills   230
Staying Patient and Modeling Self-Regulation Skills   232
Using Visual Prompts for Self-Regulation   233
Sample Scenarios for Teaching Your Child
  Self-Regulation Skills   234
    Tiny Turtle Explains How the
      Calm Down Thermometer Works   234
    Tiny Turtle Explains How to Calm Down   236

Parents Reflections about Promoting Children's Self-Regulation   237
To Sum Up....   238
Spotlighting: Building Children's Self-Regulation Skills   239

**CHAPTER EIGHT: Using Praise and Rewards
to Motivate Children**   **241**

Introduction   241
Face-to-face Praise   242
Praising Gentle Behavior—Labeled Praise   243
Rewarding Self-Regulation Practice with Sensory Activity   246
Motivating Children   248
Using Picture Prompts of Rewards   251
Encouraging Your Children to Praise Themselves and Others   252
Taking Care Of and Rewarding Yourself   254
Parent Reflections—Using Praise and Rewards   257
To Sum Up...   257
Spotlighting: Praising and Rewarding Your Child   258

**CHAPTER NINE: Spotlighting Your Limit Setting
and Managing Misbehavior**   **261**

Introduction   261
Positive Reminders   262
Transition Warnings   266
Using Picture Schedules to Help Children Understand Requests,
   Know What is Expected, and to Encourage More Independence   268
Mini Picture Scheduled   268
     Whole Day Schedules   270
     Household or Classroom Rules   271
Clear Limit Setting & Follow Through   272
Using Visual Prompt Cards to Help Your Child
   Understand Your Request/Instruction   276
Household Jobs   277
Spotlighting: Teaching Children to Understand and Follow
   Commands/ Requests   278
Requiring a Response   279

Waiting for a Response   281
Using Distractions   282
Managing Misbehavior   284
Effective Ignoring   288
Re-engaging and New Learning Opportunities   289
Limit Setting and Redirecting   292
Ignoring and Attending   294
Coping with Tantrums   295
Differential Attention   297
Handling Misbehavior   299
Ignoring and Taking a Break   300
Spotlighting: Ignoring   302
Parent Reflections about Managing Misbehavior   302
To Sum Up…   303
Spotlighting: Positive Discipline Helps My Child Feel
   Loved and Secure   304

CHAPTER TEN: Promoting Children's Joint Play with Peers   307

Introduction   307
Encouraging Joint Play   309
Encouraging Social Peer Communication—Asking
   and Answering   311
Encouraging Social Peer Communication—Listening   312
Teacher-Directed Practices—Asking and Sharing   314
Using Visual Prompts to Enhance Lunch Time Language   317
Using Snack Cards to Promote Social Communication   319
Using Dramatic Play to Prompt Verbal Social Interactions   322
Getting Joint Play Started   322
Setting Up Playdates   324
Prompting and Scaffolding Joint Play   325
Promoting Verbal Expression of Ideas   327
Modeling and Spotlighting Intentional Communication
   to Promote Sharing   330
Promoting Peer Communication   333
Prompting Peer Sharing and Praising   334

Coaching, Listening, Asking and Sharing   335
Coaching Waiting for a Turn   337
Promoting Cooperative Play   338
Promoting Cooperative Play   341
Using Picture Play Scripts to Promote Shared Joint Play   343
Using Picture Play Scripts to Promote Social Confidence   346
Encouraging Social Interactions with Picture Activity Scripts   346
Social Coaching on the Playground   348
Social Coaching—Asking to Play   349
Teacher Reflections about Hudson   352
Teacher Reflections about Amelia   353
To Sum it Up...   354
Spotlighting: Coaching Children's Social Peer Interactions: Model, Prompt, Coach, Imitate, Reward, and Use Intentional Communication   355
Series Summary   357

Appendix   361

Parent or Teachers Strategies Questionnaire   361
References   365

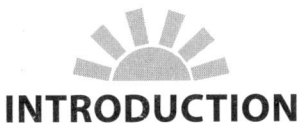

INTRODUCTION

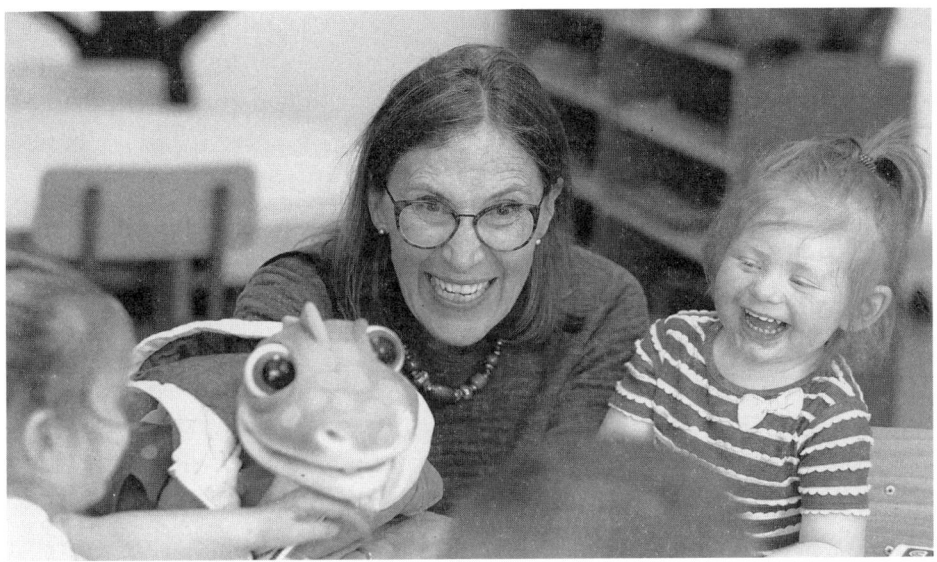

At this late stage in my career I am often asked, "What prompted you to develop the Incredible Years (IY) programs? More recently, why did you decide to develop a parent and teacher program specifically for young children on the autism spectrum? What was your motivation for the collaborative group approach and video mediated methods you used in your intervention programs versus the more traditional one-on-one therapy approach?"

As I look back now on my life journey, I confess there never was a master plan to become an academic professor or researcher, or to develop a business training others. Rather, just the opposite, my primary goal was to become a better clinician to help families and children, and I didn't want to have to charge families for providing these services (my Canadian socialized healthcare upbringing). I often explain that the growth and development of the IY programs seems to have come about because of personal experiences, a particular passion for photography and visual learning, positive research results from my first randomized control group-based video-based parent intervention program (1980), continued NIH grant support for further program development, parent and teacher feedback, and ultimately a measure of serendipity.

Forty-one years ago, I developed my first IY parenting program for parents who had children (ages 3-6 years) with behavior problems. At the time, the predominate child diagnoses for children that I worked with was oppositional defiant disorder or conduct disorder. Over the subsequent decades, I learned that this population included children who often had multiple diagnoses and developmental issues including attachment disorder, pervasive developmental disorder, attention deficit disorder, obsessive compulsive disorder, internalizing problems, depression, language delays, autism, and Asperger syndrome. Each child had a unique developmental and birth history as well as a varied family stressor history. Many children had experienced multiple childhood stressors, now known collectively as Adverse Childhood Experiences (ACEs). These stressors may have included physical and sexual abuse or neglect, poverty, severe accidents, death of a parent or important relationship figure, parental divorce, or other environmental traumatic events.

Over the years, with the generous support of National Institute of Health grants, I developed and researched what became known as the Incredible Years Series including prevention and treatment parenting programs for parents of babies, toddlers, preschoolers, and school age children. I also developed classroom management intervention programs for teachers of young children as well as a social emotional curricula (aka Dinosaur School) to provide direct intervention or prevention programs to children in small groups or classroom settings. From my clinical experiences delivering these programs, I have learned a great deal from the parents, teachers, and children as well as the professionals who I subsequently trained to deliver these IY evidence-based programs. Together they all have been the inspiration and fuel that continues to provide me with insights about what approaches work or don't work in each particular situation and how IY intervention program principles can be tailored to meet participants' goals and child development needs. I have watched with delight as parents fall in love with their children again, feel more competent and empowered about their nurturing parenting approaches, and develop their personal support networks. Additionally, I have rejoiced seeing teachers being supported by other teachers and realizing how crucial they are to the eventual success of their students' social, emotional, and academic development. It has been a privilege to be part of supporting these parent-teacher partnerships leading to children's optimal development.

My interest in autism came about because approximately 10-15% of the children who originally came to my University of Washington parenting clinic with the diagnoses of Oppositional Defiant Disorder (ODD) and language delays displayed behaviors that would likely have led to an autism spectrum disorder (ASD) diagnosis if they were assessed today. While these families seemed to benefit from the Basic IY parenting program with its focus on child-directed play, social and emotion coaching methods, and group support, I was prompted to adapt the Basic parent program further for this population of children on the autism spectrum ages 2-5 years.

In particular, two personal experiences led to my decision to develop the Incredible Years Autism Program for Parents and Teachers. The first inspiration came from some parents whose children had ASD and who attended one of my IY Parent Programs. While this program was not specifically intended for parents of children with ASD, working with these families taught me a lot about their goals and concerns for how to connect with their children in ways that would support their development of language, social, and emotional regulation skills. At the end of this training program, I asked them for evaluations and while they said they learned a lot from the program, they reported they would have liked to see videos of children more like their own children with autism. I responded spontaneously by saying, "would anyone be interested in being videotaped with their children to make some video examples?" To my surprise, several of the families volunteered for this, saying they would like to support other parents who had children with ASD by doing this. I am so indebted to the parents of Hudson, Amelia, and Kalani for inspiring me to make these videos and for their incredible parenting skills. The modeling they provide in the program videos continues to help many other parents and teachers. This program wouldn't exist without them!

My second inspiration came from a child who was attending a small group child dinosaur treatment program I was evaluating for children diagnosed with ADHD ages 4-6 years. One of the six boys in the group who also was diagnosed as having autism was completely dysregulated by the energy, volatility, and noise of the child group. Instead of benefitting from the group like the other children, his behavior became increasingly dysregulated, and he alternated between complete withdrawal and agitated, uncontrolled, and aggressive outbursts. I took him out of the group and worked with him individually, using my large life-size puppet. He was immediately engaged with the puppet and demonstrated empathic and caring behavior and language towards the puppet that I would never have imagined possible from my observations of his behavior in the child group. My puppet modeled, prompted, and taught this boy some social and language skills. Once I had established a trusting relationship with this boy, I brought in one other child for coached peer play experience. I used my puppet as a calm, prosocial, and supportive peer friend. In this safe and supportive setting with the puppet and a peer, the boy who had struggled in the group setting was able to practice the new social skills successfully. This experience prompted one of my doctoral students to pilot a small group dinosaur program just for 4 children with autism. While this was not formally evaluated, it helped me learn how we could work with children on the autism spectrum using coached child-directed play skills individually and with their peers, video vignettes, puppets, and small group practice activities.

These two experiences mobilized me to develop the autism programs for parents and teachers of children aged 2-5 years. In addition to filming Hudson, Amelia, and Kalani with their parents at home, I was also given permission to video these children and their peers in the classroom. This gave me the opportunity to see how their behavior was the same or different at school versus at home. I am so grateful to these children's teachers for their openness and willingness to be filmed in their classrooms and for the interviews they provided. These are incredibly talented teachers who provide models of child-led coached play interactions that are invaluable. Their interactions with the children help to illustrate the key behavior management principles and modeling critical to cultivating joint attention in order to promote children's language, social, and emotional development.

Thus, to answer the original question of why I did this, I would say the development of the IY autism program came about because of these personal experiences and the support, resilience, and willingness of these parents and teachers to share their successes and obstacles.

GOAL OF BOOK AND IY GROUP-BASED AUTISM PROGRAMS

Group Discussion Approach

The goal of the book is to provide parents and teachers who love and care for children on the autism spectrum with the strategies and support to help optimize these children's growth in their language, social,

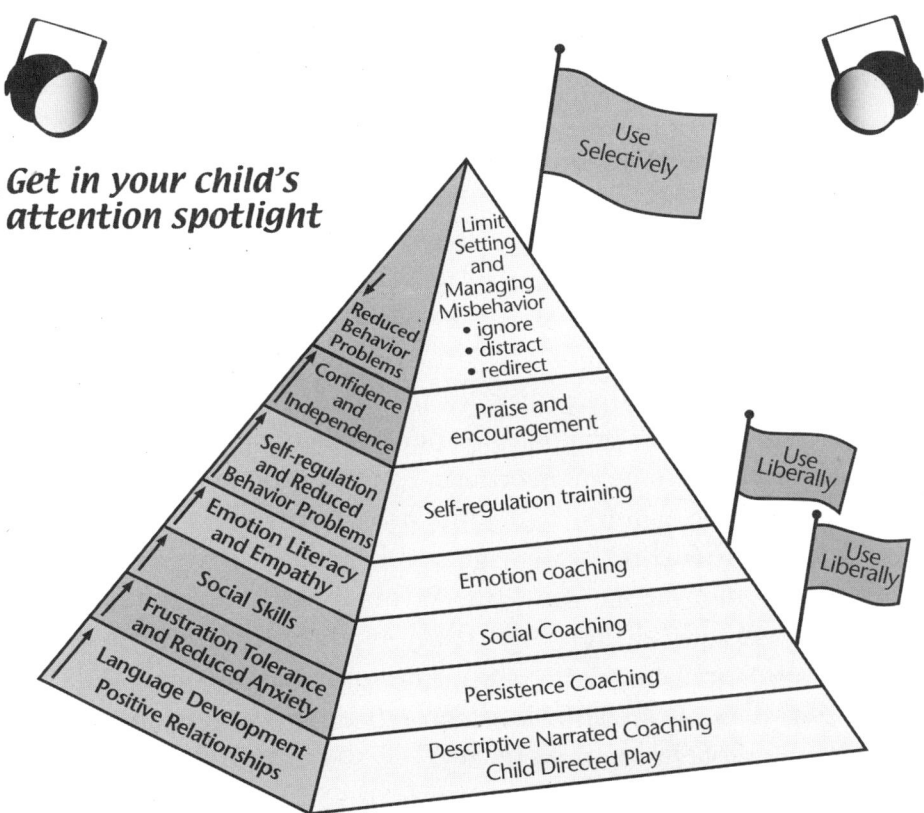

Autism Program Pyramid

and emotional development. This book is meant as a companion guide to the Incredible Years Autism Parent and Teacher group-based video training programs. The *Autism Spectrum and Language Delays Parent Program* is delivered weekly by trained IY group leaders in 14-15 two-hour sessions with 8-10 parents of children with ASD ages 2-5 years. The *Helping Preschool Children with Autism: Parents and Teachers as Partners Program* is delivered weekly in six three-hour sessions for 8-10 teachers of children with ASD. It can also be delivered to parents who have previously completed the parent autism program. The program is offered in a group format to help parents and teachers know they are not alone in their feelings, questions, and concerns about how to best promote their children's social, emotional, and language development. The group discussion approach provides support between group members and also fosters home-school connections to help parents and teachers use consistent intervention interactional approaches between home and school. Between group sessions group leaders also make home and/or classroom visits to support and provide individual coaching on parents' or teachers' use of the IY child-led interaction play and communication strategies.

Like the other Incredible Years programs, this collaborative group-based approach uses video vignette examples of parent- and teacher-child interactions to trigger discussions, problem solving, and understanding of the ABCs of child learning. It uses many of the same relationship building and attachment-based approaches and cognitive social learning principles included in the evidence-based IY parent and teacher programs for neurotypical children. It expands on this with more emphases on using visual prompts, gestures, imitation, tailored coaching, and joint attention methods to mediate and enhance the child's language level, pretend play, social skills, and emotion self-regulation skills. While a single video vignette is unlikely to exactly mirror the behaviors and goals of your specific child or student, I hope the many example scenarios here will provide a framework from which you can reflect upon, share, and discuss your own approaches with your child or student. Together with the IY group leaders and other participants in your group, you will make a plan for how your own tailored language, gestures, visual prompts, coaching, child-directed play skill principles, and joint attention spotlighting strategies will be tailored to meet your unique child's goals and positive developmental path forward.

Will this book be helpful if you are not in a group?
For those of you reading this book without the benefit of a parent or teacher support group and/or without being able to view the videos, I have provided naturally occurring scripts of the parent- and teacher-child video scenarios and have provided sample visual prompts. It is hoped that these scripts will give you ideas for how to get in your child's attention spotlight so that you can successfully communicate, model, prompt, and set up joint attention practices in your everyday activities to enhance your child's language and communication skills. I believe you can teach your child how to enjoy social exchanges with you and, eventually, expand your child's attention spotlight to include others and to benefit from these interactions.

Outcomes
As you become more confident and empowered in using these child-directed methods, you will see how your child becomes more responsive to new, naturally occurring learning opportunities in everyday activities. The change will be slow and gradual, but you can have confidence that eventually you can make an enormous difference in your child's learning and developmental outcomes. We know, from brain research conducted over the past 2 decades, that the child's brain has great plasticity in the first years of life. Parents and teachers have the potential to scaffold or shape the child's brain architecture with parent or teacher child-led, enriched interactive practice experiences that can greatly shape and enhance children's social and language development. Not only will you find that your child can overcome many of their social and language challenges but can become an engaged, motivated, and creative learner. Moreover, you will find that your feelings of frustration, stress and uncertainty are replaced with optimism and wonderment at these Incredible Years and your child's meaningful journey. Part of your pleasure will be knowing you are an incredible part of your child's successes (see references at the end of this book for studies with the IY basic and teacher programs and beginning research with this IY autism program.)

Why these Video Images?

The photographs of this book are taken from the videos used in the Incredible Years group training programs for parents and teachers with children (ages 3-4 years) on the autism spectrum and with language delays. I include these pictures in this book because parents or teachers who have attended the IY parent or teacher groups will recognize these adult-child interactions from their group discussions of the IY video vignettes. This will help you remember what you have discussed and learned from these amazing videos of parents and teachers using child-responsive spotlighted and scaffolded interactions with their children.

CHAPTER 1

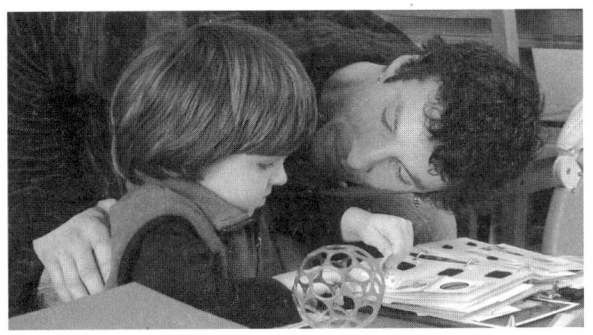

Getting to Know Your Child

Every child on the autism spectrum is unique. Autism specialists will often say if you've seen one child on the spectrum, you've seen one child, as they are all so different. The term Autism Spectrum Disorder (ASD) is used here to describe a diverse group of children who have some similar characteristics in the way they process information, communicate, and behave. Other terms may be used to describe these children such as Asperger Syndrome, Pervasive Developmental Disorder, Communication Disorder, or Language Delayed. No matter what label these children are given, they are unique individuals with their own particular strengths and special social and communication needs. Regardless of the diagnoses, the strategies discussed here are likely to help children develop their own language communication, social, and emotional potential.

SIGNS and Characteristics of Children with Autism Spectrum Disorder (ASD)

Social and emotional interaction and verbal communication is impaired with peers and adults. This may be first noticed in babies who have a delay in their babbling, recognition of their name, early use of words, or eye contact. Toddlers with ASD often have delayed language and do not seem to follow or understand simple adult commands or words. They may repeat what adults say in an echolalic way without understanding the meaning of the words. Preschoolers with ASD may show social delays, seem withdrawn from peers, have flat affect, be unaware of or uninterested in others, or show anxiety when around others. They don't readily tune into others, or imitate and learn from modeling of social interactions. Emotion words are especially hard for these children to understand. They may become easily emotionally dysregulated because they don't understand or are overwhelmed by a response from others, or because of a particular sensory sound, taste, smell, or tactile event.

Imagination, pretend play, ideas, and creativity in these children is reduced and play is unconventional. While they may be drawn to objects, they may not be adept at playing with toys in varied and typical ways. They may seem locked into obsessive and repetitive play which is solitary and copied. Attempts to add novelty or a change to this ritualistic play often causes the child to be further stressed and anxious. These children seem to enjoy the safety and predictability of the solitary and repetitive play.

Gestures and nonverbal communication are limited. Such children may not wave hello or goodbye, give eye contact, or know how to point to communicate. They do not use pointing to show something they want, or show an object to someone else, and they don't understand how to follow or "read" another person's pointing prompts. In general, they often fail to understand the meaning of other people's facial or behavioral gestures.

Narrow range of interests, routines, and repetitive behaviors. Many of these children have repetitive rituals such as flapping their arms, body rocking, spinning, finger flicking, or flipping some object around. They dislike change in routines and have difficulties with transitions.

Sensory likes and dislikes for sounds, sights, smell, touch, and movements can be peculiar. Some children seek out repetitive movements such as spinning, rocking, jumping, swinging, and running. Others may be oversensitive or fearful of certain movements or experiences such as escalators, elevators, swings, or teeter-totters. Some children seek out specific touch or sensory experiences such as being wrapped in blankets, putting objects in their mouths, or squeezing into tight spaces. Others don't like certain touch or textures such as sticky playdough, paint, certain clothing textures, getting their hair washed, or eating crunchy food. Some children crave music and certain sounds while others dislike or are overly sensitive to sounds such as the vacuum cleaner, blow dryer, or school bell. Others seek out visual sensations such as flicking lights on and off, moving fingers in front of their faces, and lining things up. Some children have sensitivity to certain tastes or smells. They may reject tastes of particular foods or foods of certain colors or textures or smells, while liking to chew or eat plastic or dirt. Many children seem under-sensitive to speech and don't respond to it but will respond to songs.

In addition to these SIGNS of autism, sleep problems are also common. It is estimated that over half of the children with ASD have a sleep problem such as difficulty falling asleep, night wakening, and reduced need for sleep. Another common medical problem experienced by children with ASD is gastrointestinal distress such as diarrhea, constipation, and abdominal pain. As noted above, feeding problems are also common among these children.

Parents and teachers of children with ASD have a wide range of feelings in response to these SIGNS of autism. Some may feel frustrated because they don't know how to connect with their children and may believe these signals are signs of a lack of attachment when their child avoids eye contact, or seems not to pay attention to them. Some parents and teachers feel rejected when children don't want to play with them or push them away. They don't understand that children withdraw because they don't know how to be part of joint play and don't understand the adult's language or instructions. All parents and teachers want to help their children to communicate and make friends, but many are unsure of how to go about this in a productive way. They lack confidence in their responses. Many parents feel a sense of loss, grief, and anxiety over the hoped for "neurotypical" or imagined child and are uncertain how to navigate and support their child's progress towards better social and emotional communication and a stronger relationship with them, other family members, and their peers. All of these feelings and reactions are normal as each parent or teacher learns how to respond to the challenges these children present. Fortunately as with any grieving process, these anxious and sad feelings will subside and are replaced with the love you will feel for your child as well as your parenting confidence in how to promote your children's optional social, emotional and language learning.

In this chapter we will start by learning how to identify each child's unique strengths as well as assess their stage of communication and play level. Understanding your child's developmental abilities and specific delays will help you know what to expect from your child and to determine what their needs and goals are. You will learn some of things that you can do to turn your everyday routines and play activities into opportunities for communication learning and joint attention as well as for building stronger attachments, joy, and confidence when interacting with your child. While children on the autism spectrum are different than neurotypical children, they are interesting, loving, observant, creative, and capable people. They can have deep and meaningful relationships with others and their way of interacting with the world is unique and valid. The goal is not to change their personalities or to make them neurotypical. Rather this book will provide ideas for ways that parents and teachers can make connections with children on the ASD spectrum, understand them better, and help them communicate and interact with the people and world around them.

GETTING TO KNOW HOW YOUR CHILD IS INCREDIBLE
Understanding How and Why Your Child Communicates

The first step is getting to know how each child is unique; that is, what we term "Incredible". This means carefully observing your child's stage of communication; how and when they communicate and the intent or why of that communication. As noted in SIGNS of autism above, most of these children have some impairments in language and social communication with peers and adults. Of course, there are many ways to communicate, through the child's nonverbal actions (reaching and pointing), facial gestures, sounds, showing pictures, and using words. The communication checklist provided here can help you to observe your child's communication and how and why it may be different in different situations. Sometimes your child's communication may be just experimenting with using their voice and practicing repeating or imitating words or sounds. They may have no intention of speaking to anyone but are just using words for the joy of it or as a self-regulation strategy. Other times, your child may be communicating with intention because they have learned that their language or gestures can influence others and can indicate wants or dislikes. Eventually, as your child's communication develops, they will learn that it can be used to get what they want, to ask questions, connect with others, and to be sociable.

The child communication checklist asks you to notice what your child does when they want something such as a food item or specific toy. Do they look at you with eye contact and point, pull your arm and drag you to the wanted object, or use sounds, a word, or multiple words in a way you can't quite understand? If you ask your child what they want, do they repeat your question without understanding what it means? If you say a word or phrase, does your child repeat it back? This known as "echolalia" and is a common feature of children with ASD. Echolalia is an early step in the development of communication. How does your child tell you they want to keep playing or conversely that they want to stop an activity? Are they able to gesture, say a word, or show a visual picture to indicate "more", "no more," or "all done"? How does your child respond when you give directions to put away the toys, put on their shoes, wear a seat belt, wash their hair, or to stop an activity and move on to something else? Do they cry or scream? Do they seem not to understand verbal language? Do they respond better to a one- or two-word request with a gesture or to a visual prompt, rather than a lengthy instruction? How do they respond when you give them a choice of what to do? Do they respond better if the choice is

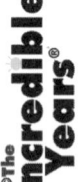

Child Communication Checklist (With Parent)
by Carolyn Webster-Stratton, PhD

Reason Child Communicates	Doesn't understand/ ignores/blank stare	Looks at parent	Protests/ Refuses/ Tantrums	Pulls parent arm/ gestures	Points/ Reacts/ Nods	Uses visual pictures	Shares/ Offers things	Makes sounds	Immediate Echoes/ copies	Delayed echoes*	Uses 1-3 words/ signs	Whole sentence/ signs
Wants something from parents (food, toy, help, play etc.)												
Wants to continue playing/reading/singing with parent												
Not getting what s/he wants												
Wants to stop activity												
Response to parent one-step direction												
Response to parent multi-step direction												
Response to parent offering choices												
Response to parent greeting (hello, bye-bye)												
Feelings expression												

*"Delayed Echoes" defined as copies from TV shows, common expressions

Child's Name: _____

Date: _____

Getting to Know Your Child   31

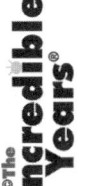

Child Communication Checklist (With Peer/Sibling)
by Carolyn Webster-Stratton, PhD

Reason Child Communicates	Doesn't understand/ ignores/blank stare	Looks at child	Protests/ Refuses/ Tantrums	Pulls child's arm/ gestures	Points/ Reacts/ Nods	Uses visual pictures	Shares/ Offers things	Makes sounds	Immediate Echoes/ copies	Delayed echoes*	Uses 1-3 words/ signs	Whole sentence/ signs
Wants something from peers (food, toy, help, play etc.)												
Wants to continue playing/reading/singing with peer												
Not getting what s/he wants												
Wants to stop activity												
Response to peer request												
Response to peer initiation												
Response to peer greeting												
Feelings expression												

Child's Name: _____

Date: _____

*"Delayed Echoes" defined as copies from TV shows, common expressions

paired with gestures, eye contract, or saying the word of the activity? How does your child communicate feelings to you? Do you know when they are sad, unhappy, anxious, happy, calm, or excited? Do they show signs that they understand how others feel? How is their verbal and nonverbal communication different with you compared with siblings, peers, or with other adults?

The first communication checklist is for you to assess how your child communicates with you and the second one is for how they communicate with peers. These responses in the two contexts can be quite different. Observing how your child communicates with you and with others will help you build on their strengths and identify communication goals. It will help identify forms of communication that are easier and less frustrating for your child as well as point you in the direction of a next logical communication step to teach. For example, learning to say "no" or shaking head and gesturing "no", rather than throwing a tantrum. In other cases, it may be more effective for your child to use a picture prompt to request something they want rather than pulling your arm in a struggle. Parents and teachers will also learn more effective ways to communicate a request such as through gestures, modeling, picture prompts, and specific words. Start by observing your child and completing this communication checklist to understand how and why your child communicates the way they do in different situations with you or with peers.

Understanding Your Child's Likes and Dislikes

Another part of understanding how your child is incredible is being aware of their sensory likes and dislikes. Keeping track of your child's sensory preferences: that is, what sensations your child seeks out and which ones they avoid is important because it will make it easier for you to understand your child's behavior and to know ways you can promote, motivate, and prompt your child to practice certain nonverbal and verbal communication. Some children make it clear what they like and dislike. For others it can be more difficult to discern. Observing what your child does repeatedly is a good tip for knowing his preferences. For example, does your child love physical sensory movement such as running back and forth, jumping on a trampoline, or being spun around?

Do they enjoying crawling into small, tight spaces, or being wrapped cocoon-like in a blanket? Do they like to flap their arms, put objects in their mouth, smell or lick objects, listen to music and particular songs, or line things up? In addition, make a list of your child's dislikes. What causes them to get upset or have a meltdown? For example, is your child oversensitive to physical sensations such as sticky things on their hands, the texture of certain clothing, having shampoo put on their heads, or sitting on the toilet seat? Are they oversensitive to certain sounds such as the toilet flushing, the vacuum being turned on, the school bell, or certain music? Do they dislike certain tastes or smells such as fish, spicy food, the smell of perfume, or frying food?

On the lists on the following pages, write in your child's auditory, visual, tactile, smell, oral, and physical proprioception (awareness of the position and movement of the body) sensory likes and dislikes. These preferences are what we will call the "motivating antecedents", the "A" in the ABC child learning sequence. When communicating with your child by using one of their likes, you may find your child can pay attention longer and you can prompt practice of a desirable behavior because it is more motivating. Similarly, you may use your child's wish to avoid a disliked item or event to prompt and teach them to communicate the request to stop or take it away. This Antecedent (A), behavior (B) and consequences (C) sequence for prompting target behaviors will be discussed in more depth in the upcoming chapters.

Knowing Your Child's Play Level

The next aspect of knowing how your child is incredible is observing their play developmental level. Play for these children often is described as unconventional. Usually this means the child's play is repetitive, ritualistic, and solitary without the typical interest in a variety of objects. The child may seem unaware of or uninterested in what other children are doing in play and may be obsessive in their exploration of the toy they are playing with. The child may not understand pretend play or how puzzles work. Neurotypical toddlers will continue to develop their play skills as they learn how to use play in a functional way; that is, realizing that Legos can be put together to make something. As they become aware of other children and what they are making with Legos, they often

BRAINSTORM/BUZZ
Sensory Likes

Write down your child's sensory likes in each of the sensory categories listed below.

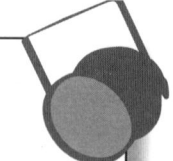

Auditory

Visual

Tactile

Smell

Taste/oral (chewing/sucking)

Proprioception (body space/balance/ need for movement/stillness)

©The Incredible Years®

BRAINSTORM/BUZZ
Sensory Dislikes

Write down your child's sensory dislikes in each of the sensory categories listed below.

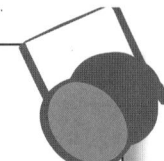

Auditory

Visual

Tactile

Smell

Taste/oral (chewing/sucking)

Proprioception (body space/balance/ need for movement/stillness)

copy and imitate what others are doing. Eventually they understand that they can play with a specific goal in mind such as to build a castle, tower, or dinosaur and become interested in involving other children in such projects. Around age three, most neurotypical children begin to engage in symbolic or pretend play. Through the use of puppets or characters, they begin to imagine themselves as someone else and to take their perspective. Developmentally, this pretend play helps children develop a sense of empathy for other viewpoints and more interest in playing with others. Finally, neurotypical children move from this "preoperational" phase of cognitive development (ages 3-5 years) to a more concrete thinking phase and eventually become obsessed with games following the rules of play. They will be upset if others break the rules.

Children on the autism spectrum may be stuck in any of these early play levels and are frequently delayed in joint play and pretend play. Because they avoid playing with other children and may be anxious about how to initiate play with others, they are often alone in solitary play. This means they are not watching peers and learning how to play by observing, imitating, or interacting with others. Understanding whether and how your child is delayed in play will help you set realistic goals for their play.

Setting Realistic Goals

Based on your understanding of your child's communication, play levels, and likes and dislikes, you will be able to set incremental realistic goals for your child. As you work with your child, continually re-evaluate, assess the barriers to reaching those goals, and problem solve how to overcome those obstacles. Set new goals as you learn what works to gain your child's attention and interest in learning.

The Incredible Years Autism Video-based Parent and Teacher Programs were designed for small groups of parents and teachers to meet with trained group leaders to discuss strategies to promote children's language, social, and emotional development. This program features video vignettes of a number of children with ASD. Among these children, three are shown more frequently: Kalani, Hudson, and Amelia. Here is a brief description of each of these children and their parents' goals. (See appendix for sample *How I am Incredible* forms)

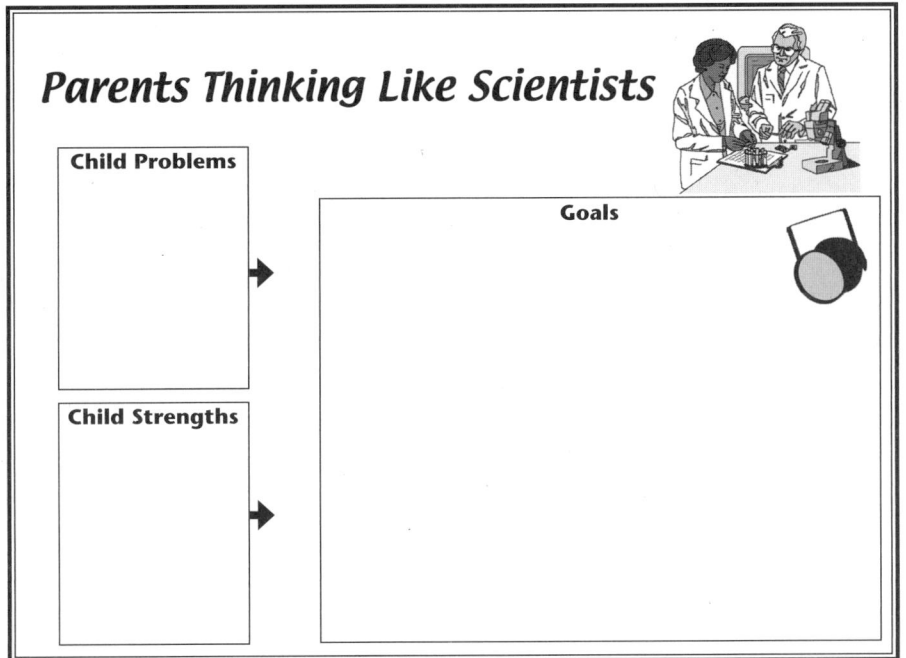

Kalani (42 months old): This boy makes sounds but has very few intelligible words. He understands words; that is, his receptive language is good, but he has difficulty saying words (expressive language). He plays alone and interacts with his parent briefly, smiles at times, and rarely interacts with his sibling or peers unless prompted by his parent. He likes play with songs, books, and functional stacking toys.

His mother's goal is to help him use more nonverbal gestures and signals to communicate his preferences and needs to others and to interact more with his 9-month-old baby sister.

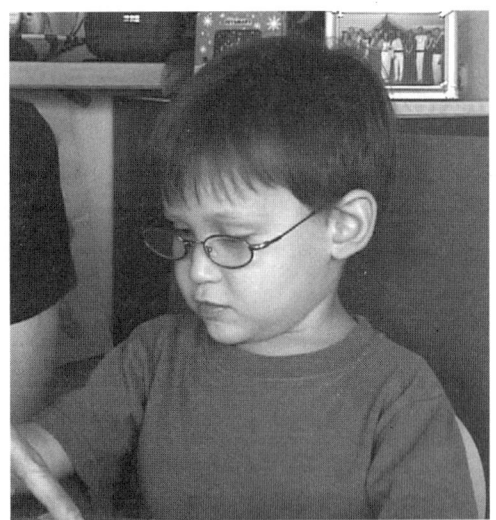

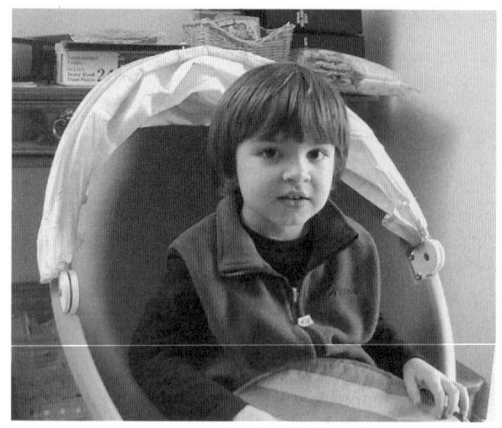

Hudson (46 months old): This boy uses 2-3 words to communicate when he wants something, echoes parents' 3-6 word sentences or questions, uses some visuals to make requests or pulls his parent's arm, and communicates with longer sentences with his parent when prompted with his favorite activities. At school he is anxious and withdraws from any contact with peers. He distances himself from other children physically, by sitting in the corner. He avoids eye contact with adults and peers. His favorite play includes spinning or chase games with his parents, and he enjoys some emerging pretend play with puppets with his father. He flaps his arms when excited and throws tantrums when he doesn't get what he wants or has to stop spinning.

The parents' goal is to promote more verbal language with eye contact, teach Hudson to request something with words, engage in more verbal back and forth communication, and learn how to calm himself down when dysregulated.

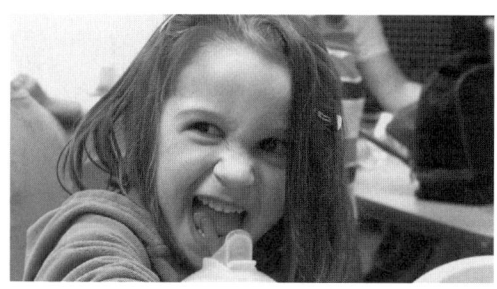

Amelia (46 months old): This girl has 5-6 word sentences, a rich vocabulary, is able to make requests and indicate choices verbally. She asks her parent questions and understands language. She likes play that involves running in circles, jumping on pillows or on her trampoline, tickling, and turn taking games. She enjoys pretend games with puppets where she shows some beginning empathy. She spins a long leaf-like plant frequently and, when prompted, has social skills such as turn taking and sharing in play interactions with her parent. However, at preschool she is more anxious, avoids initiating social interactions with her peers, and will gravitate to be alone and not communicate. Nonetheless, she does seem interested in playing with others and, when coached, seems to enjoy this. She avoids fine motor activities that are difficult and her teacher says she gives up easily.

Her parents' goals are for her to engage in more joint and cooperative play with other children and to be less anxious with peers.

For the parents of these three children, as well as for most parents with children with ASD, their primary play goal is to be able to connect with their children in fun ways and help them broaden their interests and ways of communicating. By enhancing their child-directed coached play skills and getting their children to pay more attention to them, they learned how they could make their play interactions more rewarding to their children, how they could model, prompt, and teach new communication and social skills, and how they could give their child a reason to communicate with others.

This book provides real life scripts of these parent-child interactions during videoed play interactions after parents had participated in an Incredible Years Parenting program. While these children and their goals will be different than your child, it is hoped that these actual interaction scenarios might give you some ideas for how to approach your own child. All of these children do have some language, so if your child has little or no language, suggestions will be provided for ways to use gestures and visual prompts to enhance your child's ability to communicate nonverbally. Since you are the expert on your child, you will know them best and can use the approaches that enhance your ability to help your child develop their social and emotional potential.

HELPING OTHERS KNOW HOW YOUR CHILD IS INCREDIBLE

It is important for parents to let family members and friends know how their child is incredible. Here you see the "How I am incredible" house template for you to write in key things and information you would like to share with others about your child's language level, how they communicate with others, their level of play, their favourite play activities, their sensory likes and dislikes, their strengths and your goals for them. Helping other family members know these clues about your child and the meaning of their behavior can help them to support your child's developmental progress and build a relationship with your child. Your child's teacher may also complete this template about your child at school so that parents and teachers can develop a plan for mutually agreed upon goals and strategies.

How I am Incredible!

©The Incredible Years

Child's Name and Age: _____

My Support People:	My Language Level *(e.g., no spoken language, visual language, 1-2 words, echolalic, good language)*:
My Play Level *(e.g., play alone, anxious or withdrawn, want to initiate play with others but don't know how, initiate but inappropriate)*:	My Sensory Likes *(e.g., trucks, swinging, music, water play, bananas)*:
My Sensory Dislikes *(e.g., loud noises, certain smells)*:	My Parent's Goals for Me: *(e.g., make a friend, more words, follow directions)*:

©The Incredible Years®

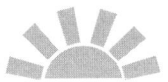

To Sum Up...

In this first chapter we have focused on ways to watch and learn how your child is incredible, that is, to understand how and why your child communicates and plays in different ways in different situations depending on who they are interacting with and what captures their attention. Observing your child using the Communication Checklist will help you identify the stage of your child's communication and what factors affect their receptive understanding of language as well as their verbal and nonverbal expression of language. This knowledge will help you gain insight into how to set realistic goals for your child and adjust your communication approach and ways of playing to help you connect and support their learning. For example, if your child is not talking, you likely will want to progress from using gestures, to using picture prompts, and then to saying a word to get what they want. If your child is talking, you may be eager for them to communicate and initiate two-way connections and interactions with yourself and others. We also talked about being aware of your child's likes and dislikes and preferences and appreciating their unique personality so that you can help others know and develop relationships with your child. Sharing this knowledge with other family members and friends will allow them to provide you with emotional support and to interact with your child in ways that are predictable, loving, and effective.

CHAPTER 2

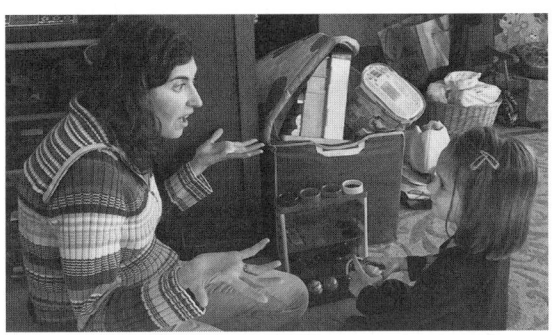

Getting in Your Child's Spotlight with Child-Directed Narrated Play

INTRODUCTION

All children benefit from child-directed play with adults because it provides them with a supportive way to learn who they are, what they can do, and how to relate to the world around them. Without parent interaction and play to stimulate growth and development, children's instinct toward creative and imaginative play and their language development will be reduced. Research indicates that even neurotypical children do not engage in positive social play with others by instinct. In fact, without some responsive, joyful parental play interactions, nurturing and coaching,

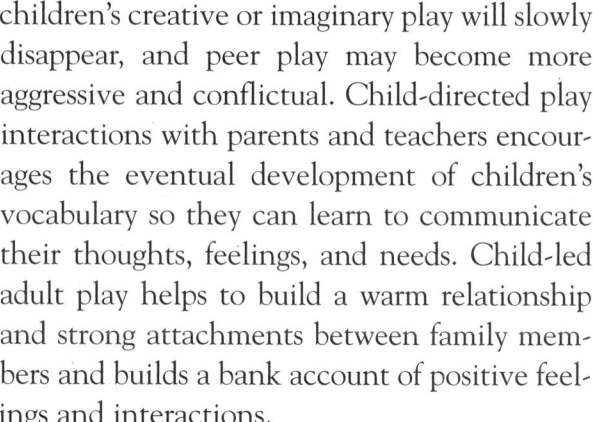

This spotlighting child-directed approach, focusing on your child's likes and choices, means your child will be more sociable and interactive with you.

children's creative or imaginary play will slowly disappear, and peer play may become more aggressive and conflictual. Child-directed play interactions with parents and teachers encourages the eventual development of children's vocabulary so they can learn to communicate their thoughts, feelings, and needs. Child-led adult play helps to build a warm relationship and strong attachments between family members and builds a bank account of positive feelings and interactions.

For children on the autism spectrum, child-led play is even more important. It is a way for parents and teachers to build a connection and a positive relationship with a child who at times seems to reject them, prefers being alone, or just does not know how to play. During play, they may not give the same positive feedback to adults that neurotypical children provide. Consequently, parents and teachers may feel unconnected with these children or worry they are doing something wrong. They may stop trying to play with their children because they believe that their play time is not worthwhile, or they may become overly directive, thus causing further withdrawal or opposition. Indeed, playing with children on the spectrum can be quite challenging! Many parents find their childs' repetitive, ritualized play to be boring, but if they try to interject a new play idea, the child may throw a tantrum or withdraw. This response discourages parents from trying to expand their child's play repertoire and reinforces their experience that playing with their child is not productive or pleasurable.

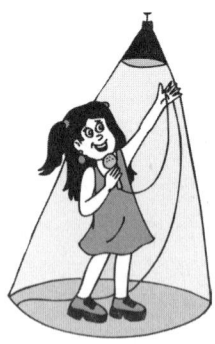

In this chapter you will see some examples of parent-child play interactions that offer pointers on how to overcome common pitfalls and barriers to playing with your child on the spectrum. You will learn how you can be more strategic in your efforts to join your child's favorite (perhaps unconventional) play activities by getting in your child's attention spotlight. You will learn how to make your joint play more rewarding, leading to benefits both for you and your child. This child-directed spotlighting approach, focusing on your child's likes and choices, means your child will be more sociable and interactive with you. Your child will learn that they can affect other people around them and don't have to redirect their focus of attention away from their desired play to what others want. In short, by entering your child's world, rather than forcing them to enter yours, you can build a stronger relationship connection. As your child becomes interested in this connection, there will be opportunities to gradually stretch and extend their spotlight to include more social and emotional communication with yourself and others.

Being Child-Directed and Getting in Your Child's Spotlight

Children on the autism spectrum are often more interested in interacting with objects than with people. They are also less able than neurotypical children to shift their attention from objects to interpersonal interactions. Since very young children's key language and social learning comes from watching, imitating, and interacting with people, one goal is to increase these children's attentional focus to others by making their play interactions with people more rewarding. Parents can do this by following their child's lead and interests and by describing their actions and what they are paying attention to. By linking your child's favorite activity to social interactions with you, your child will be more motivated to interact with you. Thus, you will be creating more opportunities for them to learn from you.

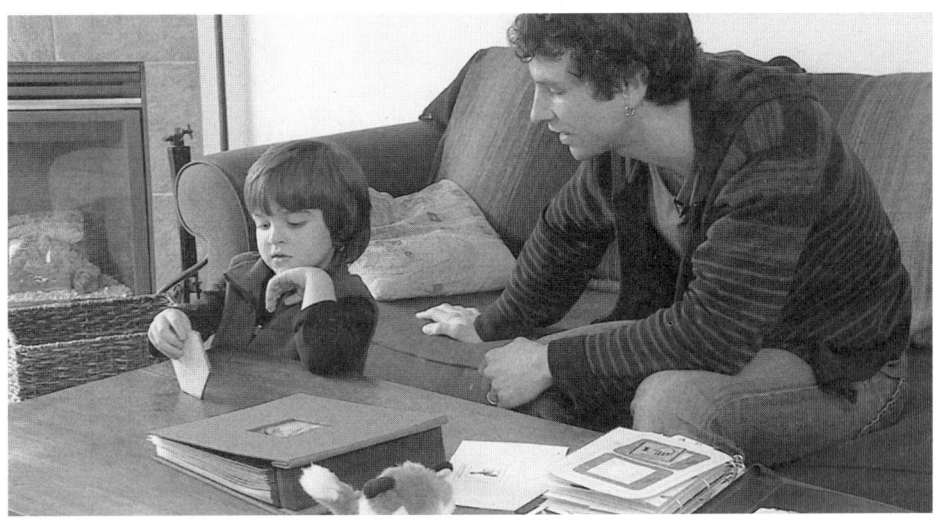

The interaction below describes how a father tries to do this with his son. In this parent-child interaction scenario, a father is playing with his almost four-year old son, Hudson, who is on the autism spectrum. Hudson is playing with two wooden hexagons on a coffee table while the father is sitting on the couch. Notice the way this father follows his son's lead and gives attention to his interests. Think about the benefits for Hudson's learning from his father's verbal narration and interactions.

Hudson: (playing with two hexagons and not looking at father)
Father: Can you say I'm excited? Say I'm excited (tickles boy's neck).
Hudson: (looks at father and continues manipulating hexagons)
Father: (enthusiastic tone) Well you are really interested in these coasters... aren't you? Hexagons, you have two hexagons. Two hexagons. Now they're stacked up. They're moving together. It's like they are hexagon friends. Oh hexagon is rolling. Rolling like a ball and fall down - CRASH!
Hudson: (rolls them off the table and they crash on floor)
Father: Oh hexagons fell off the table. Down onto the floor. One of them came back up again. Is he balancing? Looks like he is balancing!
Hudson: (not looking at his father but makes some unintelligible sounds)
Father: Yes, hexagon is balancing.(acts as if he understands)
Hudson: (drops hexagon again on floor)
Father: (delighted tone) Rolling, rolling hexagon. Oh fell down...CRASH!
Hudson: (looks up at father again with brief eye contact)

Considerations

Did you notice how the father follows and spotlights his son's attention focus and interests and describes or narrates exactly what his son is doing and feeling using rich action and emotion language words such as hexagon, balancing, rolling, and excited? He repeats the word hexagon seven times and uses the word "crash" with enthusiasm to express his delight when they fall down on the floor. Despite little eye contact or verbal response from Hudson, the father continues to use engaging, joyful, and fun language. Describing the objects the child is playing with as well as the actions of his movements increases his attention to his father's presence, motivates him to respond with some language and brief eye-contact, and consequently provides more opportunites for language connection, joint attention, and social learning.

When possible, play next to your child and imitate their play using similar play objects. See what happens below when Hudson's father tries this: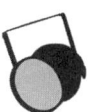

Father: (picks up two hexagon tiles and starts to imitate Hudson). I have two rolling hexagon tiles. They are rolling, rolling, rolling. Right off the table. Crash! (*imitates what Hudson did previously*)

Hudson: (looks off the table to see where his father's hexagons have landed)

Father: My hexagons crashed just like yours. Now the hexagons are going to come back up and stack up. Can they stack on top of yours? (Hudson has a hexagon on the table and his father adds another hexagon).

Hudson: (stacks another hexagon on top of his father's).

Father: You are stacking. I will stack another one too. Our hexagons are making a stack together.

Hudson: (takes the top two and starts walking them across the table).

Father: (imitates Hudson's movements). Off the stack and now the hexagons are walking together. Or, are they rolling?

Hudson: (rolls his hexagons over towards his father's).

Father: Yours are coming to see mine! Hello hexagons!

Hudson: (brief smile).

Hudson's father has stayed in Hudson's spotlight by imitating Hudson's actions. He does not try to change what Hudson is doing but instead draws attention to their joint actions by imitating him and narrating what they are both doing. He follows Hudson's lead by rolling, stacking, and then walking the hexagons as Hudson changes activities. Hudson participates briefly in stacking with his father and then moves his tiles near to his father's tiles and briefly connects with a smile! Here the idea is to imitate exactly what your child is doing and to start and stop the action at the same time as your child. After you have been imitating for a while, you could add a small variation in the action such as walking the hexagons more slowly and then perhaps changing the action altogether. For example, Hudson's father could bang the hexagons together and say "bang, bang." It can be helpful to connect your extension actions with other behaviors that are already in your child's repertoire (earlier, Hudson banged his hexagons together in response to his father's singing). Wait to see if your child imitates your action. If they do, praise your child enthusiastically, and then go back to imitating their actions. Then try again with the same extension action (bang bang). Eventually this can turn into a mutual imitation actions game.

Imitation and Sound Exchange Games: For children who say very few words and sometimes say words or sounds which are not understandable, parents can begin by imitating or echoing these sounds and encouraging expression of different sounds. One of the most effective strategies a parent can use is to respond to these vowel and consonant sounds as if they are understandable words and answer with something that sounds like what the child said. Hudson's father did that effectively. Another approach is to imitate the child's sounds and see if the child responds in a back-and-forth sound game of verbal exchange. It doesn't matter that the words or sounds don't make sense, because the child is beginning to learn about how to have a reciprocal verbal exchange. Don't worry if your child doesn't imitate your sounds back. Verbal turn taking is a new skill and it may be hard for your child to try the sound right away. Instead repeat the sound again several times and wait to see if your child will try to imitate you. Try again later. As it becomes easier for your child to make that sound,

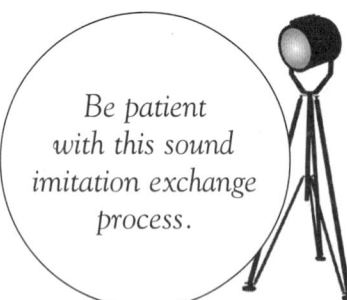

Be patient with this sound imitation exchange process.

you will get more imitations going. Be patient with this sound imitation exchange process. As your child begins to increase their vocabulary of sounds and is imitating in a reciprocal sound game with you, you can think about adding a word that is similar to the sound they are making. For example, if your child is saying the 'b' sound as you are playing with bubbles or blowing a balloon, you can say the word "balloon", "blow", or "bubble," emphasizing the "b" sound several times. Be sure not to imitate crying, screaming, or whining sounds.

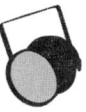

Playing this way will take a leap of faith at first. Initially your child may not respond at all and may not even seem to notice that you are there. It can be hard to maintain enthusiasm and interest and keep imitating your child without any feedback. It may take many play times before your child acknowledges your presence in some way or starts to imitate you. Indeed, it is theorized that children with ASD have decreased motivation to imitate words, gestures, or actions. This may be one of the reasons for their developmental delays, because imitation (or modeling others) is one of the most important ways that children learn. Be patient and keep trying. It's okay to keep the playtimes short (5-10 minutes at a time). You can get into your child's attention spotlight by repeatedly imitating your child's actions, gestures, and sounds. This will eventually lead to an interpersonal connection that will motivate your child to imitate you more, enjoy the interaction, and, thus, learn more from you! Most children enjoy the game of having their parents imitate them. Modeling the skill of imitation is also teaching your child how to imitate others. This provides them with a new way to learn on their own.

Adding Interactive Interest to Play

Sometimes your child's play actions will become repetitive because your child doesn't know what else to do. When this happens, and if you lose interest in what they are doing, your child will likely lose interest in the interpersonal part of the play, stop interacting with you, and

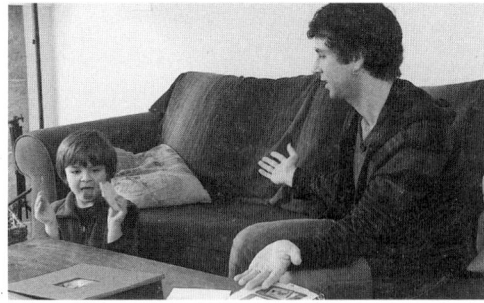

revert to safe and predictable solo play. To keep your child engaged in joint play, you can subtly add variety to the play theme. You might suggest a new color or different favorite activity, or you might change the action you are imitating slightly or add a fun sound effect. This will keep you both engaged socially in the joint activity. In the next scenario notice how the same father attempts to continue to motivate his son's interaction with him by offering a new idea for thinking about the hexagons and their actions. This results in them imitating each other. Think about the benefit of this approach for Hudson's learning.

Hudson: (finds another hexagon under table and picks it up)
Father: (narrates what Hudson is doing with hexagons) Oh there you've got two again... those hexagons are pretty fun. You can do all kinds of things with those. Now they're stacked up. One on top of the other. You're opening them. Oh they are over-lapping. These are kind of like doors. You can do like doors on the bus. These doors on the bus are hexagons. (*gestures with his hands opening and closing and sings*): "doors on the bus they open and shut, open and shut"...
Hudson: (makes hexagons go open and shut and imitates father's hand actions)
Father: Open and shut (claps hands shut when Hudson claps hexagons together and sings) doors on the bus, they open and shut. Can they go round and round like the wheels? Hexagons on the bus go round and round (sings and changes hand gesture to show his hands going round and round).
Father: (sings) Wheels on the bus go round and round, hexagons on the bus go round and round.
Hudson: (does not imitate, seems to lose interest and does not watch)
Father: (stops his action) Now they go on the table. Kind of like they are walking around like feet.
Hudson: (still seems disinterested)

Considerations

This father uses a familiar bus song Hudson has learned at school and rhythmic hand gestures to show his enthusiasm and interest in what his son is doing in order to sustain their joint play activity. This serves to keep them engaged socially with each other. Children with language delays or who are on the autism spectrum are often attracted to simple repetitive sound and action games and songs that are usually sung to younger children, such as: "Wheels on the Bus," "Ring around the Rosy," "This Little Piggy," "London Bridge," and "Row, Row, Row Your Boat". These simple songs with repetitive words will help children develop more sounds and eventually words and learn about the social interaction aspects of sounds. More details about the power of singing songs to get in your child's attention focus will be discussed in Chapter Four.

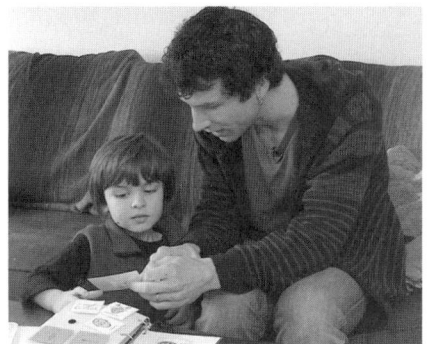

Transition to a New Interactive Activity

As the play scenario continues, the father realizes that Hudson has lost interest in the hexagons. Notice how the father offers him a way to transition to another joint play activity that he knows Hudson enjoys.

Father: (gestures all done with this hands) All done? All done with hexagons?

Hudson: (doesn't reply verbally but looks up)

Father: Okay, all done (repeats all done sign and puts hexagons away)

Father: Want to look at baby Hudson pictures? (Opens photograph book.) Let's see here. Here's little baby, that's when you were a tiny, itty bitty baby. Who's that?

Hudson: (points)

Father: Who are you with there? Is that your mama or your papa?

Hudson: (disinterested)

Father: You don't want to look at the baby pictures? Not right now. (uses all done sign)

Hudson: (picks another book of picture prompt laminated cards)
Father: What's that? Looks like you found the hand, that says wait one minute.
Hudson: Wait one minute.
Father: Wait one minute.
Hudson: Wait one minute (picks another picture).
Father: What's he doing?
Hudson: What's he doing?
Father: He's pushing the…(*partial prompt*)
Hudson: He's pushing the…
Father: What's that?
Hudson: He's pushing the…what's that?
Father: (turns to touch wall) What's this here?
Hudson: He's pushing the wall.
Father: He's pushing the wall. That's right, it's called wall push ups.

Considerations

It is helpful for children to learn to communicate that they are finished with an activity and are ready to do something else. When Hudson's father noticed that his son was losing interest, he prompted him to indicate the end of the play activity by saying, "all done" and by using an all-done gesture with his hands as well as the words. Pairing the words "all done" or "all finished" with the end of an activity will teach children to communicate their wish to stop an activity. It also provides a way for parents or teachers to communicate when it is time for the child to transition to something new. Picture symbols can also be used to indicate "all done." If a child is using a picture board, a picture symbol to indicate "all done" can be one of the options on the board. The

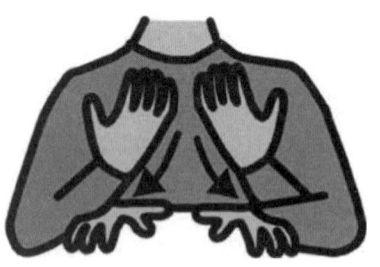

adult can turn a picture of the toy over or put in a box to reflect its completion while saying "all done". More information on using picture boards will be presented later in this chapter.

In the above scenario, this father's modelling of the words "all done" helps Hudson learn the words and/or gesture to communicate that he is finished playing with something. This father is well prepared with several of Hudson's other favorite activities to transition to when Hudson loses interest. This allows them to stay connected in their joint attention and play. With the next activity the father continues to be child-directed and waits to see which picture prompt cards Hudson is interested in looking at. He imitates his son's words and prompts him to use words by offering partial sentences (known as partial prompts) with the option for Hudson to verbalize and complete the end of the sentence by saying "wall". When Hudson does this the father shows enthusiasm for his word use.

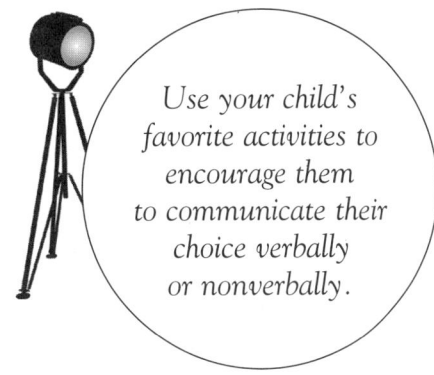

Use your child's favorite activities to encourage them to communicate their choice verbally or nonverbally.

Waiting for Your Child to Indicate Choice

You will know your child's interests by watching what objects and activities they pay attention to and that make them happy. Because children on the autism spectrum don't usually use clear signals to communicate their wants and needs, you might be tempted to make decisions for them. It is better to avoid doing this because it can delay language development. Ask your child what they want to do by providing some suggestions of their favorite activities, or by showing them the actual activity (e.g., ball) or the activity choice card and then wait for a verbal response or nonverbal gesture before proceeding. The idea is for you to use your child's favorite activities to encourage them to communicate their choice verbally or nonverbally.

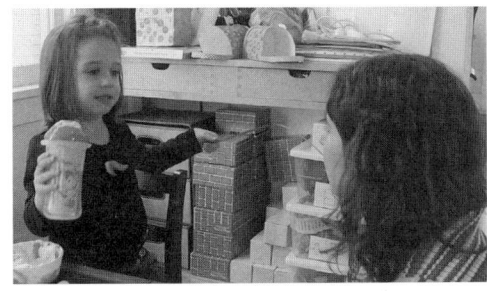

In the next scenario a mother offers her almost 4-year-old daughter, Amelia, a number of different suggestions for a play activity. Notice how the mother is child-directed; encouraging and waiting for her daughter to indicate her decision. She is responsive to what Amelia wants to do. Think about what Amelia is learning from this approach.

Mother: What would you like to play today? We have our doll house, or we could play pretend doctor or ice cream shop. Is there something you want to play today? (mother waits for a reply)
Amelia: Ice cream.
Mother: You want to play ice cream shop?
Amelia: No just ice cream.
Mother: Just ice cream, okay.
Amelia: I want to play Sneaky Squirrel (board game)…
Mother: Oh, you want to play Sneaky Squirrel.
Amelia: Who will go first?
Mother: Who's going to go first? Do you want to go first?
Amelia: Yeah.
Mother: Okay and we'll take turns. That's great. So let's get Sneaky Squirrel out? Do you want to play Sneaky Squirrel or ice cream first?
Amelia: Sneaky Squirrel first.

Considerations

This mother does a great job of encouraging her daughter to make a choice of what she wants to do and waiting for her to decide. She is child directed in that she offers three activities which are items on Amelia's "likes" list. By offering Amelia some of her favorite activities she knows she will keep her socially engaged with her. It can be tempting to save time by choosing the activity for your child, however, this misses an opportunity for your child to learn how to communicate their preferences.

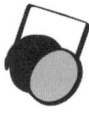

Pause to Wait for a Response from Child: Amelia clearly understands language and her mother is helping her by waiting and giving her time to express her wants verbally. All children take longer than adults to process and answer questions. Children on the spectrum often have verbal processing difficulties and will need even more time. If your child doesn't respond immediately, don't assume that your child didn't hear or didn't understand. Instead, give your child time to respond (some children need as much as 30 seconds!). If there is no

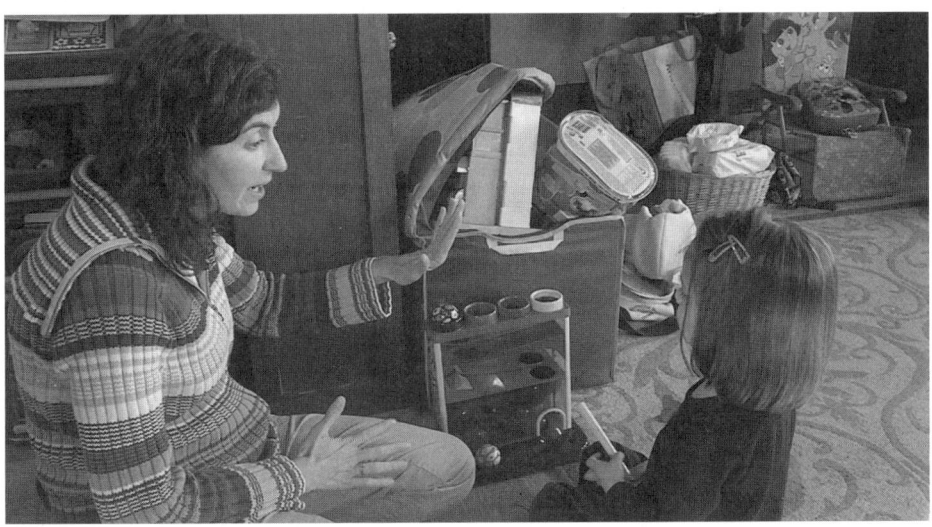

response after 30 seconds, then ask again, adding a prompt (provide a word, picture, or help the child form a gesture such as pointing). If your child responds to the prompt in any way with a look, gesture or sound, immediately reinforce the response by giving them what they wanted and acknowledging their good choice and cooperation. This patient cycle of providing opportunities for children to respond to choices is teaching them to use gestures, signs, or language to express their needs and wants.

Tailor the number of activity choices to match the child's language understanding level. Amelia is almost 4 years old, quite verbal, with good receptive language, so her mother presented three verbal choices. For a child with less language understanding than Amelia, the choices should be reduced in number and complexity. For example, simpler language might be to use only one or two words: "ice cream or sneaky squirrel game." For children with little understanding of language, it will be helpful to show the actual object or game item as you name it. For example, show the Sneaky Squirrel game and ice cream toy (or pictures of these objects) while offering the verbal choice. When prompting a response from a child who has more language and is echolalic, it is best to model the request the way the child would say it. Rather than asking, "Do you want the ice cream or the Squirrel" the adult should say, "I want squirrel" and the child will eventually repeat this request in the appropriate way. Otherwise, the child may mimic or echo the question: "Do you want the…." Below we will discuss further how you can use pictures to give children another nonverbal way of indicating their choice of activity.

Getting in Your Child's Spotlight by Following Your Child's Lead and Directions

Children on the autism spectrum frequently have unconventional or repetitive play choices, or use objects in atypical ways, or in a repetitive manner. You may want to redirect your child's play to something more typical, but this will likely result in your child's frustration and efforts to push you away. To be child directed means to get in your child's spotlight. This metaphor means the parent or teacher strives to enter into the child's world view or spotlight of attention by joining in their preferences in games and following their lead in play and preferred activities. 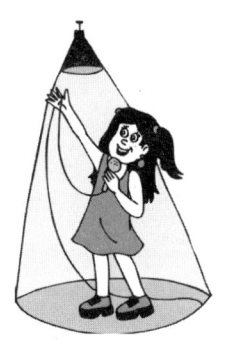 Think of the attention spotlight like a theater spotlight that directs the audience's attention to the important action on the stage. It is important to do this even when the child's spotlight of activity many seem unconventional, repetitive, and narrow. Adults can get into their child's spotlight by imitating what the child is doing in play; narrating their actions and limiting their questions; using gestures, sounds, and words; and by engaging in physical games or songs the child enjoys. When parents and teachers do this, they will capture their child's attention and interest and the social interaction will become as or more engaging than the child's normal repetitive play. This spotlighting approach helps the child know what is important to pay attention to, to model, and engage in and what will result in your applause and enthusiastic attention.

This spotlighting approach helps the child know what is important to pay attention to, to model, and engage in.

As your child becomes more interested and secure in these child-directed interactions, there will be more opportunities for them to observe and learn from the behaviors or words that you are modelling. The goal is to promote your child's social interactions and interest in playing and communicating with you. Once your child feels safe including you in their spotlight, you can eventually expand the child's spotlight to include new ways of playing. This might include imaginary play, helping them notice what others are doing, including others in their play and learning, and by imitating the actions or words modelled by you or others.

In the next scenario, notice how Amelia's mother gets into her spotlight in their play interactions with a game that involves hammering down some balls.

Amelia: Let's play ball hammer today

Mother: (sitting on floor next to Amelia smiling and giving her eye contact) Great asking a friend to come and play. Can I play with you? (*praises social play request and models verbal request to play*)

Amelia: Yeah, but I'm going to have…but I'm going to have hammer…you do like that (slaps hand on toy)

Mother: With my hands? I'm going to push them down with my hand? (motions action) (*imitates child's hand actions*)

Amelia: Because I'm going to do the hammer

Mother: (sounding enthusiastic) Okay, that sounds like a good idea. Let me come over and do it with you. So, you are going first. You get yellow.

Amelia: Where do you put this one?

Mother: (looks at block) I'm thinking I'm going to put the red and yellow ball in the red hole.

Amelia: (puts ball in purple spot) Here

Mother: Oh you put it in purple (*describes child's actions*)

Amelia: (moves ball to green spot)

Mother: Oh you changed your mind and put it in green (*follows child's lead*)

Amelia: (bangs all balls down with hammer)

Amelia: There is one left.

Mother: There is one left. Should I bang it? Should I do it like this? (*imitates child's words and offers her another choice to make a decision and take the lead*)

Face-to-Face Joint Activity

Amelia: Yeah
Mother: With my open hand
Amelia: Yup
Mother: Wham! Down it goes. There's one stuck. I wonder how to get it out. I wonder how I can get it out (jiggles toy). Help, I can't quite get it all the way out (*prompts her helping response*).
Amelia: (tips toy)
Mother: You're helping me tipping it one way. Hmm, tipping it the other way maybe. (*describes child's actions*)
Amelia: (tips it sideways)
Mother: That's tipping it in the front. Can you tip it to the side? (*points*), Oh it's coming. You helped get it out!

Considerations

Face-to-face positioning: The first step to getting in a child's spotlight is positioning. The adult should sit so the child can see them. This means sitting in front of your child at the same level so there is face-to-face contact and the child can see your face, eyes, and gestures. This can make it easier for a child who finds it difficult to make eye contact. Faces provide important social information that help a child understand what you are saying. In the scenario presented above Amelia's mother consistently positions to allow for face-to-face and eye contact when she is talking to Amelia. This enhances their social communication. Amelia can see her mother's face "talk."

Descriptive commenting and prompting: Amelia's mother is child-directed and engages her daughter in social interactions. She continually describes her daughter's actions (push, bang, tip, wham, switched), positions (down, in) and colors of the balls. In talking this way while her daughter plays, she is building her language as well as showing her how interested she is in what Amelia is doing. She is in Amelia's spotlight using an enthusiastic tone of voice and motivating her child's interest in playing with her and therefore increasing her learning opportunities. Amelia's mother also adds prompts to encourage Amelia to expand her play repertoire and social interactions. She prompts Amelia's helping behavior by telling her that she is not sure how to get the ball out. This prompts Amelia to try to help her and encourages more social interaction and communication.

The type of language this mother is using is called descriptive commenting and is one of the most important ways to help build children's language. Descriptive commenting means to describe exactly what the child is doing by labeling developmentally appropriate actions, objects, and concepts. "You are putting the yellow ball in the hole and banging it down." For children with less language than Amelia, parents would tailor their comments, using 1-2 words to describe important actions or nouns. For example, "ball up" "ball down" "ball in." In Chapter Three we will explain more about simplifying and pacing your commenting and using gestures to help your child understand spoken language.

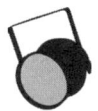

It is important to avoid distractions for the adult and child during these play interactions. Turn off cell phones, TVs, and background music. Avoid toys that make sounds or mechanical movements and limit the number of toys in the child's spotlight. This can mean putting extra toys in closed containers or boxes or behind a curtain. These can compete with the child's attention to social or verbal interaction. At first, the spotlight should be limited to one adult and one child; including others in the interaction will also be distracting for the child. More learning will occur in a spotlight with fewer distractions.

Imitation and Face-to-Face Play Interaction Games to Turn on Your Child's Voice

We have discussed the importance of noticing what your child is doing, following their interests, and joining in or spotlighting their attention focus. Amelia's mother has done this by enthusiastically describing what her daughter is doing using simple words and short phrases without interrupting or changing Amelia's focus. Children learn language much more readily when parents talk about what they are already paying attention to and doing. Be sure to set up your play times so that your child has a clear view of your face just as Amelia's mother has done. In addition to describing the actions and the objects the child is playing with,

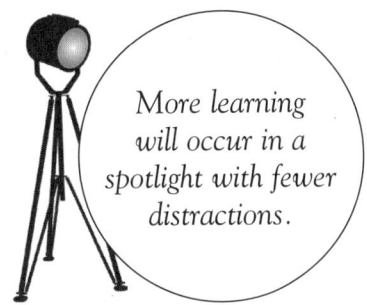

More learning will occur in a spotlight with fewer distractions.

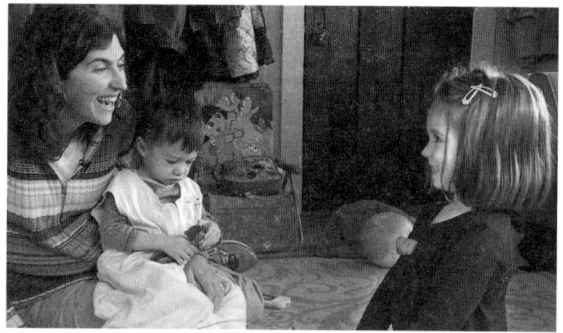

try imitating your child's actions, gestures and words. Imitation is a powerful teaching tool. By imitating your child, you will gain their attention, show you are interested in what they are doing and also motivate them to imitate you. This will enhance language development and foster empathy. In the next scenario notice how Amelia's mother uses imitation in a fun game and encourages her daughter's use of eye contact when they are communicating. Think about the benefits of this approach for their relationship and for Amelia's learning.

Amelia: Oh no
Mother: (smiles)
Amelia: I say "oh no" because now I licked it
Mother: Because now you licked it. Oh no!
Amelia: Oh no!
Mother: Oh no!
Amelia: Oh no!
Mother: Oh no!
Amelia: Oh no!
Mother: Oh yes!
Amelia: Oh no! (smiles and looks at mother)
Mother: Oh yes!
Amelia: Oh no!
Mother: That's great looking at me Amelia
Amelia: (looks away) Oh no!
Mother: Now you're being silly. (imitates her and looks away) Oh no! (looks back with big smile)
Amelia: (looks away several times) Oh no, Oh no!
Mother: (looks at her closely)
Amelia: Oh no! When I said, 'oh no', am I looking at you mama?
Mother: I can't find your eyes. Where are those beautiful eyes? Where did they go? (Sings) Where or where is my

	little Amelia? Where or where is my little Amelia? Where or where…
Amelia:	(turns back)
Mother:	There she is.
Amelia:	I'm not Amelia. I'm not Amelia.
Mother:	That's right you are Mia. Thank you for looking at me to tell me.
Amelia:	I'm Mia.
Mother:	I forgot. You're Mia. I forgot. Where or where is my little Mia? (sings) Do you know where she is? (looks under table and searches) Is she under the table? No , is she in the kitchen? No! Is she in the chair? (laughing) There you are…I found you
Amelia:	It is tickle time
Mother:	Tickle, tickle, tickle oh tickle on my back. I'm having so much fun with you. I love it.

Considerations

The "oh no" imitation game at the beginning of this interaction is a powerful way of engaging Amelia in reciprocal communication leading to a fun game to support her understanding of the importance of eye contact, which is one of this mother's goals. It is clear that this becomes a playful game where Amelia is experimenting with giving her mother eye-contact and is enjoying her mother's responses. Playing back and forth games like this one and others such as peekaboo, "I'm going to get you" chase, and hide and seek with exaggerated and silly facial expressions are great games to encourage social communication and motivate children to give parents eye contact when they talk. Moreover, the more fun your child is having attending and interacting with you, the more learning opportunities you can provide. You will also be increasing your child's internal motivation to interact with you. The goal is to increase your child's experience of pleasure in social interactions with you so they can learn more from you.

By imitating your child, you will gain her attention, show you are interested in what she is doing and also motivate her to imitate you.

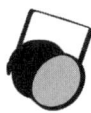 This mother is working on Amelia's understanding of using eye contact by playing a game. However, this target behavior and goal is introduced after Amelia has already learned a lot of language. Did you notice that the mother kept the game playful and was not requiring eye-contact? For children with less language, you may want to include a visual prompt to show them when they are giving you eye contact. However, for some children, eye contact may be less helpful or important than using some other communication strategy such as a gesture, or word, or visual prompt. Some children will find eye contact too distracting and overwhelming, and it may interfere with their ability to listen to what is being said or make the gesture. The important thing is to target a simple play interaction communication goal that is realistic and achievable and will help your child feel supported in their efforts to interact with you. Children with less verbal language than Hudson or Amelia need first to be able to learn to make gestures and sounds in response to an adult's language or sounds (*reciprocal responding*). In Chapter Three we will talk about how to tailor your verbal language and gestures for these children.

Target a simple communication play interaction goal that is realistic and achievable and will help your child in their efforts to interact with you.

Value of Imitation: We've talked about getting into your child's attention spotlight by imitating their play. You can also capture your child's attention by imitating or mirroring their vocalizations, sounds, words, and noises. Amelia's mother did this by repeating her words: "oh no!" Amelia was clearly intrigued with this and repeated the words many times, to see if her mother would respond. This kind of verbal imitation will attract your child's attention and shift it to you as a social partner. Pretty soon you will have a reciprocal dance like Amelia and her mother.

Encouraging Verbal and Nonverbal Communication

At times, children on the autism spectrum may seem unaware that communication is even occurring between two people. They are less likely to use nonverbal communication signals such as eye contact, facial expressions or gestures to communicate their needs. They are also less likely to understand the meaning of such gestures from others. In the parent-child scenarios just discussed, we have talked about how parents can model, prompt, and praise their children for using nonverbal signals such as smiles, hand gestures, or eye contact during social interactions. For example, Amelia's mother says, "great looking at me" when Amelia gives her eye contact because that is one of her goals. Parents can also make their responses more socially interesting by exaggerating their interactions with smiles, excitement, speech sounds, and gestures. In the next scenario, think about how Hudson's father uses a bubble wand to get in his son's spotlight and then prompts his son's use of basic verbal and nonverbal communication. See if you can pull out the ways he sets up this game as a learning opportunity for Hudson.

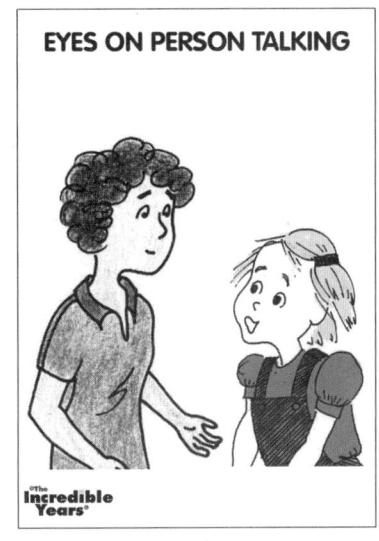

Father: Ha, ha. There's the bubble thingy. (*introduces one of Hudson's favorite activities, blowing bubbles*)
Hudson: Ha, ha. There's the bubble thingy.
Father: There it is.
Hudson: Ha, ha. There's the bubble thing
Father: There it is! Okay, what do you want me to do with it? (*prompts child response and waits*)
Hudson: Blow it blow.
Father: (*holds bubbles next to his face smiling*) Blow bubbles. Okay. (*imitates and waits for child response*)
Hudson: (*looks at father*) Blow the bubbles. Blow the bubbles.
Father: Blow the bubbles. (*imitates words and blows some*) Bubble, boing, boing, boing (*makes fun sound effects*). We have 2 bubbles. (*father waits for response*)
Hudson: Boing, boing.

Father:	Boing, boing. (*imitates*) Do you want to ask for something? (*prompts ask and waits*)
Hudson:	(flapping) I want you to blow the bubbles.
Father:	(smiling) Blow the bubbles. Okay. (*imitates child's response and blows*)
Hudson:	A really big bubble.
Father:	Okay, you want me to blow a very big bubble?(*prompts response*)
Hudson:	A very big bubble.
Father:	Okay I'll try. This is kind of small (blows bubble)—a little bigger –was that big enough?
Hudson:	(flapping) Was that big enough?
Father:	Even bigger than that? (*prompts a response*)
Hudson:	I want it even bigger than that.
Father:	Even bigger bubble. What should I do again? (*imitates child response and prompts asking practice*)
Hudson:	Blow blow a big bubble.
Father:	What are you going to do? Are you going to pop it? (*suggests different idea*)
Hudson:	No pop.
Father:	Hudson, are you just going to watch it? Okay. (*affirms child's choice*)
Hudson:	(flapping) I 'm just going to watch it.
Hudson:	More blow the bubbles. Blow the bubbles. Blow the bubbles please.
Father:	Okey dokey. I'm going to blow a bunch of bubbles. It will be easier WHEEE….(*reinforces child's use of language*)
Father:	This time do you want one bubble or a bunch of bubbles? (*Prompts a response*)
Hudson:	A bunch of bubbles
Father:	Can you look at me with your eyes? (*expands response*)
Hudson:	(gives eye contact) I want a bunch of bubbles
Father:	(with enthusiasm) Okay good eyes WHEEE …. (*reinforces child's request and eye contact*)

Considerations

In this fun bubble play interaction, the father uses several important ABC (Antecedant, Behavior, Consequence) teaching strategies. First, he gets into his son's attention zone or spotlight by presenting one of his favorite play objects – the bubbles, and he pairs this rewarding object with his smiling face to get his son to look at him. Second, he prompts the words for Hudson to use to request the activity and then waits for his son to verbalize and ask for what he wants before blowing the bubble. Third, he imitates or mirrors his son's verbalizations to encourage further imitation. Fourth, he follows his son's lead and rewards his verbalizations by doing what he wants. And finally, he expands the learning opportunity by prompting him to give him eye contact when he asks again. We will be discussing more details of the ABCs of child learning in the next chapter.

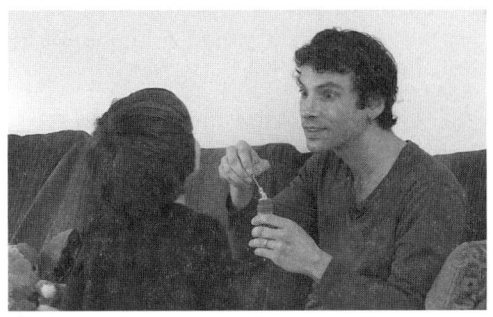

Wait and Direct Spotlight on Child Response: Here it is important to notice that the father pauses and waits a bit for Hudson to tell him what to do before doing anything. This forces Hudson to use his language to express his desires and keeps their interaction mutual. Once Hudson verbally tells him what to do, the father reinforces him by immediately doing what he wants. He repeats this interaction creating multiple opportunities for Hudson to practice asking for what he wants. Later, when the father has been successful in getting Hudson to verbalize his requests, he adds to the challenge by requiring that he look him in the eyes when he makes these requests.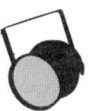

For children with less verbal communication than Hudson, focus on using a gesture, point, head-nod, or initial letter sound ('ba') to help your child indicate what they want. There is so much more to communication than verbal speaking. Exaggerate these other body signals such as: your gestures, eyes, facial expressions, actions, body position, and sounds. Through your body language your child will come to understand what you are trying to communicate and that you can understand their thoughts, feelings, and interests. They will also begin to imitate

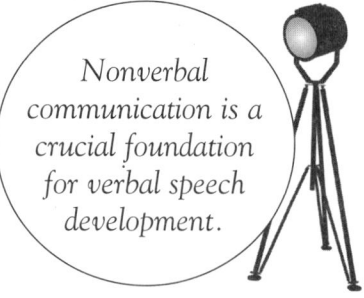

Nonverbal communication is a crucial foundation for verbal speech development.

some of this body language and may look at you, point, or make a sound as a way to communicate with you. Nonverbal communication is a crucial foundation for verbal speech development.

Go back to the communication checklist in Chapter One and choose a communication strategy that is developmentally appropriate for your child to be successful. And remember, for some children asking for eye contact can be too much information to process and it may be best to start with a simple hand gesture or head nod.

Prompt, Model, Gesture, and Imitate Language in Play

Children on the autism spectrum have fewer gestures than typical children and seem unaware that they can use gestures to indicate their wants. Parents and teachers can model gestures and prompt and teach their children to use them. Learning to point is an important communication landmark because a child can use pointing to communicate their interests or needs to you. Once your child has learned to point, you can name the object as they point. Your child will learn to anticipate and expect this verbal response from you. After that, you can pause and wait for your child to make eye contact before you name the object. This approach is also helpful for children with language delays. After playing the point-and-name language game, you will find that your child will start to imitate or model your

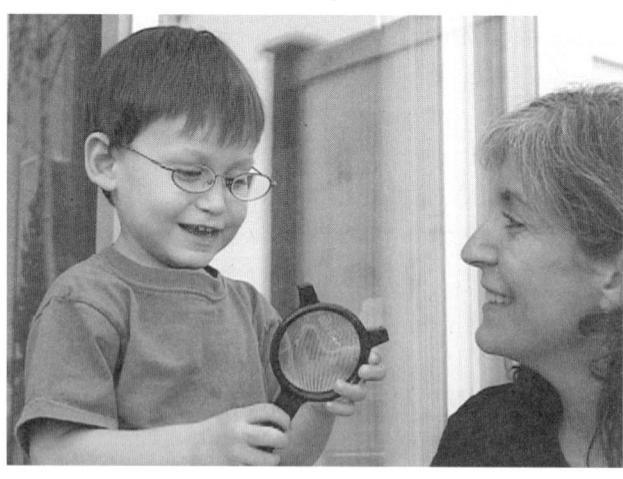

words or sounds, and you will have developed a strong base for further language learning. In the next scenario another mother is playing with her 3½ year old child, Kalani, with water, rocks, and some kitchen tools. In this case the mother takes advantage of her son's pointing gestures to prompt, model, imitate, pause and reward her son's gaze and beginning 1–2-word request language use.

Kalani: …(points to something) mumbles…this one
Mother: Which one?
Kalani: This
Mother: You want the cup? The little cup? Or the strainer? *(offers choices)*
Kalani: (points at strainer and mumbles some words)
Mother: Good pointing. This one .. the strainer ..say, strainer please *(models word for object and prompts request language)*
Kalani: …(tries to repeat what mother said) strainer please
Mother: Yes, good asking! (gives him strainer) *(reinforces language use paired with giving him object)*
Kalani: (points frantically trying to say something) This… that one…
Mother: Do you remember the name? Do you know what that one is? You can say 'strainer please.' *(models and prompts language use)*
Kalani: Strainer please
Mother: Okay, nice asking. Here's the strainer. Ooo the water goes right through—Let's see. Should we try an experiment? Here can you hold it over the bucket? And let's pour some water in it. Ready let's see what…
Kalani: more water
Mother: (gives him water) You do it and let's see what happens. Can you pour it in here?
Kalani: (pours water through strainer)
Mother: Oh—oh oh—it went right through!
Kalani: (puts his feet in the water)
Mother: Oh no, they're wet.
Kalani: More water
Mother: More water, please. *(prompts request with one extra word)*
Kalani: More water, please.
Mother: Nice talking, now do you want Mommy to do it, or you do it? *(gives choice)*
Kalani: (points to strainer and bends over to pick up strainer)

Mother: There you go! That's one way to get it. You figured it out. You went in and got it. Here are you going to try the experiment now? Okay.
Kalani: (takes the cup of water and pours it beside strainer)
Mother: Are you getting wet?
Kalani: More water
Mother: More water, please. *(repeats prompt for 3-word request)*
Kalani: More water, please.
Mother: Nice asking. Are you going to stay in or do you want to come out?
Kalani: In
Mother: In—okay.
Kalani: Water—water
Mother: Water-water there's more—into the bucket—oh boy, that's a lot of water.
Kalani: More water
Mother: More water please
Kalani: More water
Mother: More water please, okay. (gives water)
Kalani: More water
Mother: More water, please.
Kalani: Water please
Mother: Thank you!

The "one up rule;" that is, when prompting and modeling language for your child, add one more word than they usually use.

Considerations

In this scenario, when Kalani points to something he wants, his mother waits for eye contact, then names the object and prompts him to use his words to ask for what he wants. For example: saying, "strainer please". Once he imitates her words, she repeats what he is saying and rewards him by responding with what he wants. When he says, "more water," she expands his two words to a three-word sentence by saying, "more water please" and rewards him by giving more water. This is called the "one up rule;" that is, when prompting and modeling language for your child, add one more word than they usually use. So, if your child normally asks with a point, model adding one simple word to the pointing gesture: "ball". If your child already uses a word to ask for something, add a second word: "want ball". Add a third word to a 2-word request so that "want ball" would become "want ball please" or "Kalani want ball." Children figure out what to do by observing what others say

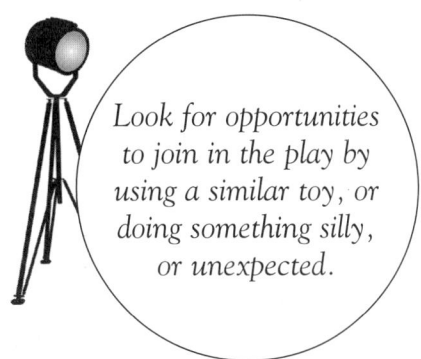

Look for opportunities to join in the play by using a similar toy, or doing something silly, or unexpected.

and do. This mother is helping her son explore the use of the strainer and play with water. At the same time, she is teaching him that his pointing gesture and language is a powerful tool that is imitated and rewarded by her responses. She combines prompting, modeling, and repetition to enhance his language for how to ask for something he wants. Did you notice that she doesn't force him to say please but models it frequently? It will take many, many learning practice trials carried out in this fun, playful way before Kalani will spontaneously say please.

Gentle Intrusions: Some children may resist narrated child-directed 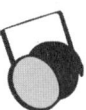 play at first. It is not unusual for children to seem to want to play alone or to be reluctant to play with you. Remember they are doing this because they are uncomfortable and don't know how to play with you. Don't get discouraged! Look for opportunities to join in the play by using a similar toy, or doing something silly, or unexpected. For example, if your child is playing with cars, begin by imitating their motions with a similar car. Your child may notice and start playing in parallel. If your child tolerates you playing next to him, then try introducing a new element or variation in the activity such as making your car do something different. For example, crashing your car into theirs and saying, "beep, beep!" or, "crash, crash"! Watch for their reaction. Some children may resist if you add a new element to the play because of their discomfort with change from their predictable and repetitive play sequence. Don't worry. This resistance is to be expected. If your child resists, don't give up; continue getting in your child's spotlight by being child-directed. Return to imitating their play, staying near and engaged, show your enthusiasm, and then try again patiently and gradually to introduce a new element or something unexpected. Eventually the new element will become familiar and will be tolerated and even welcomed by your child. Watch for your child's cues to see what new element works best (for some children new sound effects will be fun, for others new motions or actions will be more appealing). Your child will soon learn it is more fun to play with you than to play alone.

When not to follow your child's lead: If your child is behaving in inappropriate ways such as throwing blocks in anger, do not turn this into a child-directed game. Instead, tell your child firmly, "stop" or "no throwing" and briefly remove the toy and provide a distraction. For children with less language, use a "stop" visual prompt to reinforce your intent to stop this kind of play. Once you have communicated the "stop" message, try briefly turning your body away to give your child a chance to regulate their emotions. If your child begins to settle down or stops the inappropriate behavior, immediately turn back and give your attention back. If your child's dysregulation escalates, you may need to temporarily end the play activity. Later chapters will give suggestions for how to effectively distract, redirect, or ignore this kind of aggressive behavior.

Since children with limited language do not have effective ways to communicate their desires, they often whine, cry, or tantrum when they want something. Attentive adults have often learned to interpret these cries and respond by giving the child what they want when they hear the cries. In effect, cries or tantrums have become an effective way of communicating their wishes. If your child has learned to cry or tantrum to get what they want, it will be important to try to break this cycle by anticipating your child's wants and teaching them an alternative communication strategy. For example, if you notice your child is beginning to get frustrated and is heading for a tantrum to let you know that they want something, offer the object but keep it out of reach. Put words to the request: "Want train?" Then wait to see if the child looks, points, puts out their hand, or makes a sound. As soon as you see any of these forms of communication, reinforce your child immediately by giving them the object. Repeat the words: "want train!" Because you are giving the desired object right after your child's gesture, they are learning this is one of the nonverbal body cues that will get them what they want and has a more predictable response than a cry or whine. In Chapter Nine we will discuss further how to manage misbehavior during play.

Use Visual Prompts and Gestures as a Way for Less Verbal Children to Indicate their Choice or Request for Play Activity

Many children are visual learners. This is especially true for children on the autism spectrum. Why is this? Perhaps children with ASD or language delays have more difficulty processing verbal language because auditory information is presented quickly, is transient, and is more complex. Pictures, on the other hand, are fixed images so the child can take as much time to process the information as they need. Seeing it, rather than just hearing it, can help the child process and retain the information.

You can make a favorite choice activity cue card for your child to help them understand what choices they have and to indicate and gesture their choice.

Cards are personalized with your child's favorite activities such as playing with blocks or Legos, playdough, cars, bubbles, art activities, board games, reading books, singing songs, going to the park, throwing a ball, or having a special snack. Picture line drawing communication symbols (PCS) like the ones shown here and many other free line drawing printables can be found online by Boardmaker (Mayer-Johnson) or other companies. Look at the list of your child's "likes" or favorite activities that you made earlier in Chapter One. Then you can either find free pictures of these activities on-line, or

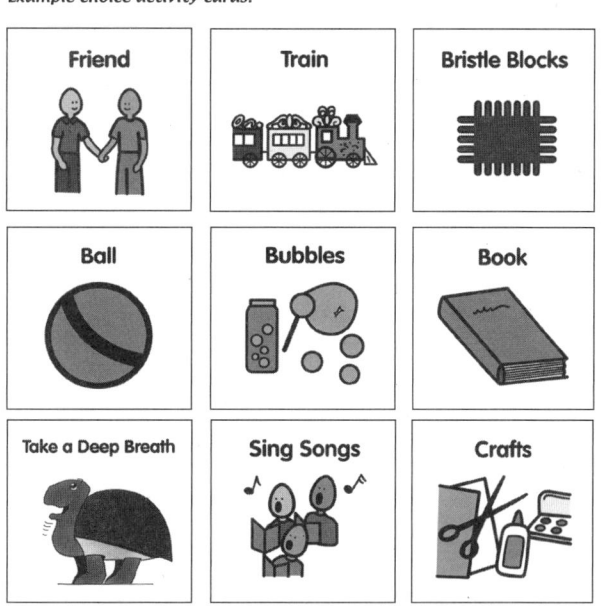

Spotlighting
Sample Choice Activity Cue Cards

If parents have access to the program BoardMaker™ or a similar symbol generating program, they can use this to create their own activity boards customized to their child's particular interests.

Example choice activity cards:

The Picture Communication Symbols ©1981–2010 by Mayer-Johnson LLC. All Rights Reserved Worldwide. Used with permission. Boardmaker™ is a trademark of Mayer-Johnson LLC

> *The child learns that pictures, like words, stand for a real thing.*

make your own drawings of the activity, or, better yet, take color photographs of your child actually engaged in these favorite activities. From these photographs you can make a customized activity choice board or book for your child. If you decide to take your own photos, make sure your picture is of the specific toy or activity and doesn't have any other unnecessary information.

These choice activity picture boards can be used to encourage your child to initiate communication on their own by pointing to or exchanging a picture of what they want rather than pulling on your arm or crying with frustration because they don't know how to indicate their needs or wants. These activity pictures can also be used to suggest other ideas for activities the child could do if they are at a loss for ideas. The child learns that pictures, like words, stand for a real thing. These choice pictures are not meant to be permanent alternatives to speech, but to assist in the child's development of speech and ability to plan activities. Visual supports such as written schedules and calendars help most adults keep track of our days and activities. These communication boards serve a similar purpose for young children on the spectrum as well as to promote their independence.

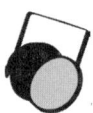

Teaching children How to Use Picture Prompts

Nonverbal children will initially need adult assistance and help understanding what each of the pictures represent before they can use the picture as a communication aid to express their wants. Parents or teachers start by matching the real object or activity with the picture. This helps the child understand that a picture can be a representation of an object or activity. For example, when starting an activity, such as playing with playdough, the adult shows the playdough picture and names it. As the child plays with the playdough, the adult may repeat saying, "playdough" and again show the picture. With time, the child begins to understand what the picture represents. Eventually the child will be able to point to the picture of playdough to indicate their choice of activity, or they may bring the picture to the adult to indicate what they want to do. After the child points to the picture or hands it to the adult, the parent or teacher enthusiastically responds with a gesture and words, "You want playdough! Here is some playdough."

To reinforce the child's learning, the parent or teacher only offers the child a small amount of playdough so that the child has another opportunity to point to the picture again or use words to ask for more. This time when the child points, the adult responds, "More playdough?" and when the child nods yes, the parent nods and smiles, "Yes more playdough." and gives the child a bit more playdough. With practice and repetition, the child eventually will repeat what the adult says by saying, "more" or "playdough" and the parent will respond with enthusiasm, "more playdough, good words." The child is reinforced for using their pointing gesture and the visual aid, and for any verbal sounds or words to indicate their choice of activity. It is important that the parent or teacher say the same words every time a visual prompt is used and that the written word of the object or activity is placed on the picture. The ongoing repetition of the same words will eventually reinforce the link between the word and the picture's meaning and your child will repeat the words to make a request.

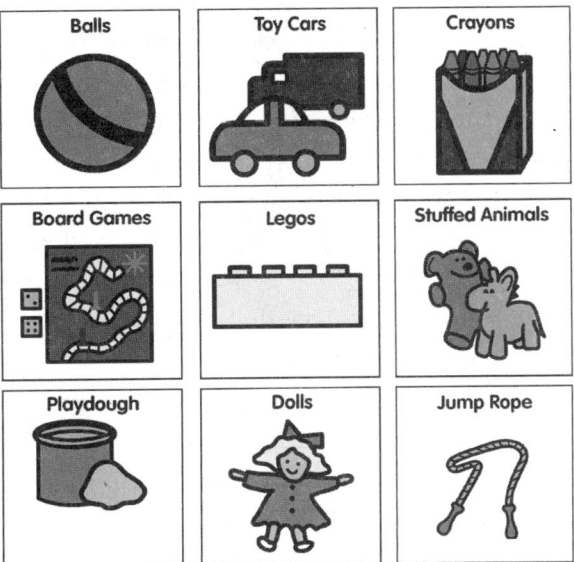

The Picture Communication Symbols ©1981–2010 by Mayer-Johnson LLC. All Rights Reserved Worldwide. Used with permission. Boardmaker™ is a trademark of Mayer-Johnson LLC

At first, the picture will take the place of words for your child. Next the picture will prompt your child to say the words, and eventually the picture will not be needed,

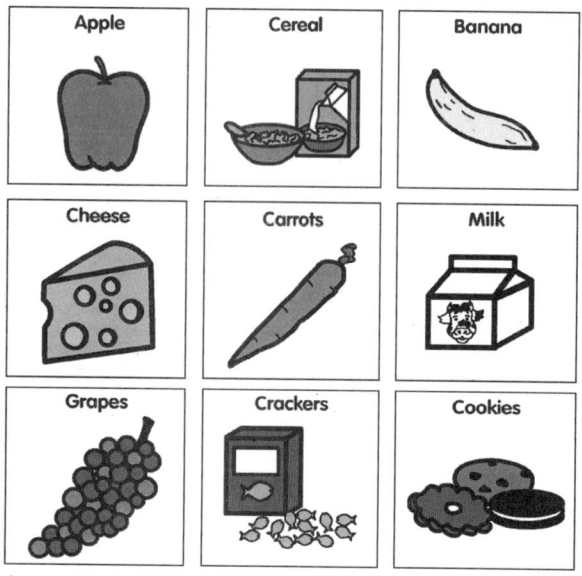

The Picture Communication Symbols ©1981–2010 by Mayer-Johnson LLC. All Rights Reserved Worldwide. Used with permission. Boardmaker™ is a trademark of Mayer-Johnson LLC

and your child will use the word directly to express their wants. Adding the written word to the picture helps expose the child to printed words and will enhance pre-reading skills.

Other lists of visual prompts can be made for the child's favorite foods or snacks such as cookies, drinks, fruits, vegetables. Again, the parent or teacher first pairs the actual food (banana or apple) along with the picture, so the child learns the relationship between the picture and the specific name for the food. Once the child has learned the meaning of new pictures and how to point to them, these visual aids expand the child's ability to let the parent or teacher know their preferences in play, singing, or eating. For a child with 1-2 word sentences, picture cards can be used to expand the child's language to 3-4 word sentences by adding an "I want" picture card. If the child has requested an apple by showing the apple picture card and saying "apple", the adult responds, "I want the apple" and shows the "I want" card. It is important for the adult to model asking for the object the way the child would say it. Rather than asking, "Do you want the apple?" the adult should say, "I want apple" and the child will eventually repeat this request in the appropriate way. Otherwise, the child may mimic the question: "Do you want the apple?"

How many objects or pictures can be put on a choice board? This will depend on the level of communication your child has, how many pictures they have been taught, and how helpful you find the visual prompts are to enhancing the child's language. If the child has no words or little understanding of words, start with just two choices of favorite activities or foods. After these visual prompts have been learned, more pictures and their meanings can be taught and added.

The "No" visual signal: Sometimes a choice on an activity board is not available. For example, no more apples or cookies are left. Or, the child has had enough computer time, and this is no longer an activity option. The parent can let the child know that an activity is not an option by putting the "No" sign (circle with slash through it) on top of the picture. The sign should be paired with the verbal information: "Cookies all gone" or "no more computer" to explain what this signal means.

Helping Children Learn How to Say No: Giving children choices also means helping them learn to say "no" to a suggested activity. The parent or teacher can teach this by deliberately offering a picture of something the child dislikes *before* offering one of their likes. For example, a child who doesn't like the feel of playdough is first offered this playdough picture as a possible choice activity. When the child looks at the other picture but looks distressed or doesn't respond, the adult says, "no thank you" shaking their head no and putting the refused playdough picture away. The adult says, "playdough gone", and then offers a picture of the child's preferred activity (toy cars) nodding yes and saying "Yes, please, car" when the child points to the car picture. Once the child has used a verbal or nonverbal communication strategy to indicate the car is their choice, then the adult gives the child one car (holding back the other cars for repeated practice interactive opportunities for asking again).

Using Sequenced Visual Prompts to Help Children Broaden their Play Activities

Children on the autism spectrum often show limited play repertoires. They may repeat an action over and over in a ritualistic way. Sequenced activity pictures can be helpful for expanding a child's play repertoire and giving new ideas about what to do with an unstructured play activity. For example, for a child who likes blocks and always

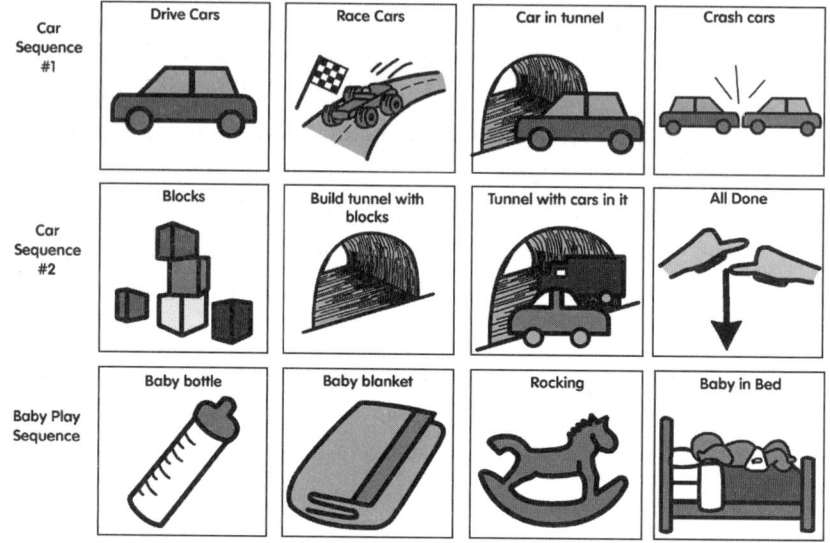

Spotlighting
Sample Picture Play Sequence

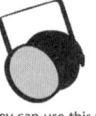

If parents/teachers have access to the program BoardMaker™ or a similar symbol generating program, they can use this to create their own play sequence boards customized to their child's interests and designed to add variety to their play interactions.

The Picture Communication Symbols ©1981–2010 by Mayer-Johnson LLC. All Rights Reserved Worldwide. Used with permission. Boardmaker™ is a trademark of Mayer-Johnson LLC

makes the same tower over and over the same way, the parent or teacher can present 3-4 pictures of different things that can be made from blocks, such as a tower, bridge, or road for racing a car (another favorite activity) under the block bridge. For a child who just rolls playdough in the same way over and over, pictures of different things that can be made from playdough rolls can be provided to offer some different choices.

Many play activities can be pictured and be provided to expand the child's play options: for example, how to play with a baby doll by showing pictures of feeding baby, rocking baby, dressing baby, singing to baby, and putting baby to bed. Often children withdraw from play or repeat play the same way because they don't know what else to do. These visuals prompt them with other ideas. This approach is still child-directed because the child makes the choice of what they want to do.

In the next scenario the teacher uses some sequenced picture cue cards with Hudson to help him learn other things he can do with

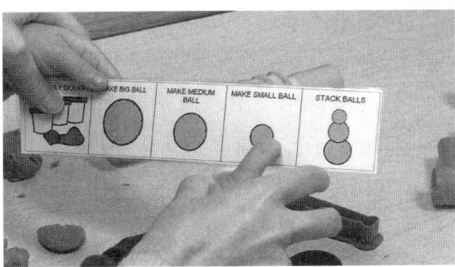 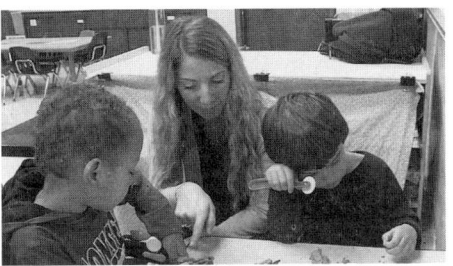

playdough besides rolling a snake. Notice how the teacher still tries to be somewhat child directed by showing him pictures of some other playdough options and letting him make the choice of what to make.

Teacher: What do you want to do first? Hmm? Which one?
Hudson: (points to picture of snake)
Teacher: Oh, you're telling me. I know, you can say "I want to roll." *(prompt and model actual words)*
Hudson: Roll
Teacher: Yeah. It's rolling. You have a snake, cool, nice job. You made a curly snake. Nice job. You rolled it! (Hudson flapping his arms.) Okay. Hey, Hudson, let's make a choice. (shows him picture cue cards of playdough options.) Hudson, do you want to make a person? Or do you want to make a snowman? *(prompt new idea with picture choices)*
Hudson: (points to snake on picture.) You made a snake. We're going to make something different. Do you want to make a person or a snowman? *(promotes choice)*
Hudson: Snowman.
Teacher: Oh, good choice. We're going to make a snowman. Okay, you got the playdough. We need to make a big ball.
Hudson: (looking at pictures of making a snowman.)
Teacher: Can you make a big ball, like this? *(prompt idea)*
Teacher: (rolls playdough.) Can you roll in a ball? Now your turn.

Hudson: (breaking up playdough into little pieces.)
Teacher: You're making little pieces. I'm going to help you. I'll take these ones. Let's do this. First is, make a big ball. Can, do you like this? (*models rolling a playdough ball on table*) Your turn.
Hudson: (Rolls playdough into a ball.)
Teacher: (*enthusiastic praise*) Oh, look at that. Nice. Now we need to make a medium ball (points to picture)
Teacher: Let's make a smaller one. Can you roll, like that? Your turn. There you go, nice. Almost... (shows him picture card). Good job. Last one, we need to make a small ball. Let's make a small one. Which one shall we do? (shows him two options of playdough.)
Hudson: (points to ball of playdough he wants)
Teacher: Oh, that one. Okay. Look at that. You made a snowman. Nice, Hudson. Good job, you made a snowman. Do you want to make another snowman? Or do you want to make a different choice? Which one, Hudson? Do you want to make another snowman, or do you want to make a different choice? (*offers another choice*)
Hudson: I want...
Hudson: (points to snowman on picture.)
Teacher: Oh, you're going to make another snowman. Good idea. Okay. Your turn. You can do it. What's first?

Considerations

This teacher has focused on helping Hudson learn a different way to play with playdough besides making snakes. It is hard for him to try something different from rolling snakes, but the pictures help him make a decision and then know what to do to make the snowman. The teacher describes and models the process of making different size balls: big, medium, and small. Hudson imitates her actions and is also learning the language for the size words. It is important to balance being child directed with gently prompting children to expand their play. At first this change in routine will be hard for Hudson, but eventually, with coaching and support, he will become more comfortable and will have widened his options for what he can do with playdough. When Hudson took the risk of trying the snowman, his teacher supported him through the steps. Notice that when she offers the choice of making another snowman or trying something different, he chooses the snowman. This has now become comfortable to him, and he wants to try again. This time the teacher reinforces this choice and agrees that it is a good idea to try another snowman. If she had pushed to have him try a second new task, that might have been too much change, too fast. Did you also notice that after she modeled how to roll a ball she said, "now your turn"? In addition to expanding his play choice options, she is also helping him understand what it means to take a turn.

Think about what picture sequences you would make to promote different things to do with cars, blocks, playdough or Legos.

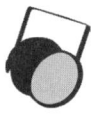 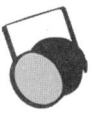

SPOTLIGHTING
Tips to Using Visual Prompts for Promoting Child-directed Play Choices

We all rely on visual prompts or supports such as calendars, daily schedules, checklists, stickie notes, or street signs to make sense of the world, to know what is expected, and to keep ourselves organized. For children on the autism spectrum, picture visuals will help reduce some of the confusion of understanding verbal input. Visuals provide information in a way that is easier to process. Better understanding provides children with security, a sense of predictability, understanding of the rules, and what activities are available to them. Visual prompts give children another way of communicating their preferences and needs to their parents, teachers, and peer group. They will help the child to be calm and more relaxed and also

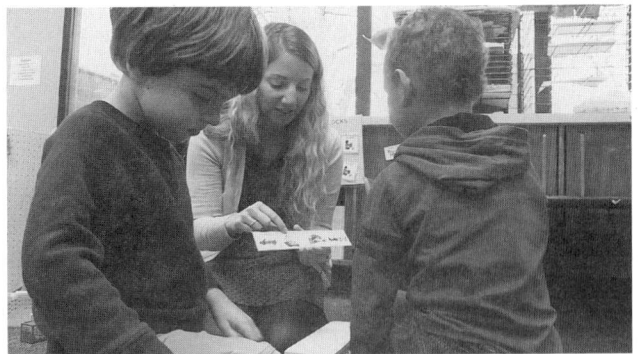

help promote language development, joint attention, and expand the child's play options. Here are a few tips to remember:

Visual Prompts, Pictures

- Put visual or picture prompts of activity or food choices or objects in places where they can be easily found, seen and used by the child and adults. For example: on a key ring, on a Velcro board, on the refrigerator, or on a low table.
- Target which activities or play sequences you want to start with; stay simple and avoid using too many new visuals at the same time.
- Use real objects to pair with pictures when teaching what the visual prompt represents.
- Add the printed word to the visual prompt.
- Use the same words for the picture every time. Don't use too many words. Be simple and clear.
- Prompt the child to look at the picture, wait for their response, and then imitate or repeat their response.
- For sequenced pictures, preview the sequence by pointing and saying each step. "First, big playdough ball (point to picture), "then medium ball " (point to picture). Then review by pointing to each step as the child is engaging in that part of the activity.
- Actual photographs of the child doing the favorite activities or behaviors can help the child make sense of what will be happening.
- Add more pictures to the picture routine schedule, or requests, or activities as the child's understanding of the pictures increases.
- Provide multiple learning trials for communication by providing small parts of the activity or item at a time. For example, if the child asks for a banana, apple, or cookie or points to a picture of the food item, just give a small piece so they can ask again for the next piece. If they ask for cars, just give 1-2 cars to start.
- Use the visual prompts to cue or prompt a child to understand an adult's request, make a request, indicate a choice, understand what will happen next and what to do, try a self-regulation strategy, point out an emotion, or practice a targeted social interaction.

Using visuals for teaching emotion literacy, social skills, emotional regulation, and rules or commands will be discussed in later chapters.

In Chapter Three we will talk further about how to strategically use your language during child-directed play, for children with varying language levels.

Father Reflections about being Child-Directed

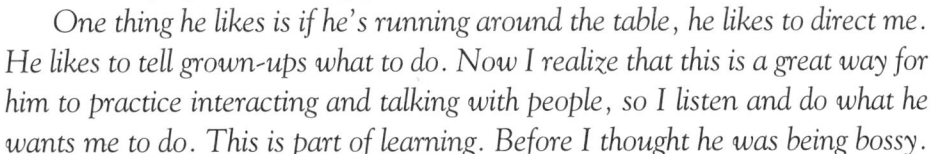

Being child-directed, was something I did frequently, but I didn't necessarily take advantage of it as a teaching situation. I wasn't thinking of it that way. When I was always trying to draw Hudson back to something I wanted to do, it just got frustrating because he didn't want to me to lead him. When I go along with what he's doing and focus on him having a good time, it's easier to keep him engaged. Then I can slip in the ways to connect with him or work on our next goal. If we're playing, like knocking a balloon around or something, I'll generally do what he's doing. I'll join him in on whatever activity he's doing, but I'll change my language to comment on what he's doing, or I'll prompt him to ask me to play before I keep playing. He will do that because he's having fun.

One thing he likes is if he's running around the table, he likes to direct me. He likes to tell grown-ups what to do. Now I realize that this is a great way for him to practice interacting and talking with people, so I listen and do what he wants me to do. This is part of learning. Before I thought he was being bossy.

Mother Reflections about being Child-Directed

I was very concerned at first, how am I going to be child-led when I know I have to direct Amelia in doing A, B, C and D because she can't do it on her own. How am I going to put those two things together? And then, over time, I started to realize that I could use lots of different coaching strategies to help her to become interested in certain things and then use her child-directed favorite preferred things as rewards for that ability to kind of expand her skills.

Teacher Reflections about Using Visual Prompts

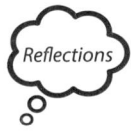

To help support Hudson's and other children's language learning, we use a lot of visual supports in our classroom. During mealtimes we have what we call snack talks that are cards that prompt conversation around a particular topic. It starts out with the teacher modeling how to use it but then quickly we encourage students to use it between themselves to start a conversation.

Hudson's language has come a long way. His receptive language is definitely much stronger than his expressive language. He has a lot more language than he is comfortable sharing in the classroom. So, the big challenge is helping to both build up his confidence and build up his use of expressive language to get his needs met. We are working to help him start to do it more independently. Then we are able to back off our supports to the point where he is using his expressive language on his own.

Second Teacher: *We use visuals all the time with Hudson. We have found it be a very successful support for him. So, I use a visual for certain kinds of play scripts for expanding his play. I see his growth in that area of more dramatic play through the use of visual supports like our play scripts. This is pretty simple one of get some blocks, make a tunnel, drive the car through the tunnel and then, you are all done. So, it is kind of making a less structured activity into a more structured activity, a closed ended activity for him.*

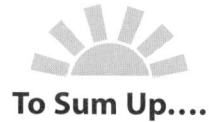

To Sum Up....

When you play and interact with your child in this child-directed way, you will find that being in your child's attention spotlight results in your child realizing you are interested in what they are doing because you are imitating and narrating their actions and words. Moreover, you are giving them both verbal and visual ways to tell you what they want or don't want to do and are helping them make choices and do things independently. This reduces their sense of confusion, increases their confidence, and strengthens their feelings of attachment and joy in your relationship. At times this repetitive, imitative, descriptive, and strategically paced commenting and gesturing on your part may seem uncomfortable, slow, or even boring, but this is merely the awkwardness anyone feels when doing something unfamiliar. You may worry you aren't making progress because your child is not yet imitating your gestures or words, and you don't get the same kind of immediate feedback from your child as you might from a neurotypical child. However, if you are persistent and patient in your child directed spotlighting and strategic verbal and nonverbal communication approach throughout all your child's daily activities, you will find that your child will come to love having you in their attention spotlight. This will allow you to increase the number of learning opportunities for language communication and social play skills.

SPOTLIGHTING
Getting in Your Child's Attention Spotlight During Play and Other Activities

- Position yourself carefully in your child's spotlight so you have face-to-face contact with your child without too much distance.
- Reduce distractions by turning off TV, computer, phone; limit other people present and put extra toys out of sight or in boxes so they are not attracting attention.
- Be child-directed and play your child's favorite activity.
- Follow your child's focus of attention or theme during play.
- Observe and respond to your child's nonverbal initiations; avoid instructions, corrections, and questions—curb your desire to give too much help.
- Describe and narrate what your child is doing with simple words or short phrases and animated expression (like a sportscaster).
- Model and imitate your child's actions, words, and sounds with enthusiasm and entertainment; have some toys similar to the child's toys for imitation; offer to help.
- Pace your child-directed play times. Several shorter sessions may be better than one longer session. It takes a lot of social energy for a child on the spectrum to engage with others, and after a while your child may need a break to recharge.
- Encourage your child to look at you by putting a desired object next to your face and wait for a response E.g., "what do you want me to do now?"

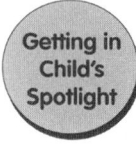
Getting in Child's Spotlight

- Reinforce your child for looking at you with smiles, gestures, praise and by giving them the desired object. However, do not force eye-contact if your child resists.
- When your child stops interacting with you, seems disinterested, or is engaged in repetitive or obsessive actions, offer another favorite joint activity or change the action slightly with a new idea, song, funny gesture, or sound effects and sensory routine.
- When you feel your child has lost interest or seems exhausted with the joint play activity, end the play with a predictable routine of putting things away, making transition clear with and "all done" gesture, and making a new choice.
- Be an "enthusiastic audience".

Remember your child is not deliberately trying to exclude you. They just don't know how to interact in play yet.

 Shine a Light on Your Child During Play Time

CHAPTER 3

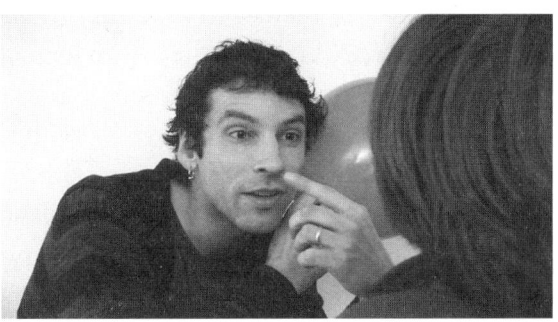

Descriptive Commenting and Coaching Promotes Language Development

Shine a light on your child's nonverbal and verbal language during play time

Introduction
In Chapter Two we talked about getting into a child's attention spotlight during play by body positioning to have face-to-face contact, reducing other distractions, being child-directed, using the child's favorite activities, and spotlighting the child's focus of attention or theme during play. We discussed the importance of observing and responding to the child's nonverbal initiations with gestures, imitation, and sounds. We also talked about the value of using visual prompts to

give children choices and waiting for your child's verbal or nonverbal response before talking again. We learned that prompting, modeling, and imitating your child's actions, sounds, and word responses with enthusiasm adds to your child's interest and motivation to be involved in joint play with you. All of these child-directed play approaches will strengthen your relationship and sense of joy, connection, and bonding with your child.

In Chapter Three we will build on that relationship foundation spotlight and discuss ways to "coach" your child to build their verbal and nonverbal language development, prepare them for school, and help them persist with a difficult learning activity even when frustrated or anxious. The definition of coach is not quite the same as a sports coach who is preparing the athlete for a competition. Rather, the parent or teacher coach supports and nurtures the child learner, praises their strengths, and models and prompts language communication and social interactions. In a coaching role, you will set up practices according to your child's particular goals and language and play developmental level.

In this chapter you will learn about three kinds of language coaching. The first is called descriptive commenting. This is when you show interest in what your child is doing by simply describing and providing supportive comments and gestures about what your child is doing. We will talk about how to tailor this language to first describe and imitate the child's beginning vocalizations and sounds and then add some basic words for the child's actions and the objects they are playing with. As the child's receptive language and words begin to emerge, we will discuss using Pre-academic Coaching. At this stage you can turn up the volume of your communication and attention to describe pre-academic concepts such as the colors, shapes, names of objects, numbers, letters, and positions of the things your child is playing with.

A third type of coaching is Persistence Coaching. This language and gesturing is used to help scaffold your child's ability to stay focused and persist with a difficult learning activity even when frustrated or anxious. Pairing pre-academic and persistence coaching with your child's favorite activities will expand your child's language development and school readiness skills and help reduce their anxiety by increasing your child's confidence in their abilities.

Assessing your child's communication level will help you decide which kind of coaching your child is ready for. Children with little or no language will benefit from narrated descriptive commenting with simple words used repeatedly, gestures, and labels or visuals for basic objects and actions (e.g., walk, run, eat, dress). You will not move on to pre-academic or persistence coaching until your child understands and is using 2-3 word sentences.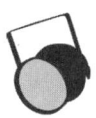

Using Descriptive Commenting to Turn on Your Child's Voice

Often parents ask children questions when they are playing such as, "what animal is that?" or, "what are you making?" or "what is that called?" and will correct their children's word efforts or pronunciation. While parents' intentions are to help their children use more verbal communication, all too often this approach has the reverse effect, causing children to become more withdrawn and confused, especially when they don't understand or know the answer to the questions. Instead show your interest by using child-directed descriptive commenting. This means narrating your child's play by labeling actions and objects and imitating their sounds or language attempts. Children who hear this type of focused and attentive narrative language from adults are absorbing and learning important things about language use as it relates to their own interests and actions. Gradually, they will start to link the words with their meanings, and without the pressure to speak or perform, they will be more likely to experiment with using the words and sounds to narrate their own play or to communicate with you.

For children on the autism spectrum, the pacing and use of language needs to be deliberate and matched to each child's goals. The IY Child Communication Checklist from Chapter One can help you determine the appropriate developmental goals for your child. Children with very little verbal language can be overwhelmed by adult fast-paced narrated play or descriptive commenting. Language that is too complex or rapid can result in the child feeling anxious and withdrawing from the play. It may seem to the parent or teacher that the child is

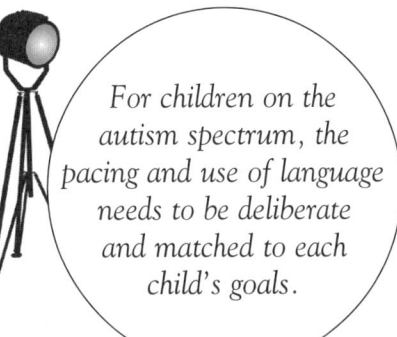

For children on the autism spectrum, the pacing and use of language needs to be deliberate and matched to each child's goals.

rejecting them, when in fact, the child has stopped listening because they are unable to process or understand the words they are hearing.

For these children, the descriptive commenting and coaching process must be slowed down and simplified. This means using a few targeted words, highlighted with a higher level of enthusiasm, more repetition, gestures, and persistence. Imagine you are lost in a country where you don't speak the language and you ask someone for directions. The more unfamiliar words the person uses to give you directions and the faster they speak, the more confused you become. However, if they are patient and positive, slow down and use fewer words and more gestures, draw a picture, show you a map, or even take you to your destination, you will understand more and feel less anxious or intimidated. Parents and teachers can act as a communication translator for their child, by limiting the number of words and using gestures and visual prompts to enhance their child's understanding. They can help the child realize that they can turn on their voice with sounds, gestures, and pictures to indicate their wants and needs to others. Eventually their sounds will turn into meaningful words.

Act as a communication translator by limiting words and using gestures and visual prompts to enhance understanding.

For Children with Less Language
Model and Imitate Simple Sounds

Children with less verbal language need to first learn to make sounds in response to an adult's language or sounds *(reciprocal responding)*. Children with ASD produce fewer sounds than neurotypical children. Hard consonants like "ba, da" are more difficult than soft consonant and vowel sounds like "zip, zap, zee." Parents and teachers can start by frequently modeling simple and exaggerated vowel sounds. When the child vocalizes back, repeat and imitate their sounds with delight, wait for another sound from the child, and repeat, making this into a fun back and forth vocal turn taking game. Most children will need time to learn to vocalize a new sound, and parents and teachers must patiently model the new sound multiple times, allowing the child to listen and learn before imitating. With repeated practice, the adult is gradually turning on the child's voice and helping them realize their sounds promote an interesting response from the adult.

Most people naturally speak this kind of "parentese" with babies, and continuing this language approach is crucial for older children on the autism spectrum who are learning to use reciprocal language. Parents can do this sound imitation game by making fun exaggerated sound effects during play with cars (vroom! or beep, beep, crash, or wheee), animals (moo), or objects such as a train (choo, choo). Children love these sounds and will repeat them just to hear their parent or teacher say them again. Songs with simple, repetitive rhythms such as, "Old MacDonald has a farm" are also good ways to reinforce the fun of language, emphasizing the animal sound effects in each verse. Parents and teachers can make silly fun noises during any daily routine such as getting ready for bed, mealtimes, lining up for recess, or hand washing. Combine simple words and sounds with gestures, actions, and songs. Children love the rhythmic social action routines that accompany songs such as "Row, row, row your boat" and "London Bridge". Pause these songs and action midway through to see if the child will fill in the blank with a word, sound, or gesture (partial prompt). To encourage interaction, the adult imitates any child initiation and can add a gesture, additional sound, or word. Treat your child's efforts to communicate as if they make sense!

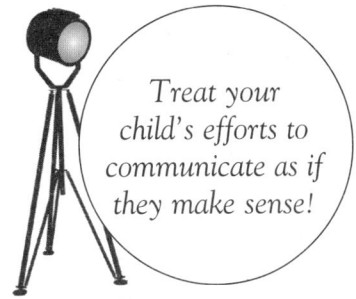

Treat your child's efforts to communicate as if they make sense!

Gesturing

Using gestures to help children communicate is useful because they help make meaning for the words that are not yet understood by the child. It can be useful to teach some specific gestures that can be used when prompting behavior in the child. Gestures that include a desire for social interaction and joint attention include: waving hello, smiling, reaching out with arms up to indicate wanting to be picked up, clapping, high fives, thumbs up, reaching your hand out to indicate "you," or patting your chest to indicate "me," and waving good bye. Use these gestures repeatedly. For example, every time the adult leaves or returns, wave hello or good-bye in an exaggerated way with a big smile and a wave. If the child doesn't wave, you may gently take their arm and wave it *(physical prompt)*. Repeat these greetings multiple times each day. You can also use puppets to model these greetings. After a few weeks, your child will likely respond to the greetings with a wave, eye contact, a sound, or word.

Naming objects and actions when using request gestures
Children who have single word language are ready to expand the range of words they know. Adults can help them learn new words by naming *objects* such as foods, toys, body parts, animals, and clothing. Don't worry about colors or letters at the early stage of learning words. Name *child and adult actions* or requests in daily situations such putting on shoes, walking, making dinner, taking a nap, going to the bathroom, stopping actions, and making requests for something such as food or an activity.

Once children know the names of objects or actions, then the next step is for parents or teachers to add a word to the simple gestures that have been taught in earlier stages. When the child gestures for an object, the adult should imitate the gesture and add a word for the object that they want. Focus first on the object or action rather than on the words or gestures for "please" or "more." This gives the child a more accurate way to convey a specific request. A child who says "app" or "apple" is communicating more clearly than a child who says "more." As with sounds and gestures, reward the child's attempts to make words by giving the child the requested object as soon as they have attempted to say the word. Even if the word is not said correctly, respond to this verbal request with enthusiasm and understanding and repeat the word several times while giving the child the requested object.

Using the "One Up Rule" for Expanding Language
For children with more words, the parent or teacher responds with the *"one up rule"*; that is, adding one more word to the child's word sentence or completing the sound with a full word. If the child has single-word responses, one more word is added to the description of what the child is doing or asking for. For example, if the child says "apple", this may be expanded by saying, "want apple". If the child is

already combining two words, use sentences that are 3-4 words, such "please give me apple." If the child echoes a whole sentence, but only produces single words spontaneously, then stick to the "one- up" rule. Echoed sentences or phrases are not generally being used by the child as communication. Keep the words simple and short; just slightly more complex than the child's existing language. Children who have more language still benefit from gestures.

Descriptive Commenting and Visual Prompts To Build Language

In the next scenario, think about what makes the teacher's use of a visual prompt along with her descriptive commenting effective for helping this girl learn language.

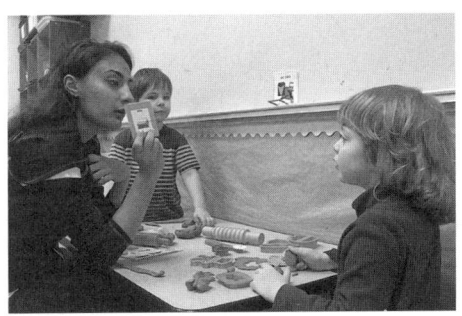
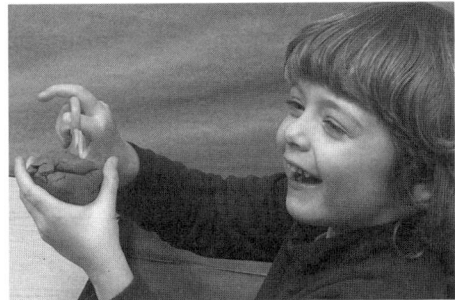

Teacher: (shows visual chart of playdough activity choices.) It looks like you made shapes.
Victoria: He's squeeze.
Teacher: That's next. Can you show me "squeeze dough"?
Victoria: (squeezes the playdough.)
Teacher: Nice! That's squeezing. (also squeezes dough and imitates her.) Good choice.
Victoria: (pokes dough.)
Teacher: Now you're poking. (points to picture of 'poking' on chart.) I see you poke the dough. Good job.
Victoria: (pokes playdough again.) It's kind of pokey.
Teacher: Yes it is kind of pokey. Nice job, you're poking. (teacher pokes playdough.)
Victoria: Now squeeze.

Teacher: (laughs.) You're squeezing it. Around your finger like this. (Demonstrates putting playdough around her own finger and shows her.)
Victoria: (copies teacher and puts dough around her finger and shows her.)
Teacher: Yeah. Oh, I like that. (laughs.) I like that.
Victoria: Where did your hand go?
Teacher: Where's your hand? (points at girl.) Ah! I see it! I see your finger. Alright, check it out. What else should we do with the playdough? (shows playdough activity chart again.)
Victoria: (points at cutting objects on chart.) Cut it.
Teacher: Great idea. Let's cut it. Check it out. What do we need?
Victoria: (points at scissors on table.)
Teacher: You're going cut it with the scissors? I'm going to cut it with the knife.
Victoria: (starts cutting playdough.) Oh!
Teacher: (cuts her own playdough.) Cut. (points at scissors.) I see you are cutting with scissors.
Victoria: We got playdough.
Teacher: You do have that playdough. Nice cutting the playdough.
Victoria: (looks at teacher and laughs showing her the scissors stuck in the playdough.)
Teacher: Nice cutting.

Considerations

This teacher is being child-directed in her use of the visual prompts. She imitates what Victoria does with the playdough and repeats what she says, letting her make the choice for what she will do with the playdough. She points to the picture of the action on the card as she says the action words (squeeze, poke, cut) and models the action herself as she watched Victoria do it.

Most children on the autism spectrum are visual learners and we can see how Victoria learns new ideas for what to do with the playdough from the visual prompts. For children who have difficulty processing speech, the picture gives them more time to receive and understand the information than just a word. Even if a child has language skills, the picture prompt improves their learning experience and understanding of what it means to "squeeze" or "cut." The teacher shows the picture of the scissors cutting and labels the words cut and scissors while Victoria is using the scissors. Thus, the picture and words cut and scissors are paired with the action of cutting. This helps Victoria understand the meaning of this action as well as the name of the tool.

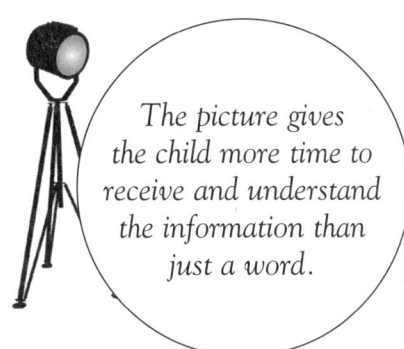

The picture gives the child more time to receive and understand the information than just a word.

Think about what visual prompts you can use to enhance your descriptive commenting. See Chapter Two for more discussion of how to use visual prompts to enhance language development.

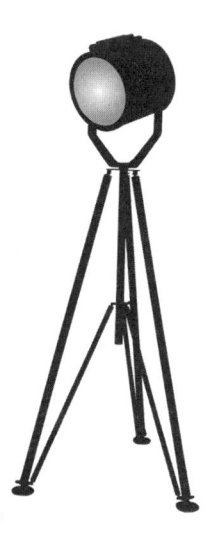

SPOTLIGHTING
Child Directed Coached Play for Children with Limited Language

- Try to get face-to-face contact and gain your child's attention before talking.
- Use simple, short words to describe what the child is doing, seeing, and experiencing. Limit instructions and questions. Follow your child's lead.
- Wait and pause for your child's turn to respond with a gesture, look, or word before speaking and narrating again.
- Imitate and repeat your child's sounds, gestures, behaviors, and words (sound effects such as animal or engine noises help promote sound production).
- Try to sustain back and forth verbal interchange as long as your child is interested, by reinforcing verbal and nonverbal responses.

- Use the "one up" rule, adding one word to your child's existing language level. Keep it simple, slow down, imitate and build repetition.
- Combine your words with nonverbal gestures, visuals, and imitate your child's words and actions.
- Narrate your child's activities with simple language during play times as well as daily routines such as mealtimes, bedtime, getting dressed, hand washing, and following your instructions.
- Use visual prompts or concrete objects along with simple words used repetitively
- Encourage your child to look at you by putting the desired object next to your face and waiting for a response.

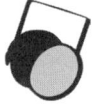

For children who are just beginning to talk, focus on labeling common objects and actions. Do not try to teach numbers, letters, colors, or shapes. These will come later, once your child can name basic objects and actions.

PRE-ACADEMIC COACHING PROMOTES SCHOOL READINESS SKILLS

Incorporating Pre-Academic Coaching into a Game

Some children on the spectrum, like Amelia, have quite a bit of language, and are ready to be introduced to pre-academic coaching. This type of coaching is when you label the objects the child is playing with (truck, block, horse), the attributes of these objects (colors, shapes, numbers, letters, textures, smells, sounds, sizes), and prepositions to describe what the object is doing (up, down, beside, next to behind). This approach will help children learn academic concepts and scaffold their attention. Pairing this pre-academic coaching with your child's favorite activities will

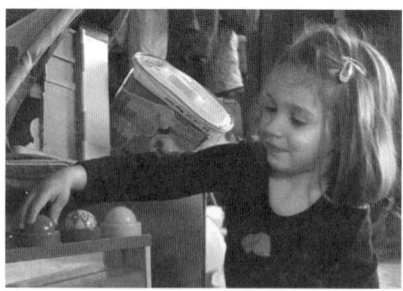

Teachers and Parents "Descriptive Commenting" Checklist

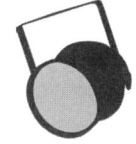

Descriptive Commenting is a powerful way to strengthen a child's language skills. The following provides some examples of actions, objects, prepositions or sounds you can comment upon when interacting with a child on the autism spectrum. Modulate the number of words and complexity of your language according to the "one up" rule. Combine physical gestures with animated language. Remember to keep your language simple, slow down, and build repetition. Write down the the verbal and nonverbal communication approaches you will use to achieve your goals.

Actions		Goals
_____ walk	_____ wash hands	
_____ run	_____ bye	
_____ finished	_____ hi	
_____ sit	_____ break	
_____ stop	_____ quiet	
_____ stand	_____ shoes off/on	
_____ wait	_____ your turn	
Objects		
_____ books	_____ clothing items	
_____ animals, puppets, or stuffed animals		
_____ transport toys (tricycle, truck, boat)		
_____ art supplies (crayons, play dough)		
_____ foods & drinks, food utensils		
_____ body parts (ear, nose, arm)		
Prepositions		
_____ up	_____ behind	
_____ down	_____ in front	
_____ inside	_____ next to	
_____ on top	_____ below	
Sounds		
_____ loud	_____ crash	
_____ quiet	_____ zip zip	
_____ funny	_____ choo choo	
_____ whee	_____ animal sounds	
_____ zoom	_____ letters	

Part 1: Promoting Language Development   ©The Incredible Years®

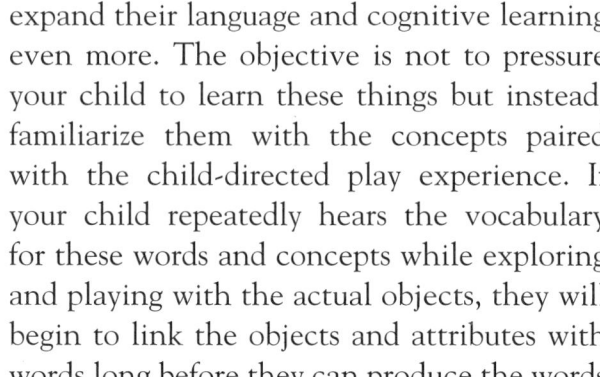

The objective is not to pressure your child to learn but instead, familiarize them with the concepts paired with the child-directed play experience.

expand their language and cognitive learning even more. The objective is not to pressure your child to learn these things but instead, familiarize them with the concepts paired with the child-directed play experience. If your child repeatedly hears the vocabulary for these words and concepts while exploring and playing with the actual objects, they will begin to link the objects and attributes with words long before they can produce the words themself. This is called "experiential learning". In the next scenario, think about how the mother is child-directed with Amelia while she uses pre-academic coaching. Notice what she describes with her language and the pre-academic concepts she focuses on.

Amelia: Where are you going to put this one?
Mother: I don't know where should I put this one? (holding purple and green ball)
Amelia: You could put it right here, you could put one (takes out her green ball to make room).
Mother: Well, I could put it there because there is green in it.
Amelia: (moves it to purple hole)
Mother: Or we could put it there because there is purple in it. You are matching purple and green.
Amelia: (bangs them all down)
Mother: You got them all down. All of them, all four of them, one, two, three, four. All four of them.
Amelia: No, one, two, three, four, five.
Mother: Do you see five? I see one, two, three, four.. is there another one somewhere?
Amelia: Yeah right there.
Mother: Right there. Can you help me count them?
Amelia: (points to all the balls and one rolls away)
Mother: One rolled away... one, two, three...
Amelia: One, two, one, two, three.
Mother: One, two, three.

Amelia: Do you want to...to bring one back?
Mother: Do you want to bring it back? You can bring it back. Let's go find it.
Amelia: (Brings it back.)
Mother: 1,2,3,4 all of them down. Whee…Humm (looking at yellow ball). Can I make it my nose?
Amelia: (shakes head no)
Mother: Should I make it part of my ear?
Amelia: No.
Mother: No it's not an ear!

Considerations

This interaction shows how the mother is being child-directed and is using pre-academic coaching to count the balls and describe the colors of the balls they are playing with. She starts by assuring Amelia is fully engaged in their play and social interactions by positioning herself face-to-face and asking for her daughter's help by saying, *"I don't know where we should put this one?"* When Amelia shows her mother where to put the ball, her mother comments on the color match and then prompts her to see another possible color match (purple). As Amelia hammers the balls down, the mother names the action and the number of balls, and Amelia imitates the numbers counted. They play a game of counting the balls and repeating the numbers as one rolls away. Finally, the mother adds to her daughter's interest and engagement in the game by suggesting that one of the balls is possibly a nose or her ear. The mother's enthusiasm, pretending, being funny, and pausing to wait for her daughter's response, enhances Amelia's engagement, pre-academic language learning (colors, numbers, body parts, positions), and lengthens their joint social interaction and communication.

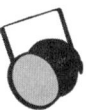

When you feel your child is stuck in doing the same routine the same predictable way and you are losing the spotlight connection, try something completely unexpected, different, or silly. Using *silliness or surprise* can keep your child's attention longer in your social interaction. In the example above we saw how Amelia's mother captured her imagination by turning the wooden ball into her nose and then an ear. Amelia responded to this silliness by correcting her mother's "mistake." Children will often delight in correcting an adult who is pretending something that is obviously wrong: pretending to put a Lego piece into a puzzle, pretending to eat a shoe, putting a hat on an elbow. When the child notices the problem, laugh with them saying, "Uh oh!" and ask for their help. Children love it when parents make mistakes or act goofy and silly. This is an excellent way to get you back in their attention spotlight zone.

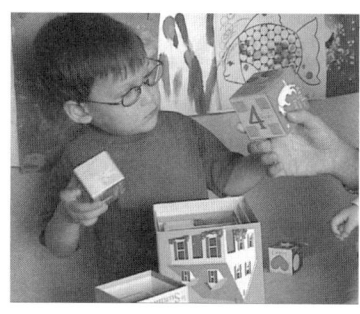

Pre-academic Coaching Combined with Persistence Coaching

In the next scenario Kalani, who is 3 ½ years old, has fairly good receptive language, but less expressive language than Amelia. Notice what the mother comments on and how she encourages him to keep playing with the blocks. Think about what Kalani is learning by her approach.

Mother: Oh there it goes Kalani, it's getting tall —you've got lots of boxes: little boxes and big boxes.
Kalani: (box fell over)
Mother: Oh, oh—it fell over? You're trying again.
Kalani: Big box (not clear what he is saying)
Mother: You want the big box? Okay here is the big box.
Mother: Yes, you are going to do a big tower with that big one on the bottom.
Kalani: Big.
Mother: Yes, big box! (*one up rule*).
Kalani: Continues playing with boxes; building and nesting them inside each other.
Mother: That's it Kalani . You took it out, Oh they are all going in. You are making them fit! You stacked them all in! Yea Kalani! You did it! I'm so proud of you. You kept trying. You got them all in. All right! High five! (*praising his persistence*)

Kalani:	(gives his mother a high five and continues working)
Mother:	Wow! You keep trying different ways, and you made the little boxes fit. Kalani that's a great way to solve your problem.
Kalani:	(looks at his mother and gives a big smile)

Considerations

This time we see the mother combining pre-academic coaching with persistence coaching. We see her using descriptive or narrated commenting by describing Kalani's *actions* (*stacking, going in, fitting*) and the names of *nouns* (*box, tower,*) and *sizes* (*big, little*). She keeps her commenting simple and repetitive. She builds on the words that Kalani uses by using the one-up rule (big box) and responds to his words by giving him what he asks for.

She also uses persistence coaching (described further below) by commenting when he tries again after his blocks fall and persists in trying to make all the boxes fit. When he succeeds, she enthusiastically praises him with a high five hand clap. She labels his success, saying that he kept trying and solving his problem. While Kalani has very little verbal language response to his mother during this interaction, he appears to be enjoying his mother's attention and her spotlight on his work. He persists at a task that is difficult for him, likely because of her attention and encouragement for his efforts. He rewards the mother at the end with a wonderful smile; indicating there was strong connection during this joint play.

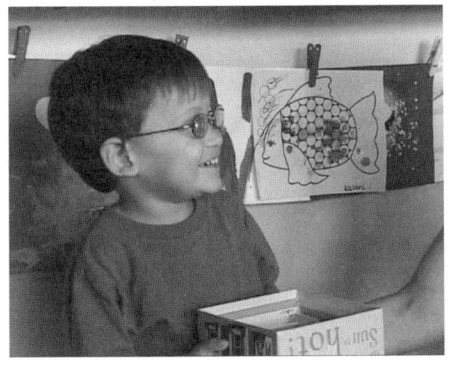
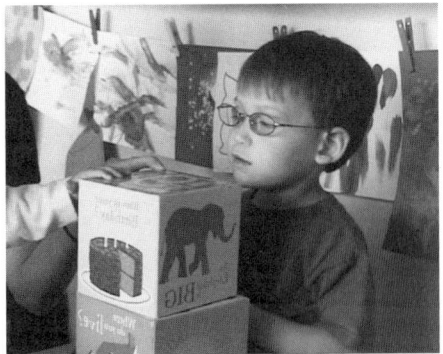

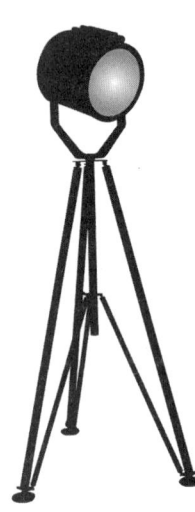

SPOTLIGHTING
Pre-Academic Coaching
Promotes Children's Language Skills

- Notice what your child is giving attention to and talk about it.
- Describe the objects, shapes, numbers, letters, and colors of things your child plays with; avoid questions.
- Listen to your child and imitate or mirror, your child's sounds and/or words.
- Talk about positions of objects (e.g., inside, under, beside, next to, behind).
- Describe your child's actions, body parts, and clothing.
- Prompt your child to communicate by modeling words for them to copy.
- Use new and more complex words to expand your child's vocabulary even if you know they won't understand at first.
- Chant, sing rhymes, and teach your child body movements that go with the words.
- Describe your own actions to your child (e.g, "I'm folding three shirts and two pairs of red socks now).
- Describe your child's actions during everyday activities such as dressing, eating, or getting ready for bed.
- Match real objects with words and pictures of objects.

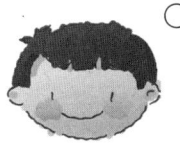

The blue block is next to the yellow square, and the purple triangle is on top of the long red triangle.

You are putting your blue sweater on top of your white sweater. This will keep your body warm.

Joint picture book reading is another child-directed activity that will increase your connection with your child, while also encouraging their attention and language development. Below are some tips to reading in a child-directed way, using the descriptive commenting and pre-academic coaching described above.

E-Care Encourages Language and Reading Readiness

Extra care reading involves providing children with autism and language delays with added opportunities for language development, joint attention, and social interaction. To start with, take extra care to choose a book with your child that is on a topic they are interested in, perhaps something from your child's "like list".

For example, if your child likes planes, trains, cooking, dinosaurs or a particular animal, pick a book on this topic. This will help you to enter your child's interest spotlight. Choose books with pictures, and very few words which are repetitive and have silly rhyming words, simple plots, and sensory activities (flaps, textures, smells, and hidden objects).

Comment strategically according to your child's language level.

The amount of commenting you do will depend on the extra-care you take in first understanding your child's receptive and expression language ability.

For a child with no language, start by making the appropriate sound effects that match the book pictures of the animals, trains, or birds and imitate your child's attempts to copy these sounds or gestures. Name and point to the object when you make the sounds and, when possible, also include the actual object that matches the picture in the book. For example, have a toy train, animal, or bird puppet while you are reading the related book. Pace slowly and repeat 1-2 words with hand signals, pointing gestures, funny noises, and enthusiastic tone. Turn towards your child so that they can see your face and emotions. Say less and simplify what is written in text.

For a child with a few more words, use the "one-up rule;" that is, make comments that are 1 word longer than your child's typical utterances. If your child communicates by saying: "bear", you might say: "big bear" or "polar bear." If your child says *"polar bear growls,"* elaborate by saying, *"a huge, polar bear growls like…."* accompanied by a growling sounds and the gesture for huge. Start with pointing and naming words of objects, feelings, and actions before progressing to pre-academic words of colors, shapes, numbers, and letters. Continue using gestures, sound effects, puppets, and songs or rhymes to stay in your child's attention spotlight. Simplify text according to your child's language level. Give your child an opportunity to show you they understand by pointing to pictures and turning the page.

For a child with more receptive and expressive language, you can ask a few who, what, and why questions about what is happening in the story, such as, what will happen next? how the character feels? or who is doing something in a picture? If they have trouble answering, you or your puppet can model an answer. Books with simple plots will make it easier to ask these questions. You can begin to read books where the pictures don't always match the text. For some stories, you can act out the story with puppets and figurines. Eventually you will start to encourage your child to notice the letters and words in the books. Read the text slowly and point to the words as you say them. Doing this will help your child understand how the printed word talks. You can add to this understanding by pointing to words on cereal boxes, to-do lists, billboards when you are driving, or menus in restaurants.

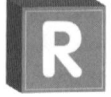

Avoid open-ended questions, pace your commenting, and repeat often. Asking questions when reading can be intimidating and cause withdrawal, anxiety, and confusion, especially for children with receptive and expressive language delays. Your child may not understand the questions or may not have the language to respond. Instead, strategically decide what words you want to encourage, allow time for your child's response (verbally or nonverbally), and then imitate their response. This will show your child you are interested. If your child repeats your sound effects, gesture, or word, imitate again so your child sees how their response affects your response. Be sure to smile and try to have eye contact when you do this. If your child refuses eye-contact, don't force it.

Respond and listen with interest. Wait and pause before talking again so your child has time to respond. When your child responds with a smile, gesture, sound effect, or words, enthusiastically respond to these responses verbally, even if your child's response doesn't make sense to you. Always act as if you understand what your child is saying! Imitate your child's gestures, sounds, and words. The goal here is to encourage your child's interest in books, to get into their spotlight, and to engage in joint attention and positive interactions.

Expand on what your child says. If your child has no language, you can use hand signals to model the action, show the actual object as you name it, or use one of your child's likes (song, touch, or favorite object) to add more excitement to the joint reading interaction. If your child has some words use the "one-up rule" and add an additional word to your child's comments. To combine social interactions with reading, read to two children at the same time and prompt language in both children. Occasionally surprise children by doing something unexpected or a add a variation on the story such as a different and humorous word, or naming the object or feeling incorrectly, and then correct yourself. *"Ooops! My mistake!"* Make games out of a book by covering up a picture with sticky notes and guessing what is under there or what comes on the next page. Sing a song using the word you are encouraging.

Expand reading modeling by including your child's favorite puppet as a reader. When you have read the book multiple times, pause periodically to see if your child can fill in the missing word. If, your child doesn't respond to the partial prompt your puppet can say the word or say part of the word and see if the child can complete it. Keep doing this pausing the sentence at the same places every time and one day you will find your child completing the word before the puppet does. You and your puppet can respond with a clap and praise, "you are reading!" End your reading sessions with the routine of an *"all done"* and hand signal.

Some children with ASD have a gifted ability to read. Even though they 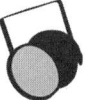 read long and difficult words, it doesn't mean they always understand what the words mean. Using the E-care reading tips will help enhance your child's understanding beyond the written words. It will help them think about the feelings and intentions of characters, connect the story to their own experience, and predict what might happen next. Exploring a book together in this way can help them discover a new way to communicate.

In the next scenario notice how Kalani's mother uses the E-Care reading principles including pointing, use of gestures and verbal language, sign language, and speech. She is child-directed and follows Kalani's attention focus and praises his word use. All of these approaches 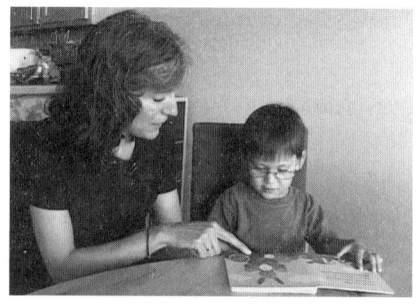 encourage his reading readiness as well as his speech development. Think about how you might use some of these reading principles with your child.

Mother: (points to picture of melon) That's a melon.
Kalani: Watermelon.
Mother: (enthusiastic tone) Yeah, you like watermelon, yummy! That's a red watermelon. Ooh (points to picture) there's a little spider. (makes spider gesture with both hands and fingers moving)
Kalani: Spider.
Mother: A spider—he's a purple spider—yeah.(Kalani turns page and claps down hands on picture of the bird) Oh see the bird (she whistles and uses a sign for bird) the bird is sitting in the tree.
Kalani: Kalani looks and smiles, but does not comment or imitate the bird sound.
Mother: Kalani, look it's raining (points to picture and then with both hands makes raining sign).
Kalani: Raining, raining, raining. (copies the rain sign)
Mother: Yeah you've been out in the rain before. (Kalani points to the cow picture). Look there's a cow. (makes cow sign)
Kalani: Cow.
Mother: Is he taking a bath? (makes gesture on chest)
Kalani: (points to a picture of sheep) Yeah, sheep – the sheep. (makes sheep sign)
Mother: Yes! Sheep, a wooly sheep. Sheep say "baaa."
Kalani: Aman. (his word for animals)

Mother: All the animals. All the animals. Yeah.
Kalani: ooo ooo ah ah (monkey sound and makes gesture under arms)
Mother: There's the monkey. He says: "ooo ooo". You know all the sounds!
Kalani: (tries to whistle)
Mother: There's the bird (uses bird gesture). "Moo" said the cow.
Kalani: Moo.
Mother: I see some shapes too (points) you've got the…what's that?
Kalani: (points to each shape and tries to say the names of the shapes—not really understandable)
Mother: (with enthusiasm, moving closer and gently touching his arm) Square, circle, triangle! Oh you've named all your shapes wow!

Considerations

Kalani has language delays and his mother encourages his language expression by naming the objects, showing him the sign language for the words, and pointing to the picture of what she is naming. You can see how Kalani modeled his mother's actions by pointing to the picture of the sheep after his mother had pointed to and named several other pictures. She is child-directed and gets in Kalani's spotlight by giving him the opportunity to direct the reading by turning the pages himself. She only comments on what he is noticing and paying attention to on the pages. She models some words and is very encouraging when he responds. She is also teaching him a love for reading by her warm tone of voice and enjoyment. It is clear he has read this book before and is beginning to memorize it and feel confident about his ability to read the book and identify the animals.

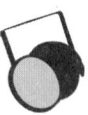

We saw that Kalani copied his mother's pointing gesture as she talked about the picture. If your child doesn't copy your pointing, you can take their hand and shape their finger into a point at the beginning. Eventually you will fade out your physical prompt, so your child doesn't become dependent on it. Kalani showed great interest in this book because he has read it many times. Some children will not be interested in reading the book, and will use it for other sensory exploration like tasting, chewing, tearing pages, or another purpose, like stacking or lining it up. If this is the case, start with books that are made of durable materials and that lend themselves to sensory exploration, with flaps, textures, and sound effects. Try to engage your child in the interactive reading and exploration of the book, but don't force it if your child resists. You can always try again later!

Keep books in a place that is accessible to your child: a low shelf or book box. Provide books to match your child's interest and developmental level. If your child is just starting to explore reading, limit the choices to a few books. As your child develops a love of reading and is comfortable with a few favorite books that they know by heart, you can add new books and expand the choices. Encourage your child to pick one new book and one old book to read together. Since trying something new can be hard, read the new book first, and use the familiar book as a reward for exploring the new book with you. Make the new book short, so your child won't have to wait long before reading their favorite book. Explore the new book together, looking and commenting on the pictures and letting the child turn the pages. Although this is not the traditional way to read to a child, this approach is building your child's vocabulary and fine motor skills (holding book and turning pages). This type of interactive reading is also beneficial for encouraging language development in neurotypical children.

Encourage your child to pick one new book and one old book to read together.

Interactive, child directed reading, will increase your child's attention span and interest in reading. Even so, your child's attention for books may still be relatively short. Sometimes children may be content to sit and read for many minutes, other times they may start squirming or reaching for another book before the first page is done. This is developmentally normal, even in neurotypical children. You can continue to encourage your child's engagement by reading in a dramatic way, adding in favorite objects or puppets or sound effects or gestures and actions. You can continue to read a few more pages even if your child has started to wander off. If your child looks at you or stops doing what they are doing to listen, you will know they are still interested. However, if your child has moved on, you should follow your child's lead and see what they want to explore. Try reading again later when your child is not so driven to do something else.

SPOTLIGHTING
Coaching Children's Reading Readiness with Extra-Care (E-Care)

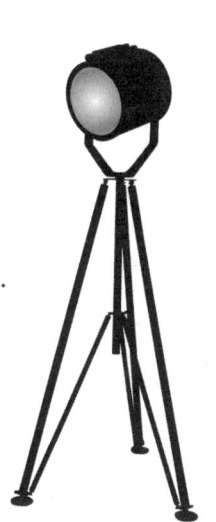

- Read at a quiet time when you are relaxed and comfortable with TV and music turned off (this prevents over stimulation).
- Read for a few minutes each day when your child seems calm and alert.
- Place your child in front of you during reading with face-to-face contact so your child can see your face and expressions.
- Keep the reading fun and simple using the "one up" principle to tailor language to your child's development. Say less and go slowly. Avoid commands and criticisms. Be child-directed in your approach. Label the picture that captures your child's attention. Don't expect to read text as written!
- Use physical hand signals, pointing gestures, sound effects, real objects, and puppets when looking at pictures to enhance your child's understanding and enjoyment.
- Respond immediately to your child's verbalization or gestures.
- Prompt and imitate your child's word use. Repeat words often.
- Re-read books your child likes many times. This is a pre-reading skill and leads to mastery and confidence. Once your child has learned the story, you can add partial prompts to see if they will fill in the blank.
- Read slowly. Be animated and enthusiastic. Exaggerate key words. Pause between words to give your child time process the information.
- Praise and give positive feedback ("that's right!").
- Sing and use sound effects during reading.

- Slide your finger under the words or letters on the page and show left to right movement. Draw attention by guiding child's finger under words you read.
- Encourage your child to turn the pages and choose a book they are interested in. Start a sentence and let your child fill in blanks. "I see a……."
- Choose books with colorful pictures and simple, familiar plots that relate to the pictures. Interactive books with flaps, buttons to push, textures to touch, and "scratch and sniff" pictures to smell can be engaging and fun.
- Make sure there is a back-and-forth quality to the reading. Don't read without requiring some response or connection with your child.
- Create books and journals for your child with photos of things they do and transcribe personal stories about these activities.
- End reading with a repetitive routine of "all done" or "all finished" signal and kiss.

Parent Reflections with Descriptive Commenting & Pre-academic Coaching

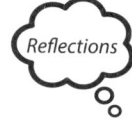

Father: *Introducing descriptive commenting for Hudson. I don't think it was too difficult. He'll tend to listen and repeat what I say. So I feel like it's a very useful way to help increase his vocabulary. Before I started the class, I don't think I was doing it that much. It's a good example of building on one of his skills. Something that he enjoys doing.*

Mother: *We've done this descriptive commenting with books where I'll read to her and I pause. She knows the book, and she'll look at me when I pause and then give me the answer because she knows the sentence. I don't think she actually is reading but has memorized the book. However, it really helps her use her language with me.*

PERSISTENCE COACHING

All children get frustrated with their attempts to learn something new or try a new activity. However, children with language delays and children on the autism spectrum may be more likely to get frustrated because they don't understand the adult's instructions, don't know how to ask for help, or are anxious about their failure. They may give up easily and revert to repetitive actions that are more comfortable.

Persistence coaching is a method of talking to your child that will help them learn to persist with difficult tasks and continue to try hard despite frustrations and difficulties. Persistence coaching means naming the child's internal cognitive state when they are being patient, trying again, staying calm, concentrating, focusing, being curious, persisting, or working hard on a difficult task. This type of coaching is beneficial to all children but is particularly helpful for inattentive, impulsive, hyperactive, easily frustrated children who have language delays. This type of coaching provides the brain scaffolding to help support such children to stay calm and persistent for a few minutes longer than they could do on their own. This approach can be used to help a child persevere with difficult tasks or some of their "dislikes" such as brushing their teeth, getting dressed, washing their hair, doing a puzzle, or learning to read. Eventually this approach will promote your child's independence and confidence.

Persistence Coaching for a Child with More Language

In the next example, Amelia's mother helps her learn to persist with opening a yogurt container. Amelia has fine motor difficulties and when something is hard to do, such as opening her sippy cup or a container, she gives up. Notice how the mother combines persistence coaching and descriptive commenting to help her daughter be successful at opening the yogurt container and stirring. Think about what makes her approach effective.

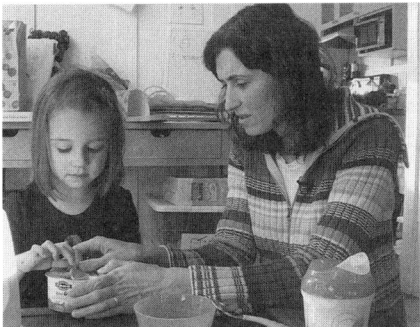

Mother: I have a brand new yogurt that needs opening, can you help me peel the foil? (hands her the yogurt to open.)
Amelia: (tries to open the yogurt top)
Mother: Good trying, you keep working on it and pulling. Pull real hard. Pull, you're getting it. It's almost there. Almost there! Keep pulling, keep going, keep going. You've got it! (foil on the top of the yogurt is

half off, and Amelia takes her hands away, looking like she is giving up).

Mother: Oh, I think one or two more pulls (Amelia, tries pulling again). That's right—you're trying again! (while Amelia is trying to open the top, her mother helps by pulling it along gently without Amelia realizing she is helping her) And maybe one more. Pull hard. Pull real hard. There! Whoo. High-five. You did it! That was hard and you stuck with it!

Amelia: Smiles and gives high five.

Mother: Can you help me put some of the fruit in? Scoop it in the yogurt?

Amelia: Yeah. (works using spoon with yogurt)

Mother: You practiced so nicely putting the strawberry in. Wonderful scooping. You're getting it all out. Okay, I think we can mix now.

Amelia: We need a little bit more.

Mother: Okay, a little bit more in there.

Amelia: Why do you need a little bit more?

Mother: Do you like a little bit more? Does that make you happy when you have more strawberry in there?

Amelia: (looks at mother and smiles)

Mother: I see a smile. I see you are definitely happy, yummy.

Mother: Okay time to mix, mix it all up. Great using two hands. I love how you are mixing it so nicely.

Amelia: Am I using two hands?

Mother: Maybe use one to hold the bowl. There you go! You figured it out. Look at that. Up and down and round and round. Up and down and round and round. Up and down and round and round. There you go, round and round.

Amelia: (tastes yogurt)

Mother: Taste good, thumbs up. You're happy, that's good.

Amelia: (tries to do a thumbs up)

Mother: You fixed your own yogurt today! You're a pretty big girl!

Considerations

Amelia has fine motor difficulties and would easily give up trying to open the yogurt container. She frequently doesn't use her spoon to eat because holding the spoon and getting it to her mouth has been difficult. Amelia's mother used to do these things for Amelia, and then she realized that Amelia needed to be encouraged to be more independent. In this scenario, you see the mother saying, *"Good trying, you keep working on it. It's almost there."* and *"You're getting it all out. There you go. You figured it out."* and *"You are mixing all by yourself. You are getting it."* These words help Amelia to persist with her fine motor skills. For children with less language, you might give a thumbs up and say, *"You are trying hard,"* or *"You can do it"*.

Notice how the mother provided some physical scaffolding (gently helping with the foil,) to support Amelia's success. It is important to practice persistence with tasks that are hard, but not impossible for children to do on their own. You might even have the yogurt container partially open to set her up for success. Persistence coaching helped Amelia stay engaged to successfully complete the task herself. Amelia experienced pride in doing something for herself!

Persistence Coaching for a Child with Less Language

Most children will need parental support to be able to persist with a difficult task without getting overly frustrated – and some children will need much more support than others, especially those with language delays and autism. In the next scenario notice how Kalani's mother uses some persistence coaching to make Kalani's child-directed play a valuable learning experience for her son.

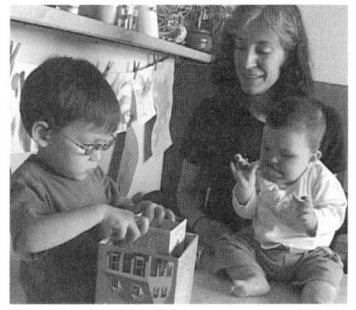

> **Mother:** You are trying hard on that. You almost have it...
> **Kalani:** (keeps trying to get small box out of big box)
> **Mother:** There you got it. You kept trying. (the little box is out.)
> **Kalani:** Three.
> **Mother:** You got all three boxes. You got three by yourself.
> **Kalani:** Big one.

Mother: Are you going to build a big tower? Oh it's getting tall. You put more and more on. You are sticking with it. (one falls off). Uh oh, it fell off, but you put it right back! It's getting taller than you are! Look how big! Oh my goodness, oh way up high (laughs).
Kalani: Little one.
Mother: The little one – where's it going to go?
Kalani: Way up high.
Mother: Way up high. Oh you did it. I'm so proud of you! You built a very big tower! You kept trying and you did it!

Considerations

Kalani's mother supports his persistence by using encouraging words like, "you keep trying" and "it is getting taller than you". When the box falls, she makes the "uh oh" sound, but then focuses on his trying again. When he completes the tower, she tells him how proud she is of how hard he worked. Other words you might use are, "I know you can do it", or "You are staying calm even though its hard", or " You are really thinking". For children on the spectrum with language delays, try to repeat the same set of words each time you coach their persistence. Mixing up the different words for persistence can make it confusing for them to match the words to their internal cognitive state. Choose one set of 2-3 words, depending on your child's language level, and repeat this phrase whenever you see your child persisting with something hard. Combining these same words with a gesture or picture, such as thumbs up, will enhance your child's understanding that that you believe they will be successful. Be sure to keep your developmental expecta-

Parent and teacher modeling calm and patient responses when the child gets frustrated is imperative.

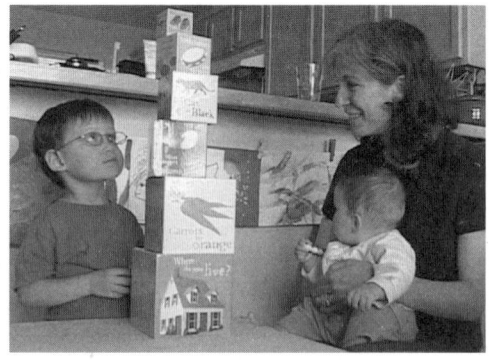

tions realistic, as each child's ability to focus and stay calm depends on the child's temperament, and their neurological, language, and brain development. There is a wide normal range for children's ability for self-control and ability to wait and persist. Children with delayed language may have more trouble with persistence and self-regulation and fostering the development of more nonverbal and verbal language skills will help them with this self-regulation process. Moreover, parents and teachers modeling calm and patient responses when the child gets frustrated is imperative. We will talk more about teaching children self-regulation skills in Chapter Seven.

Parents Reflections on Persistence Coaching

Mother: *Right as the course started, Amelia's preschool teacher said to me, "She doesn't persist in doing certain activities that are a little harder like some of the other kids do." I think that I used to do things for her, but I really wanted to be able to help her persist in activities that are difficult. I went from her being frustrated doing puzzles and just putting them down and walking away...to her literally saying, "I try and try again, and then I can do it." She actually pushes me away now, like "I can do it, I can do it." And so that is something that has been just glaringly huge.*

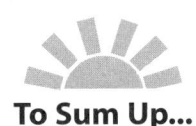

To Sum Up...

Be child-directed when you play with your child. Use strategically tailored descriptive commenting, gestures, pre-academic, and persistence coaching to show that you are interested in what your child is thinking and doing and that you enjoy being with them. This strengthens the attachment and joy in your relationship and enhances your child's language skills and self-confidence. You are also scaffolding your child's attention and helping them to stay calm despite distractions and feelings of frustration. Once your child feels you are in their spotlight with them and understand and support them, they can feel safe to explore social communication within your child-directed approach.

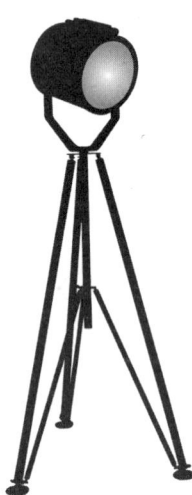

SPOTLIGHTING
Persistence Coaching Promotes Children's School Readiness Skills

- Describe when your child is working hard, concentrating, being calm, or staying patient when doing an activity.
- Describe your child's persistence with a frustrating activity by labeling that they are: trying again, sticking with it, thinking of a new way to do it, staying focused.
- Use a gesture such as "thumbs up" signal to show you are pleased with your child's persistence.
- Listen carefully and try to understand what your child is telling you about their thoughts, ideas, and discoveries.
- Comment and praise your child for listening to you or a peer or sibling.
- Encourage your child to discover, explore, experiment, and provide support when mistakes are made.
- Try not to give too much help; encourage your child's verbal and/or non-verbal responses to other children or adults.
- Practice encouraging persistence with "just right" tasks. Pick things that your child can do independently with a little extra effort. If the task is impossible, then provide some physical support or scaffolding, but don't take over.

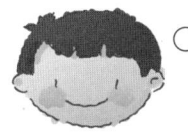

You are working so hard on that puzzle and thinking about where each piece will go. You are concentrating!

You are so patient and just keep trying to use your spoon.

You have figured our how to put on your shoes all by yourself.

You are staying calm and trying to ask him for the truck again.

Teachers and Parents "Pre-Academic & Persistence Coaching" Checklist

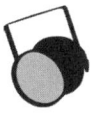

Pre-academic and persistence coaching are powerful ways to strengthen a child's school readiness skills. The following is a list of academic concepts and behaviors that can be commented upon when playing with a child. Modulate the number of words and complexity of your language according to the child's language development. Combine physical gestures with animated language. Remember to keep your language simple, slow down, and build repetition. Write down the the verbal and nonverbal communication approaches you will use to achieve your goals.

Academic Concepts	Goals
_____ colors _____ number counting _____ shapes _____ letters _____ sizes (long, short, tall, smaller than, bigger than, etc.) _____ positions (up, down, beside, next to, on top, behind, etc.)	
Persistence Skills (Preschoolers)	
_____ working hard _____ concentrating, focusing _____ persistence, patience _____ following teacher's directions _____ problem solving _____ trying again _____ reading _____ thinking skills _____ listening _____ working hard/best work _____ independence	

CHAPTER 4

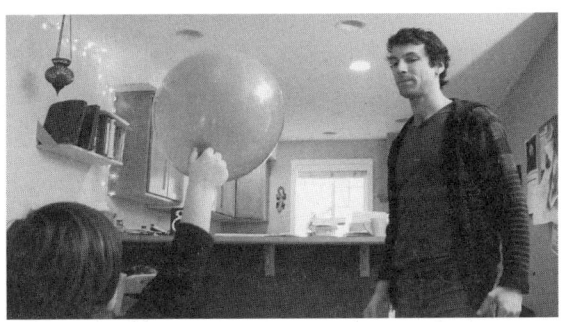

Turning Up the Spotlight on Your Child's Social Skills

Introduction

Earlier chapters covered coaching strategies for strengthening children's language development and pre-academic school readiness skills. This chapter describes another type of coaching: *Social Coaching*. The ability to share, trade, ask, help others, and take turns in social interactions is fundamental to children's social development and communication. Making friends comes easily for some children but is especially difficult for children on the autism spectrum and for those with language and developmental delays. Such children may be unaware of another child's desire for a turn or request for help because they are less tuned in to subtle communication cues in others' eyes, face, gestures, and tone of voice. They are far more focused on exploring an object than looking at people and find it difficult to shift their attention from the object to people. The risk is that these children will continue to play alone, rather than engage with parents or peers in their play activities. This will deprive them of the chance to learn from the regular social interactions that neurotypical children experience in their day-to-day encounters with others.

In this chapter you will learn how to turn up the volume of your joint attention social interactions by using social coaching, gestures, visual prompts, sensory routines, and songs. You will learn the importance of modeling social skills and prompting your child's social behavior and awareness of others in your play interactions. You will practice setting up ABC learning opportunities with your child to help practice social skills and broaden your child's spotlight to include recognition of others. This chapter builds on earlier language strategies, by adding social coaching methods to your tailored descriptive commenting, pre-academic and persistence coaching methods.

Turn almost any interaction or activity into an ABC joint attention learning opportunity.

Six Steps to Using the ABCs to Set Up Social Learning Opportunities

The ABCs for learning social behaviors include identifying the antecedent which motivates the child (A), then choosing the developmentally appropriate behavior (B) or target goals for the child to learn, and providing a rewarding consequence to the child (C) for using this behavior. The ABCs will be tailored to each child's current language and play development levels as well as their target social behavior goals.

Parents and teachers will model, prompt, scaffold, and engage in carefully crafted ABC scenarios designed to use a child's motivating antecedent (A) to elicit the child's developmentally appropriate target behavior, which will then be reinforced by something important to the child. Once parents and teachers understand the ABCs, they will find they can turn almost any interaction or activity into an ABC joint attention learning opportunity designed to teach their children more age-appropriate and socially acceptable ways of behaving.

This chapter is designed to give you a little more understanding of the ABC process of learning for children on the autism spectrum. The ABCs are based on the research and science of Applied Behavior Analysis, often known as ABA. ABA principles underlie many of the scenarios you have already read about in earlier chapters. The ABC model is particularly useful for these children because it provides a rather non-directive and supportive style of scaffolding activities around the child's interests as a way to teach new behaviors that they may not spontaneously learn on their own. They often miss out on the naturally occurring social reinforcement that supports language and social development in typically developing children. For children on the spectrum, the intensity of the positive consequences and motivators for targeted social behaviors must be highlighted or spotlighted in order to increase the likelihood of the children's discovery and enjoyment of being the objects of others' attention. There are six steps to assuring success with the ABC approach.

STEP 1: Identify your child's motivating antecedents

In Chapter One, you identified your child's likes and dislikes on the "How I Am Incredible" form. Offering the "likes" and removing or avoiding the "dislikes" can be highly reinforcing and can be used to motivate your child to learn new social behavior patterns. Moreover, understanding your child's likes helps you get into your child's attention spotlight and join your child by giving your attention to the child's unique play experiences, even when the activity may seem unconventional or pointless. As we noted in earlier chapters, you can usually tell what objects and activities a child likes by observing what they do repetitively. Examples of some common likes are lining up cars or other objects, playing with a certain toy, wanting a particular food or food texture, helping with a specific household chore, reading the same book over and over, singing, playing with the dog, being held or swung, rough and tumble play, bouncing, tickling, or other sensory activities. In the scenarios that follow, we will see examples of children motivated by a spinning egg chair; playing chase with dad; blowing, popping, and chasing balloons; banging hexagons; using playdough; playing with puppets; eating a particular food; and using the cell phone.

These strong preferences for an activity or object can be used as a motivating antecedent (A) to prompt a target behavior. The preferred activity or object is then given as a reward (or consequence) when the child engages in the desired behavior. For example, in the case of Hudson, we saw earlier how the father used his son's love of blowing bubbles to encourage the target verbal behavior (B) of asking for bubbles. Hudson's asking was followed by the rewarding consequence (C) of the father blowing the bubble for him to chase. It is also possible to use a child's dislikes as a motivator. For example, if a child dislikes a loud noise, such as the vacuum, the noise may be removed if the child exhibits the desired appropriate behavior of asking or signaling the parent to turn it off.

It is important that this ABC sequence be used for developmentally appropriate target behaviors and not for misbehavior. For example, giving the child their favorite stuffed animal when they scream or tantrum will reinforce the screaming as a strategy to get what they want. Here the child will have been reinforced for screaming by getting the stuffed animal. In the same vein, if the parent or teacher stops brushing the child's teeth because the child put up a screaming fight during tooth brushing, then the child learns that protesting accomplishes the goal of ending the tooth brushing. In this case, the child has been reinforced by the removal of the aversive event (negative reinforcement). Instead, the parent or teacher will use a motivating antecedent to get the child to use a more appropriate behavior to get what he wants. For example, asking calmly for the stuffed animal, or getting to read a favorite book or getting a tickle after cooperative tooth brushing is finished.

STEP 2) Choose the developmentally appropriate target behavior to model and prompt for your child

Once you understand antecedents (A) and consequences (C) that motivate your child, the next step is to be clear and specific about the positive target behaviors you want to encourage in your child. For example, if you are working to teach your child how to ask for what they want, then unpack what "asking" means according to the child's language ability.

For a child with some language skills, the asking goal might be to work on saying, "truck please". For a child with less language, it might be just making the "T" sound combined with putting his hand out to gesture "give me". Or, if the child has no language, the goal might be to teach how to point or use a picture prompt system to indicate their wants. In this case, the first step will be for the parent or teacher to model pointing while saying the name of object wanted and then physically moving the child's hand into a point gesture (physical prompt). Later a pointing visual prompt might be added to give the child another way to indicate his wants. In each case, the target nonverbal or verbal asking behavior has been carefully thought out, modeled and then the rewarding antecedent and consequence will be employed. Choosing the developmentally appropriate target behavior is important to the success of the ABC teaching loop. The chosen target behavior should be one small step up from the child's current level. Think in small joint attention steps forward.

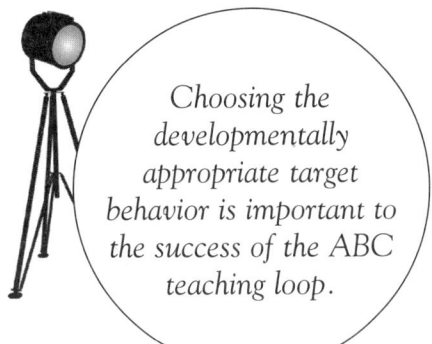

Choosing the developmentally appropriate target behavior is important to the success of the ABC teaching loop.

STEP 3: Wait for the chosen target behavior before rewarding

It is important to offer the antecedent (the thing your child wants and results in joint attention), wait for the desired behavior response (targeted communication or social behavior), and then give the reinforcing consequence. Frequently when children don't respond, the parent or teacher gives the reward anyway, either to avoid a tantrum or because they don't believe the child is capable of the response. This means they have lost the leverage to teach the child a way to communicate their needs. If the child doesn't respond, revisit the motivating strength of the antecedent as well as the developmental appropriateness of the desired behavior. Perhaps your child is not interested in the motivating consequence you are offering! Or, perhaps you are too directive and have set up a behavior goal that is too challenging. Or, perhaps you have not modelled the skill enough. Once you have made the right adjustments to establish joint attention development and engagement, the ABC sequence should work.

STEP 4 — Provide many ABC learning opportunities

One or two practices using the ABC sequence is not going to teach your child the targeted behavior. Try to set the practice up to provide many learning opportunities. In the bubble scenario, we saw how Hudson's father used bubbles (motivating antecedent), and how he blew only one bubble at a time so that Hudson would have further learning opportunities to ask him to blow again. He modelled the asking words frequently. Repetition is key. Another example of breaking down activities into small chunks for more learning practice opportunities would be to offer a small amount of a food item during snack or meal time. Instead of giving a whole piece of fruit when your child asks, give one small piece of apple or banana after each request. In this way, your child has multiple learning opportunities to practice asking (verbally or with gestures) for their favorite fruit.

Model target communication skill frequently. Avoid pressuring child to copy by saying, "you say it" or giving directives.

STEP 5 — Enhancing the effectiveness of the ABC script with imitation and repetition

In addition to setting up these ABC learning opportunities, the parent or teacher can add social value to the reinforcing consequence by joining in with the child; for example, by repeating the child's words with enthusiasm or a gesture, imitating the child's behaviors by chasing a bubble, or taking a bite of the food item at the same time the child does and verbalizing enjoyment (yum!).

STEP 6 — The added value of modeling and then prompting behaviors

You may also teach the desired social behavior by modeling the targeted social behavior. For example, if the child's target behavior was to learn to ask for something using one word, the adult could first model this behavior, asking the child to share a piece of his banana, by saying, "banana please" and modeling pointing to the banana. Gesturing and using body language along with using the word can enhance the child's understanding of the word. After frequently modelling how to ask with words and gestures, the adult can begin to try to prompt the behavior or words when the child wants something. For example, if you know your child wants some banana, you can prompt, "you can say, banana," and if they attempt the word, make a sound, point, or put out their hand, give them a small piece of the banana right away. Then model and prompt the next request for more banana. Parents and teachers sometimes find

Motivating Antecedent Behavior (child's goal)	Targeted Child Behavior	Consequence that Rewards Target Behavior	Parent/Teacher Behaviors to Promote Learning
CHILD WHO IS NONVERBAL			
Wants car	Child points to object	Child given 1-2 cars out of set of cars	Adult models pointing when asking child for something; adult takes child's hand and forms finger into pointing gesture; praises child's pointing & gives car to child; waits for another request and models or prompts again.
Wants to be picked up	Child puts out arms	Child is picked up	Adult puts child's arms out, or models putting out arms before picking up child and saying, "up".
Wants banana	Child puts out hand and says "b" sound	Child given segment of banana	Adult models saying "b, b, banana" and gestures with hand out as gives piece of banana to child.
Wants apple	Child points to picture of apple on visual card of fruit options	Child given piece of apple	Adult joins child in pointing to picture of apple, saying "apple." Adult also eats apple while saying "yummy apple." Praises child's use of visual or gesture.
Wants playdough	Child looks at playdough, points, makes a sound	Child gets piece of playdough for a few minutes	Adult smiles and imitates child's verbalizations when child points, gives child a small piece of playdough.
CHILD WHO IS SOMEWHAT VERBAL			
Wants car	Child says "ca" and points	Child given 1-2 cars out of set	Adult points and imitates saying "car" several times. Waits for another one-word request to imitate and praise.
Wants to be picked up	Child says "up" and puts up hands	Child picked up	Adult models additional word "up please" while picking child up.
Wants banana	Child says "nana please"	Child given segment of banana	Adult says "banana please", gives banana, and also takes a segment of banana and says "yummy banana" while eating. Praises good talking. Waits for another request or models and prompts it occurring

CHILD WHO IS SOMEWHAT VERBAL (continued)			
Wants apple	Child says "want apple"	Child given piece of apple	Adult gives child 2 pieces of apple and praises "nice asking". Then models by gesturing to self and asks, "Mommy wants apple please."
Wants playdough	Child says "playdough"	Gets small piece of playdough	Adult models and imitates child by adding a word. "want play dough?" Plays alongside child, saying: "fun to play with playdough." Waits or prompts further request for more playdough.
Motivating Antecedent Behavior (child's goal)	Unwanted Behavior/Target Replacement Behavior	Consequence that Rewards Target Behavior	Parent/Teacher Behaviors to Promote Learning
Stuffed animal	Grabbing/Asking or Pointing	Grabbing does not get stuffed animal/ asking does	Adult holding stuffed animal says, "you can say teddy please". Wait till child asks to give the stuffed animal to child.

it helpful to make an ABC table outlining the possible antecedents and consequences and the specific target behavior for their children. The table above is an example of this.

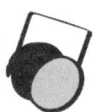

Cautions: Be sure you are not reinforcing undesirable behaviors by withdrawing demands or giving in when the child tantrums. If the child is engaging in unwanted behavior that is not harmful to another person, it can be ignored. When the unwanted behavior ends, if feasible, provide an opportunity for the child to use the positive opposite behavior to achieve the desired outcome (prompt the child to ask, gesture, for what they want). For example, the child is tantrumming for a cookie at snack time. The parent prompts child to say, "please cookie" and models pointing. If child calms down and uses a signal to ask or gesture, the parent can give the child a cookie and praise the child for asking calmly. This will not be appropriate in all situations. There are times when the child's desired outcome is not something that the parent can or should do even if the child asks appropriately. If the parent has set a limit "no cookies before dinner" or "time to turn off the screen," then the limit should be enforced, even if the child asks politely. It is important that children also learn to manage disappointment and see that your limit setting is consistent. Chapter Nine will provide more information about managing misbehavior.

Sometimes it can be tempting to avoid problem behaviors by giving children the desired item without requiring the child to communicate the request. Parents may jump to appease the child by always anticipating the child's desires ahead of time; for example, providing the stuffed animal, toy, or game, or food item before the child has "asked" for it. This takes away a possible learning opportunity. If the child doesn't have to do anything to get what they want, then there is no opportunity for learning to ask, or to response to the interaction. Instead prompt, model, and coach the target request behavior that you have identified for the child.

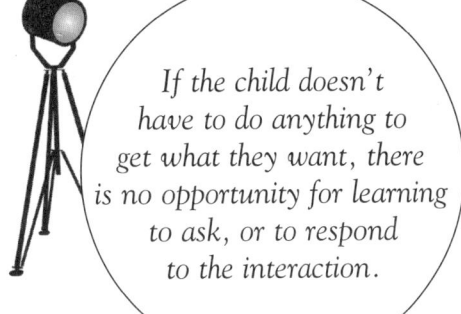

If the child doesn't have to do anything to get what they want, there is no opportunity for learning to ask, or to respond to the interaction.

Getting In Your Child's Attention Spotlight with ABC

In the next scenario we will see how Hudson's father engages his son's attention and gets in his spotlight by offering a red balloon, another one of this boy's favorite games. This shared activity may look light-hearted play, but it is actually serious learning about social interaction as Hudson learns to ask for a turn, share, listen, and communicate with his father. Think about how the father uses the ABC learning opportunity.

Father: (holds balloon up next to his face where Hudson cannot reach it) Do you want the balloon? What do we say? Say, "I want the balloon, please." (*prompt and model language for Hudson to use*)

Hudson: Want the balloon.

Father: I want the balloon please, papa. (*repeats what child says with added word*)

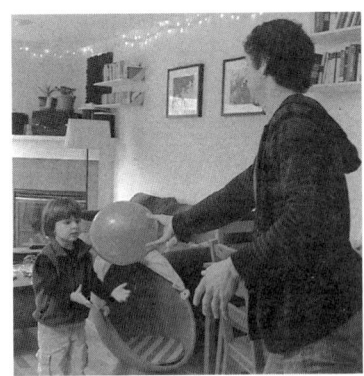

Hudson: Balloon please papa.
Father: Okay, great asking, here you go! Oh you're going to hit the balloon. Hit the balloon up in the air. (*praises language use*)
Hudson: (hits balloon)
Father: Wow you hit that pretty hard. You are strong! Up, keep it up, up in the air so it doesn't touch the ground. Here you go. Your turn. (balloon is hit back and forth between them.)
Father: (excited tone) Wooo! you got it.
Hudson: Balloon, balloon, balloon, balloon.
Father: Balloon balloon. I never heard you say that before! (Holds the balloon up high). The balloon is up here. What do you say to get the balloon? (*prompts asking*)
Hudson: What do you say to get the balloon? (echo's father)
Father: Is the balloon up here? He has to climb up the lamp post to get the balloon... right? (imitates climbing a post) Remember that? He climbs all the way up and he gets it. (reference to a book that Hudson likes: The Red Balloon) You can say: "Can I have the balloon please?" (*models the words for Hudson to say*).
Hudson: Balloon please...
Father: Nice asking, you said: "Balloon please." Here it is! You can have it. (*reinforces word use with praise and imitation*).

Considerations
Helping Your Child Learn to Make Requests

While it may be tempting to set up your child's environment to foster their independence, such as putting their favorite art activities and books on a lower shelf, it also is important to set up learning opportunities for your child to have *intentional communication* with you. This means sometimes holding back the things your child is most interested in doing. In this scenario the father has strategically engineered a reason for Hudson to have to make a request. He has put one of his favorite play activities, the balloon, up high so that Hudson can see it but has to ask to play with it. The father prompts and models the words, "I want the balloon." When Hudson imitates the words, the father repeats them and gives Hudson the balloon. This is the ABC of behavior change and learning. Hudson connects the balloon with a story, The Red Balloon, that he loves to read, and his father joins him in his attention spotlight by gesturing climbing a pole and commenting that he is climbing the lamp post to get the balloon before it flies away. By following Hudson's interest and having fun together with the balloon, we see their father-son social connection blossom.

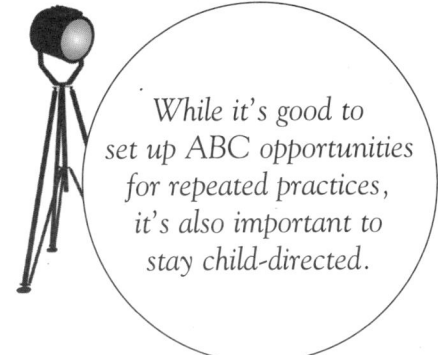

While it's good to set up ABC opportunities for repeated practices, it's also important to stay child-directed.

An extension of this activity that would add additional ABC opportunities would be to start with a deflated balloon so that Hudson has to ask his father to blow up the balloon. Each time Hudson asks, the father would blow once and then wait for him to ask again. This would provide repeated practice in asking his father to blow up the balloon. You could even add to the fun and surprise by having the balloon fly away so you start again blowing with the child practicing making requests. The idea is not to offer the child everything all at once or too quickly. Breaking the play opportunities down into small chunks it allows more joint attention learning opportunities for your child to communicate their needs to you. For example, toys such as cars, puzzle pieces, Legos, train tracks, and art supplies are easy to give out bit by bit so your child has to ask for more to complete the activity. You can add to the fun by hiding some of the pieces and make them appear as if by magic from your pocket or behind your child's ear. The surprise element always adds to your child's social engagement.

While it's good to set up ABC opportunities for repeated practices, it's also important to stay child-directed. You want your child to enjoy the interaction, to see the practice as fun, and to want to stay engaged with you. For children on the spectrum, it is hard work to gesture,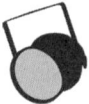

request, or maintain eye contact, and they may tire of doing these things after several tries. If you can see that your child is becoming frustrated by the repeated learning trials, take a break at the point where they are still cooperative. For example, if your child is beginning to lose focus or patience after asking for three pieces of a snack, give a larger piece after the next ask and allow them to finish eating without further practice. Ending the practice after a successful interaction will mean your child is happy to practice again at the next snack time.

Most children on the spectrum will need some time to play in their own world in their preferred way each day. It can also be exhausting for the parent to feel as if every interaction needs to be a teaching opportunity. You can alternate parent-child interaction times where you use the ABC's to encourage your child to connect with you with times when your child takes a break and plays alone with a soothing activity or with you narrating and imitating their activity. While it's true that the social interaction is important for your child's learning, you'll want to be realistic about what you can both manage and tolerate. Many small practice opportunities across the course of each day, will be better than marathon practice sessions!

Engaging Your Child with Songs, Gestures and Teaching Turn Taking

Songs and gestures are great ways to get into your child's attention spotlight and build social language. In the next scenario, the mother is sitting on the floor facing her son with her ten-month-old baby

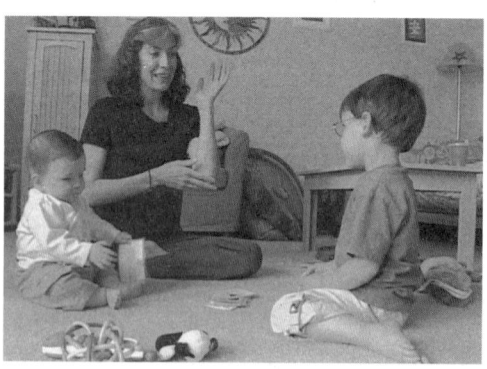

sitting next to her. She has picture prompts cards of various songs on the floor between them. Think about the way this mother engages her child in interactive play with songs, gestures, and descriptive commenting. Think about what Kalani, who has minimal language, is learning about social interactions from all the ways the mother responds.

Mother: (sitting in front of Kalani on the floor, baby Nika is next to her) Which song do you want to sing? (shows him picture cards of different songs to choose from.)

Kalani: (points and picks up one of the pictures on floor with excitement)

Mother: (Mother points) This one? This one was—do you remember this one is Skina Marinky? Can you help me do it, do you remember? (shows the gestures for the words in the song)
Skina Marinky Dinky Dink
Skina Marinky Do
I love you
Skina Marinky Dinky Dink
Skina Marinky Do
I love you
I love you in the morning, and I love you late at night (points at herself and then Kalani)
I love you in the evening when the moon is shining bright
Yay! (claps her hands. Kalani avoids looking at her but is smiling) Okay it's Nika's turn to pick. You want her to have one of those? (Kalani is holding up two picture song cards) Which one should she do? All those?

Kalani: (gives baby all the song visual cards.) (mumbles) All those.

Mother: All of those! Good sharing. Look Nika you get all of these. Which one do you want? She's gonna pick when it's her turn. Kalani had a turn, you picked Skina Marink, and Nika's gonna pick one. What song does she want to sing? (*intentional communication*)

Kalani: Mommy do it.

Mother: Mommy do it? Let's see. She picked two. Let's see what's this one... (takes one card from baby).

Mother: Twinkle Twinkle. You picked Twinkle Twinkle! (uses sign for twinkle with hands) You just did one (points to Kalani). Now it's Nika's turn (points to Nika). She picked Twinkle, Twinkle. Can you show me

	your stars? (shows both hands twinkling and sings) Twinkle, twinkle, little star, how I wonder what you are. Now it's your turn.
Kalani:	(looks at mom with excitement laughing and showing the same song card as before)
Mother:	Skina Marink again! Okay! Are you gonna help me sing this time? (looking at baby) Kalani chose Skina Marink, are you ready to sing? (looking at Kalani) Can you help me? (sings song again) (Baby in mother's lap as she sings, claps baby's hands, and laughs with delight,) Yaaay.
Kalani:	(mouths some of the words and smiles with delight)
Mother:	(song ends) Yeah! (ends arms in air and claps) Now It's Nika's turn.

Considerations

This mother begins by being attentive to body positioning by making sure Kalani can see her face as well as his sister Nika's face. She is using the song as the antecedent (A) and consequence (C) to encourage Kalani's asking behavior (B). She models social communication by using nonverbal hand gestures and exaggerated actions that match the meaning of the words in the song. For example, when she says, I love you, she points to herself for "I" and to Kalani for "you." In doing so she is helping Kalani to understand pronouns. Her tone of voice and facial gestures are enthusiastic and engaging. She is child-directed by letting Kalani select the visual song card prompt he wants to sing, giving him a sense of autonomy or independence. She also encourages his learning of the social skill to wait and take turns by naming and gesturing that it is Nika's turn to pick a visual song choice card. She helps build Kalani's cognitive understanding and empathy for his baby sister by recognizing that Nika likes a different song. When it is Kalani's turn again, he chooses the same song choice card. His mother recognizes that, with each repetition, Kalani is memorizing the words, gaining mastery over them, and will eventually be able to sing the words with her. Remember, the key to children's language learning is repetition. At the end of the song, the mother indicates it is finished by saying, "Yay!", and clapping hands with baby Nika. With these gestures, the mother is teaching Kalani the social skill of how to end a song or an activity.

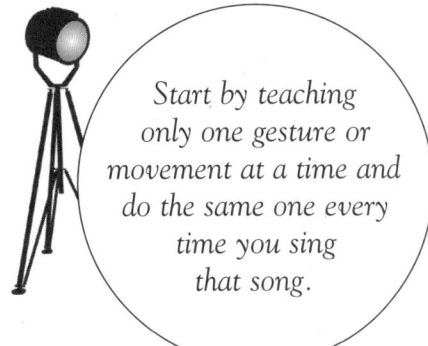

Start by teaching only one gesture or movement at a time and do the same one every time you sing that song.

Making the Most of Music

Songs are often the first place where children with ASD use words and engage in social reciprocation. Perhaps this is because songs are catchy, repetitive, and easily promote social interaction and gesture movements. For children with limited language, some songs may need to be simplified. Repeat 1-2 lines of the song, pacing it slowly. With familiar songs, it is helpful to use a "partial prompt"; that is, to pause the song at the end of the line to see if the child will fill in the last word or show the gesture. For example, "Row, row, row your_____". Your child may finish the line by saying: "boat." Be sure to pause at the same place every time as part of a fun song routine. Once your child shows that they know a song, you can insert an unexpected or silly word: "Row, row, row, your train…." to see if you child reacts to the difference.

To encourage your child to use gestures with song routines, start by modeling the gesture. Remember, it is harder for children to imitate facial movements, gestures, and sounds than physical actions with objects, so this will take practice. If your child doesn't make some attempt to imitate your gesture, you may need to prompt it by physically taking your child's hands to clap with the song or bring their hands into the air to make another motion. Gradually, with repetition, you will be able to fade your physical prompt. Always continue the song after your child makes the gesture (with or without your help). Start by teaching only one

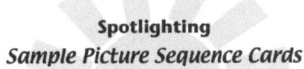

Spotlighting
Sample Picture Sequence Cards

Animal choices for singing "Old MacDonald"

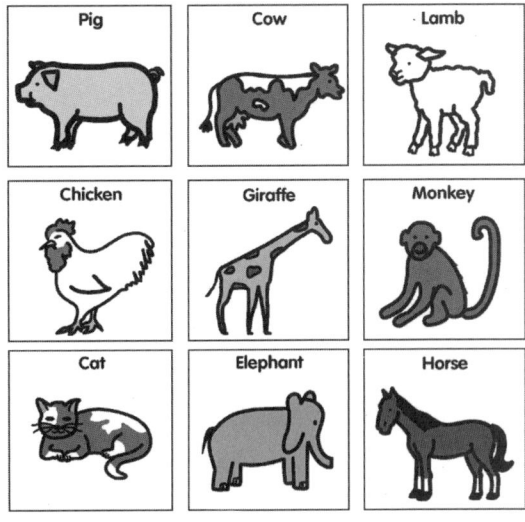

♪ We're Going On a Bear Hunt	♪ Row Your Boat
♪ We're going on a bear hunt! We're going on a bear hunt! We're going to catch a big one! We're going to catch a big one! I'm not afraid! I'm not afraid! Are you? Are you? Not me! Not me!	♪ (Sitting face to face on floor hold your child's hands and rock back and forth.) Row, row, row your boat Gently down the stream Merrily, merrily, merrily, merrily Life is but a dream.

gesture or movement at a time and do the same one every time you sing that song. When your child can produce some version of the gesture, you can add another gesture, facial expression, or fun sound effect. Be sure to pause after modeling a gesture to give your child time to imitate.

For songs with choices (like Old MacDonald), you can integrate turn-taking practice by deciding whose turn it is to name or point to the picture of the next animal to sing about.

You can also make a choice song board or cards with pictures of your child's favorite songs on them to help your child choose a song.

If your child loves motion, make sure your songs include large motor movement sensory stimulation like rocking, jumping, and bumps on your knees.

Some of the best songs are ones you make up for your child. You can target the specific nonverbal or verbal communication goals you are working on with your child and integrate the specific sensory actions and activities your child likes. Using your child's name in the song makes it even more personal. As always, your child will enjoy and engage in singing more when you follow their lead. These individualized song routines, incorporating gestures, actions, and exaggerated facial expressions, can be used throughout the day to help your child with routines such as getting dressed, eating a meal, or taking a bath.

SPOTLIGHTING
Connect with your Child through Music

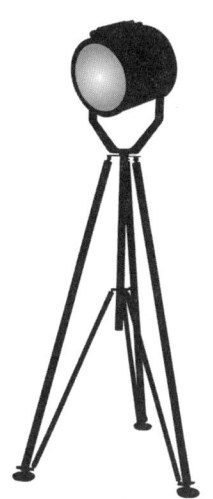

Many children on the autism spectrum are responsive to music, even if they don't react to the sound of your regular voice. Songs can be the first place your child begins to pay attention to you, uses words, and joins in activities with you. Here are some tips to using music and songs to teach your child about communication.

- Sing songs slowly and repeat often.
- Pair your song words with modeling repetitive gestures, large motor movements, and other sensory stimulation activities your child likes such as rocking, jumping, or clapping. Wait for your child to imitate. Then prompt your child to perform actions with song.
- Choose short songs with a small number of familiar words repeated over and over. For example, sing "row, row, row your boat" and mimic a rowing action.
- Sing face-to-face.
- Adjust song's number of words and actions to your child's communication level.
- Pause songs and offer your child turns with words and actions. Label your child taking a turn or show them a picture prompt of turn taking.
- Make up songs using your child's and other family member's names in your songs.
- Use song picture cards so your child can choose the song to sing.
- Use instruments and props such as a toy drum, tambourine, or harmonica when singing.
- Introduce pretend play into songs. (Example: Use puppets to sing and let them model asking for a turn and taking a turn)
- Remember to say "all done" when the singing is over.
- Remember these old stand-by songs: *The Wheels on the Bus Go Round and Round, If You're Happy and You Know It, Ring Around the Rosy, Old MacDonald Had a Farm, Twinkle, Twinkle Little Star,* and *Humpty Dumpty.*

Coaching Turn Taking and Sharing

One of the milestones for young children's social development is to learn to interact with others by taking turns and sharing. The ability to cooperate in give and take exchanges is fundamental to social development. However, turn-taking and sharing is difficult for children on the autism spectrum because they are so focused on their own activity, are oblivious to others, or are not sure what social response is expected. For example, they may not understand when someone asks for a turn or may not have the words to ask when they want a turn. As we have seen with Kalani's mother and baby sister, parents can help their children learn to shift their attention from objects to other people by expanding their joint attention spotlight to include others and their needs. We saw how Kalani's mother helped him shift his attention to his sister and learn to give her a turn choosing the next song. She is helping him to be aware of his sister and to consider her choices, a beginning step in turn taking, sharing and empathy building.

In the next scenario we will see how Hudson's father continues the balloon game and joint attention engagement by using gestures and words to teach and signal Hudson to take turns and share.

Father: (holding balloon.) My turn (*points to self*). Now it's going to be your turn (*points to Hudson*). Okay (passes balloon to him), Hudson's turn.

Hudson: (hits balloon)

Father: All right will you give me a turn now? (*holds out his arms*) Give the balloon to papa. Will you hit it to me? Okay, hit it to me.

Hudson: (hits balloon to dad)

Father: Thank you for sharing! My turn (*points to self*). Okay I'm going to hit the balloon. It's my turn. It's coming to you. Now it's your turn to hit it. Hudson's turn. (*points to Hudson*)

Hudson: (hits balloon back, but balloon falls to floor.)

Father: Okay, can I have another turn? Hudson will you give me the balloon? (*holds arms out*)

Hudson: (picks up balloon.)
Father: Bring me the balloon so I can have a turn?
Hudson: (gives father balloon)
Father: Thank you for sharing, thanks for the turn! Hudson that was very friendly. Now we can play with the balloon together. We're sharing. (praises social skill)
Hudson: We're sharing.
Father: We're sharing, there we go. (hits balloon to Hudson)

Considerations

Hudson's father uses gestures as well as words to signal what he wants Hudson to do. He names and uses gestures to label the turn taking for Hudson and himself. He prompts Hudson to share with him by saying: "my turn" and holding out his arms when Hudson has the balloon. He helps his son understand that this is friendly behavior and that this is what it means to take turns and to share. This father's approach helps his son learn about reciprocal communication, taking turns, and sharing. He makes sure that Hudson is watching him take his turn and signals or gestures "my turn" to make it explicit.

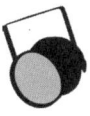

Think about all the ways you can help your child practice waiting and taking turns with yourself or others using some of their favorite activities. For example: throwing a frisbee, rolling a ball, going down a slide, turning pages of a book, playing sensory games such as chase, eating a snack, or choosing what game to play. Think about play themes that also require waiting, taking turns, and sharing such as, having a tea party, alternating putting pieces in a puzzle, pretend cooking with playdough, or reading words in a book. This turn taking joint attention play can also occur during your regular daily activities, such as having a bath, getting dressed, emptying the dishwasher, putting away toys, or leaving the house for preschool. For example, when bathing, perhaps your child gets a turn to soap his feet and legs and then you say, "it is my turn to wash your

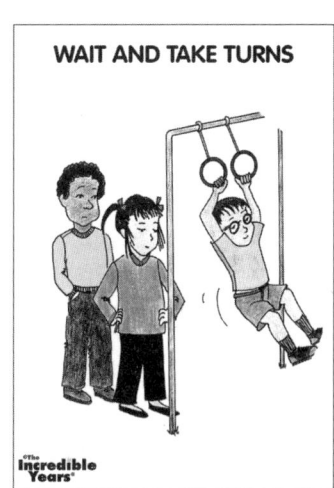

WAIT AND TAKE TURNS

arms" and then, "now it is your turn to do your tummy". Continue alternating turns as you finish soaping up all their body parts! This turn taking can continue with taking turns drying parts of their body and getting dressed.

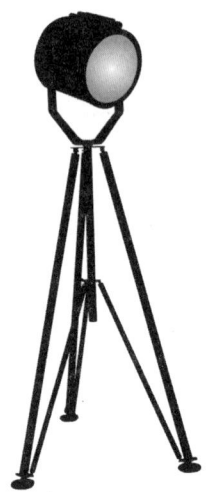

SPOTLIGHTING
One-on-One Parent-Child Social Coaching

- During child directed play or daily activities model social skills for your child such as offering to share, waiting, taking turns, asking for help, pointing or gesturing, smiling, eye contact, and praising.
- Stay in your child's attention spotlight and be sure your child is watching the social skills and gestures that you model.
- Name the social skills that you model, and name them again when your child copies. "I am sharing with you." "Now you are sharing with me!"
- Prompt your child to ask for help, take a turn, share something, or respond to a friend's request. Praise them if they try the social behavior. Let it go if your child does not respond to your prompt.
- Enthusiastically praise your child any time they (verbally or nonverbally) share, take turns, help, respond to a request, wait, or give eye contact.
- Participate in pretend and make-believe play with your child by using a doll, action figure, or puppet to model skills such as asking to play, offering to help, taking a turn, giving a compliment, calming down with a deep breath, and waiting.
- Model and prompt by suggesting the appropriate words to say. For example, "You can say, 'I want the truck, please.'"
- Use visual social prompts (picture cards) along with your verbal prompts to help non-verbal children associate the friendship behavior with the name of the behavior.

Turning Up the Spotlight on Your Child's Social Skills   137

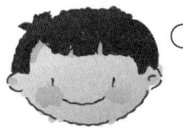

Parent Prompt Examples:

"I will be your friend (gesture to self) and share this with you." (hand out palm up to child)

"My turn with truck, now your turn"

"Help me find a blue one?"
"You are a good friend for helping me."

 Get in your child's social spotlight

Prompting Waiting, Asking and Turn Taking

When practicing turn-taking and reciprocal play, it will be easiest for your child to first practice with you. Sharing with a sibling or peer is more difficult. After your child is successful in one-on-one practice with you, then you can look for times to expand your child's attention spotlight to encourage turn taking with a peer or sibling. Amelia is able to share turns well with her mother and is ready to practice taking turns with her younger brother. In the next scenario notice how Amelia's mother uses the Sneaky Squirrel board game to model turn taking and help Amelia practice this skill. Notice how she spotlights her daughter's attention to include her younger brother.

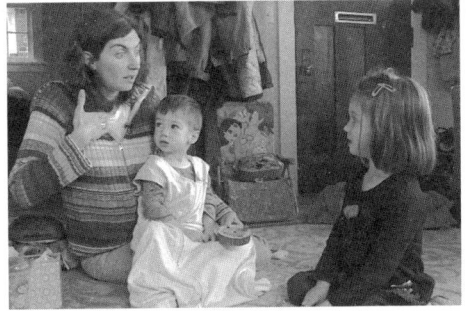

Mother: (to Amelia) Do you want to do it again? Or do you want to get a red one?
Truman: I want this one, I want this one.

Mother: Truman wants a turn. Truman is waiting. Amelia is finishing her turn. (*intentional communication*)
Amelia: I already got one.
Mother: You got red, Amelia. It was your turn. Okay, Truman's turn.(she gives him the spinning wheel).
Truman: (holds spinning wheel)
Amelia: Why does he got the Sneaky Squirrel?
Mother: Truman is taking a turn and you are waiting! Do you want to spin Truman? (*intentional communication*)
Truman: (spins)
Mother: Oh, you got it, Truman got red too. I'll help you get red Truman. (gives Truman the Sneaky Squirrel.)
Amelia: I got red also.
Mother: Yes, you both got red! Now it's your turn. (*gestures to Amelia*) Great waiting for your turn, Amelia.
Amelia: I got green.
Mother: Amelia you got green, your turn. (*gestures to Amelia*)
Amelia: (uses Sneaky Squirrel to move acorns.) Take this one, take this one, watch how I do it.
Mother: Look at that, I love how you did that all by yourself and used the squirrel to get him and used his hands to put it in, you got a green one and put it in your tree stump.
Mother: (*gestures to herself*). It's my turn now.
Amelia: (hands Mother the spinner)
Mother: Thanks for handing me that. It is my turn. (*gestures to self*) Thanks for handing me the squirrel. Thank you. (*praises social skill*)
Amelia: I catched it.
Mother: You handed it to me, thank you so much. All right, my turn.

Game continues.....

Amelia: (Truman has the squirrel). I want the Sneaky Squirrel.

Mother:	You want the Sneaky Squirrel. How could you ask your brother for it? What could you do if you want it? (*prompts the idea of asking.*)
Amelia:	(does not respond, busy playing with game pieces.)
Mother:	You could say: "May I have the squirrel please, Truman?" (*prompts actual words.*)
Amelia:	Can I have the squirrel now?
Mother:	(helps Truman give squirrel to Amelia.) Nice asking. Yeah, here you go. (*praises asking*)
Amelia:	Did I say please?
Mother:	Amelia that was so nice asking your brother for it.
Amelia:	Did I say please?
Mother:	You didn't say please but you asked for it very nicely. That was great, being very polite.

Considerations

This mother does a great job of teaching her daughter about turn taking by gesturing and labeling all aspects of turn taking: giving a turn, asking for a turn, waiting for a turn, and receiving a turn.

When Amelia doesn't respond to the prompt to ask her brother for the squirrel, her mother provides the actual words for Amelia to use saying, "Can I have the squirrel, please, Truman?" When Amelia uses these words, she helps Truman give Amelia the squirrel. This ensures that Amelia is reinforced for her polite asking by getting a turn. Her mother also praises her for asking, which provides social reinforcement. In this case the motivating antecedent (A) is the squirrel, the target behavior (B) is asking and waiting and the consequence (C) is getting the squirrel plus mother's praise.

Because of Amelia's advanced language skills, this mother is able to coach several different social skills in this game: waiting, taking turns, asking politely, and being aware of the importance of involving her brother in the game. Amelia is at the start of learning how to interact with another person in her attention spotlight. This is an important goal for Amelia. Her teacher reports that in school she withdraws, sitting alone and avoiding contact with peers rather than initiating.

For children with less language, you will want to pick one social skill to work on at a time. We saw Hudson's father began with teaching him how to ask for what he wanted by modeling the words. Or, you might want to focus on the idea of taking turns by modeling it with the "my turn, your turn game" as Kalani's mother did with the song cards.

You can encourage your child to give you a turn with a picture prompt cue, verbal cues, or a gesture. To keep your child engaged, quickly give your child their turn back again so they don't have to wait too long. You can model by showing what word to say, "your turn". You may even need to give physical support such as putting your hand over theirs (known as hand over hand guidance) and moving the object to the other person so that they know exactly what it means to give a turn. Eventually you will fade out the visual, physical, and verbal prompts so that the child learns to do this without your help. As you practice turn-taking with your child, the trick is to stay in your child's attention spotlight and keep your child engaged in the game so that they experience the rewards and joy of the reciprocal social interaction. Make sure to provide praise, encouragement, silliness, and fun as you practice the social skills. Below you will see some examples of using visual social prompts or supports.

For children with less language, you will want to pick one social skill to work on at a time.

Encouraging Sharing and Noticing Others

In the prior scenario Amelia needed prompting and encouragement to give her mother and brother turns in the game. In the next scenario, you will see that Amelia is spontaneously paying attention to her brother. This is a big step! Notice how the mother praises her daughter's social interactions and helps her understand the effect her sharing has on her brother's feelings.

Mother: Your spinner landed on purple. Let's spin again.
Amelia: (hands spinner to Truman.) Truman, Truman your turn.
Mother: Oh, thank you so much. You just gave Truman a turn! That was so friendly.

Truman: (spins)
Mother: Good spinning Truman... you got yellow or gold butterscotch, as Amelia likes to call it.
Amelia: Why's it yellow mama?
Mother: Because Truman's still learning his colors. I know you like to call it gold butterscotch, but we are trying to make it a bit easier for Truman because he doesn't know his colors like you do.
Amelia: Truman, look at my bandaid (shows Truman her finger).
Mother: Oh, great showing your brother. Truman do you like Amelia's bandaid? She has Micky Mouse bandaid. Do you like that? It's cool isn't it? Nice showing your brother.
Amelia: Did Truman like this?
Mother: I think he did, did you like Mickey Mouse?
Truman: Yup.
Mother: Yup, he did, he says. (*intentional communication*)
Amelia: He did?
Mother: He liked Mickey! You are really paying attention to Truman today. He likes your attention!

Considerations

In this interaction Amelia is learning that giving a turn to her brother or talking with him is a social behavior that will get her mother's attention and will be clearly praised and applauded. It is interesting here to see that Amelia asks her mother for feedback about what her brother thinks. Amelia is beginning to think about her brother's feelings, a first step toward building empathy. The mother also teaches Amelia about how to make the language simpler for her brother buy using the word "yellow" instead of her word "gold butterscotch." This encourages her to think about her brother's perspective and also makes her feel important as the big sister who understands more complex language.

Coaching Sibling Play

In the next play scenario notice how Kalani's mother uses persistence coaching to support Kalani's puzzle task and social coaching to expand his attention spotlight to focus on his baby sister.

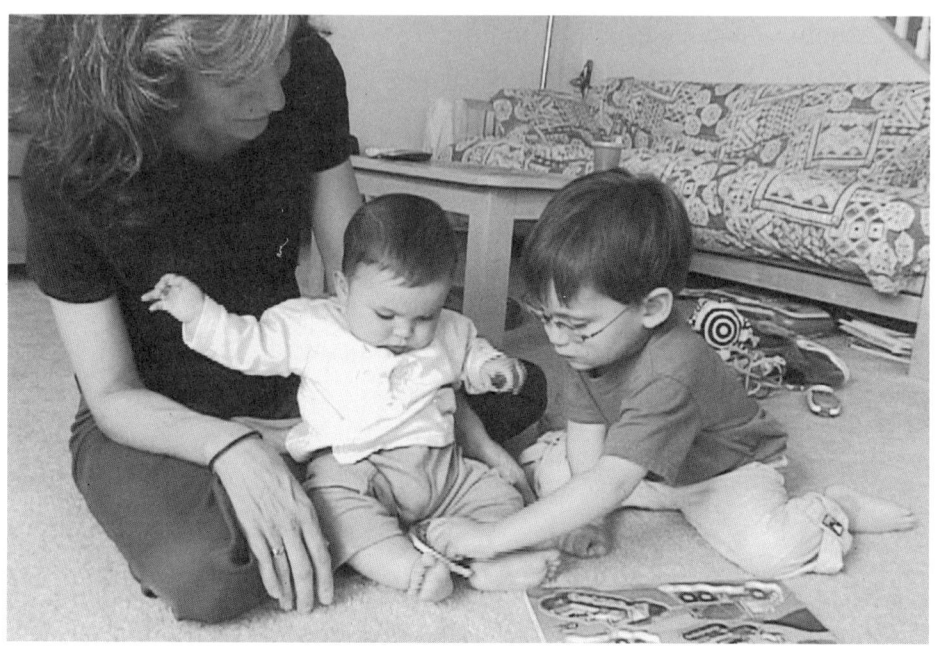

Mother: Let's try another one. Can you do the red truck? A little red truck.

Kalani: (finds a piece of the puzzle)

Mother: That is a dump truck. You're turning it and it went in! Which one's next? (*enthusiastic*)

Kalani: (finds another piece)

Mother: Blue truck and you have two. You are trying that one first. Wiggle, wiggle, wiggle, there you go. It's hard, but you are trying a different one. There you go! You got it. (*promotes persistence*)

Mother: (baby is fussing and takes a puzzle piece.) Nika wants to get this one. Can she have a piece too? (*promotes awareness of baby sister*)

Kalani: No. (he takes the piece from Nika).

Mother: (does not comment on Kalani taking the puzzle piece). Nika is ready to do something. Kalani I see you are working hard to finish the puzzle. The red one is going in – wow! You did it – you put all the puzzle pieces in. *(promotes persistence)* I think Nika wants a turn with the puzzle. Can you give her a piece? *(intentional communication)*

Kalani: (sits back watching baby touch his puzzle.) Mine.

Mother: What?

Kalani: Big one.

Mother: (gestures) You want her to have the big one? You want to help? Say: "Here Nika." *(models and prompts sharing)*

Kalani: (hands puzzle piece to his sister)

Mother: Oh thank you! you were sharing your pieces with her—two pieces for Nika! She is so happy!

Mother: (Mother pretending to be baby.) Thank you Kalani. *(models social skill)*

Considerations

Even with a 6-month-old baby, this mother manages to turn this puzzle play time into an opportunity for her son to learn about sharing with his baby sister as well as fostering his language development and persistence with completing the puzzle. She is gentle with her prompts and gives Kalani plenty of time to decide if he wants to share. She doesn't give attention to his refusal to share and waits, allowing him to decide. She helps him understand his sharing is appreciated by praising him herself and also pretending to say "thank you" from his sister, expanding his emotional understanding of another.

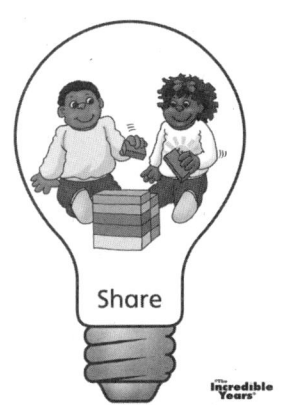

Helping Kalani understand the connection between his actions and another's feelings. When naming and praising a child's prosocial behavior it is useful to connect the social skill to the feelings of the other person. In the scenario above the mother told Kalani that his sister was

happy he shared. In doing this, she is helping Kalani connect his social sharing with another's feelings. If you are playing and your child shares with you, you might smile, point to yourself, and say, *"thank you for sharing, I'm happy."* In Chapter Five we will talk more about the value of connecting social behaviors to feelings.

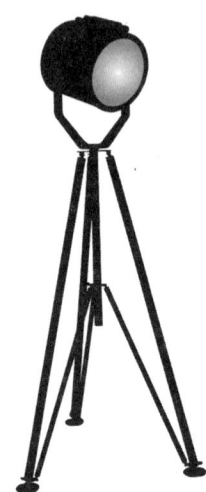

SPOTLIGHTING
Prompting Your Child's Social Awareness

- When your child is responsive and enjoys social interaction with a parent or other trusted adult, you can slowly begin to add a sibling or peer into their attention spotlight.
- Coach short play times with a friend or sibling. Start coaching just one other child, ideally a child with social skills that can be modeled for your child.
- Prompt your child to notice what the other child is doing, saying, asking, or feeling.
- Prompt your child to interact with a peer or sibling by helping them notice the other child needs help, or is asking for something.
- Help your child understand that when they share or help, the other child feels happy. This promotes the connection between their behavior and another's feelings.
- Praise your child when they initiate interactions, look at, or notice what a peer is doing, or help, or share with them.
- Use social coaching instead of asking questions.
- Coach and praise your child's friendly behaviors whenever you see them initiate an interaction, look at or notice what another child is doing, talk with them, take turns, engage in joint play, , apologize, or give praise.
- For children with less language, use visual prompts of the social behavior such as asking, or sharing, or turn taking to promote and praise their use of a social behavior.

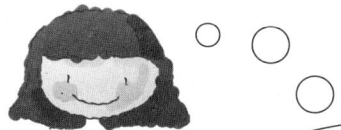

"Your friend is looking for a red block, can you help him?" (prompt)

"That's so friendly. You are sharing your cars and waiting your turn. Your friend looks happy." (connect behavior to feeling)

"You are both helping each other like a team."

"You waited and asked first if you could use that. Your friend listened to you and shared." (connect social behaviors to positive outcome)

"You both worked together to put those blocks together. That was great cooperation." (enthusiastic response)

"You could give your friend a compliment and say, 'I like your picture'." (prompt and model words)

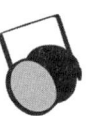

Getting your child's attention spotlight on other children!
Tailor your social coaching to your child's language level. For nonverbal children or children with only a few words, use gestures and visual prompts and reduce the complexity of your language. Remember the one-up rule.

Reading as a Joint Social Activity to Promote Social Skills
In Chapter Three we talked about reading using the E-CARE reading principles to promote children's language development. Reading together can also promote social skills such as turn taking, waiting, sharing, and helping with perspective taking. In the next scenario, Amelia's

mother uses a book entitled, *My Turn*, to teach her daughter some important social skills. Think about how she promotes Amelia's understanding of the benefits of turn taking and how it feels to wait for a turn.

Mother: (holding book towards child and face-to-face with toddler on her lap) Let's see what's happening with these guys. Oscar and Tilly found a playground. "Shall we play on the slides?"

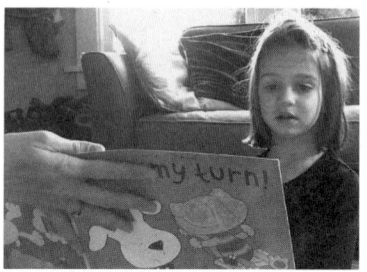

Amelia: What's this?

Mother: It says Oscar and Tilly are their names. "Shall we play on the slide?" asked Oscar. "I'll go first said Tilly", so Tilly's going to go first.

Amelia: Is this Tilly?

Mother: Yes, it looks like that's Tilly, and she's going first. Oscar wants to go next: "I'll go now said Oscar," Oh, but Tilly's not giving him a turn: "Not yet," said Tilly, "it's not your turn." I think it is Oscar's turn, it would be so nice for Tilly to give Oscar a turn. What do you think, Amelia? Is it Oscar's turn? *(prompts thinking about a social skill)*

Amelia: She's going whoo, whee down the slide.

Mother: Whee, I know somebody else who likes the slide (points to Amelia).

Amelia: I do like the slide.

Mother: You do like the slide. I know it. It's so thrilling, and exciting. You get excited going on the slide huh. Tilly is excited too, but Oscar is sad. Let's see what happens next, maybe Oscar will get a turn? *(intentional communication about characters' feelings)*

Amelia: Yeah.

Mother: "Wow that looks like fun," said Oscar, "Is it my turn now?" "Not yet," said Tilly." Boy Oscar is waiting and waiting, and he is being so patient for a turn.

	Oscar's not having any fun, because he doesn't get a turn. Tilly is using all the fun things without sharing. *(intentional communication continues)*
Amelia:	Because maybe she's bigger.
Mother:	Yes, she's bigger. What do you think, though? Do you think that she should share with Oscar? Maybe you could tell Tilly, 'you need to give Oscar a turn, He's your friend'
Amelia:	Tilly, Oscar's your good friend you can tell him…
Mother:	To have a turn.
Amelia:	To have a turn.
Mother:	Yeah, have a turn Oscar. Amelia, that is a friendly idea. I think you would be a good friend to Oscar. If Tilly let Oscar have a turn, how would Oscar feel?
Amelia:	Happy.
Mother:	Yeah, I agree he would be happy! You have friendly ideas. Should we keep reading and see if Tilly can be as friendly as you are?
Amelia:	Yeah, keep reading.

Considerations

In this scenario the mother uses the "My Turn" book to help Amelia think about Oscar's point of view and feelings when Tilly doesn't give him a turn on the slide. She positions her body so Amelia can see the book pictures as well as her facial gestures. She reads with enthusiasm using fun words like, "Whee", and helps Amelia think about the feelings of Tilly who is excited with the slide while Oscar is patiently waiting his turn. She prompts Amelia to think about how Oscar is feeling when Tilly won't give him a turn. Then she prompts Amelia with the words Tilly could say to indicate she will give Oscar a turn, by suggesting she tell Tilly, "You need to give Oscar a turn". Amelia repeats these words as if she is teaching Tilly. This pretend play practice is very effective in helping Amelia learn the words to say when sharing a turn.

In this scenario example Amelia clearly has a lot of language understanding and some beginning empathy. The mother is helping her learn the social skill of sharing and the feelings involved that include not wanting to share and what it means to share and wait. She connects the happy feeling that Oscar has when he does get to use the slide so that she can see the connection between one's friendly social behavior and another person's feelings. This is a good example of social coaching combined with emotion coaching, which will be discussed in more detail in Chapter Five.

While some children with ASD seem to have a precocious ability to read or repeat complex language, they don't necessarily understand what the words mean.

For children with less language and less interest in or attention to peer interactions, this mother's language will be too complex. Instead, you can simplify the discussion by describing the waiting and asking behaviors in the book. "Tilly slides. Oscar waits. Oscar asks. Oscar slides." You can prompt your child to practice what Tilly might say, "your turn" or what Oscar might say, "my turn please." You can repeat this practice using the same word many times as you show the pictures in the book. Practicing this social language with a book, can help children learn the words to use in a real-life situation. Remember that while some children with ASD seem to have a precocious ability to read or repeat complex language, they don't necessarily understand what the words mean or understand the social context behind the words. As we discussed in the E-Care reading tips in Chapter Three, books are an ideal place for children to learn about the meaning of words. Turning book reading into an interactive experience, as we saw in the scenario above, requires all the same strategies we have talked about in earlier chapters. This includes keeping it simple, exaggerating your words, pointing, repetition, imitation, being child directed, and giving your child opportunities to participate in interactive practices.

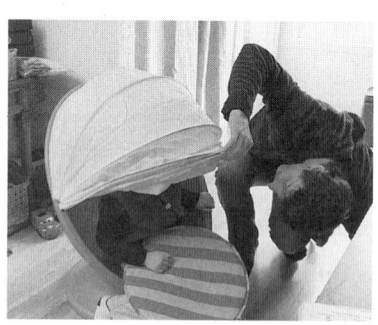

Using Sensory Physical Activities to Increase Social Interactions

Since social interactions are not as rewarding for children on the autism spectrum, finding ways to increase their pleasure in social exchanges is important. Most children on the spectrum enjoy sensory physical activities – such as dancing to music, running, bouncing on a trampoline, being chased, and swinging. These activities can serve to increase their internal motivation to seek social play interactions and engage longer in social activities. In the next scenario notice how Hudson's father strategically uses a spinning egg chair activity to foster reciprocal communication with his son. Think about what makes his interaction approach effective and what Hudson is learning.

Father: All right you are sitting in the egg chair. Are you taking a break or do you want to go for a spin?
Hudson: I want to go a spin.
Father: Go for a spin.
Hudson: Go for a spin (pulls down cover).
Father: Hi Hudson. (looks under cover.) Okay what do you want me to do?
Hudson: Faster than fast.
Father: Faster and faster (looking at him under cover).
Hudson: Faster and faster.
Father: All right shall we do clockwise, shall we spin you to the right or the left?
Hudson: To the right.
Father: To the right.
Hudson: To the left.
Father: This is the left.
Hudson: Left.
Father: Okay here we go.. Whee whee. I'm spinning you to the left now. Is that okay?
Hudson: Faster than faster.
Father: Faster and faster! Say: "Spin me faster and faster."
Hudson: Spin faster and faster.
Father: Okay here we go. Whee you are going round and round and round. It must be pretty exciting, Hudson... Is that exciting? Is that exciting? (stops the spinning.)
Father: (looks under cover and gets eye contact.) Is this exciting or pretty boring? What do you think?

Hudson: Exciting.
Father: Exciting, oh yeah.
Hudson: Faster faster. (Signals to continue.)
Father: Okay faster fast fast.
Hudson: Faster than fast.
Father: Okay this time fast to the left or the right?
Hudson: Fast to the right.
Father: Fast to the right okay.

Considerations

Since children on the autism spectrum seem not to get as much internal pleasure from verbal social interactions and don't naturally seek out these social exchanges, it is necessary to increase their experience of social pleasure with you through fun, physical sensory activities. These experiences will lead to longer interactions with you and more joint attention learning opportunities and will result in faster and more sustainable learning and memory.

In the egg spinning scenario, it was important that Hudson's father paused the spinning activity strategically and looked expectantly at his son to get in his attention spotlight with a smile and laugh. Then he waited for Hudson's signal and request to begin again. Waiting for Hudson's cues makes this a reciprocal game where Hudson is learning to respond and request the next move. If the father had just spun his son without pausing to request communication, it would have become solo and passive play and the father would have lost the learning opportunities for Hudson to express his feelings or give directions. Also noteworthy is how the father starts by getting Hudson to state his wishes, such as what direction or how fast. Hudson is learning how his words can result in a specific response from his father and keep them engaged.

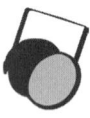
Think about what sensory routines (games and songs) you can use with your child. Typically, these physical sensory routines don't involve objects. Here are some possible sensory games to think about: tossing your child in the air, the chase game, hide and seek, being swung, jumping, rocking, spinning, running, pattycake, and peekaboo games. Add these to your child's Likes and Dislikes list from Chapter One.

Back and Forth Sensory Activities
"I'm going to get you"

Participating in your child's sensory physical routines can increase their pleasure and motivation for social exchanges, and engage and pull them back into the social world. In the next scenario you will see how Hudson's father uses another physical activity, the "catch me chase game," to engage his son and to practice balanced, back and forth movements, gestures, and communication. Notice how the father modulates the amount of activity so Hudson doesn't get over-aroused. Think about what Hudson is learning here.

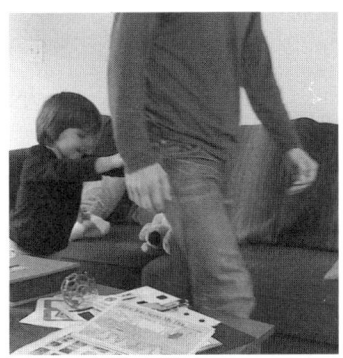

Father: What else do you want to do Hudson? (pulls up choice picture card.) Do you want to do anything from here? Do you want to do some tickles, or chase, or make a train track?

Hudson: Chase.

Father: You picked chase! All right, are you going to chase me or am I going to chase you?

Hudson: Chase and then spin.

Father: Chasing and spin. You want another spin? Okay... you can't catch me.

Hudson: I'll push you.

Father: You're going to push me, oh no.

Hudson: I'll push you.

Father: Oh no, you can't catch me.

Hudson: Help me push you.

Father: Help me push you (laughs).

Hudson: (pushes Father).

Father: (falls down on floor.) Oh I fell down! Will you help me up?

Hudson: (helps him up)

Father: Will you give me a kiss so I feel better?

Hudson: (kisses Father.)

Father: Oh thank you can I have a hug? Oh thank you.

Hudson: Push me in the bum.
Father: Don't push too hard! Okay you are just helping me go around the table. That's all right. That's a friendly. Is that a friendly push?
Father: My turn. I'm going to catch you now. I'm going to get you. I'm going to get you. I'm going to get you... get you... (catches him and tickles him).

Considerations

In this scenario Hudson is learning to make decisions about how and what he wants to play as well as how to respond to his dad's request for a kiss and hug. This fun social game keeps Hudson attending and interacting with his father so there are more learning opportunities. Remember, the more fun you and your child have, the faster the learning. However, it is important to watch for signs of overarousal or excitement that could get out of hand and to try to calm down the activity before your child gets too over aroused. Hudson's father is modulating this activity by not running too fast and reminding his son to do gentle, friendly pushes. Other types of sensory play that some children prefer are having lotion put on their bodies, soap bubbles in the bath, running in the sprinkler, playing with sand, or playdough. When introducing a new sensory routine, do it softly and slowly and remember that your child might not immediately like the new routine. Keep trying in brief repetitions. However, if your child withdraws and seems anxious, stop the game and shift to another sensory routine he likes.

When introducing a new sensory routine, do it softly and slowly and remember that your child might not immediately like the new routine.

You can weave these sensory physical routines in your interactions throughout the day such as bath time, diaper changing, mealtimes, getting dressed, or bed time.

Mother Reflections about Sensory Routines

Amelia craves some sensory-type activity. For her, it's vestibular, which is jumping or that running movement. Anything that really gets her body moving really helps her regulate herself.

If she gets angry, sometimes she needs to just run and get it out. We have a trampoline, and we have a little spot that she can run in our house. It helps if I say: "oh, you're taking your gymnastics break to help calm down. That's great." So I just describe it for her.

She also loves fidgeting with objects that are long that she can flick or tap. And so, if I need to try to redirect her, I have to give her a plan. First, we're going to do X, and then we're going to do the thing she wants, like flick a fidget toy, or stim to herself. We use the sensory activity as the reward.

SPOTLIGHTING
Using Fun Sensory Physical Routines to Motivate Social Interactions

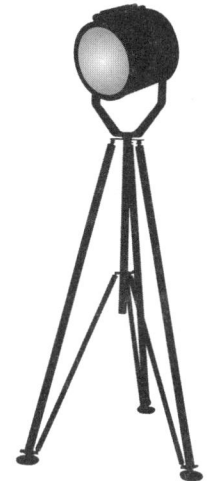

Face-to-face sensory physical routines can motivate your children to interact, laugh, have fun, and stay connected with you for longer periods of time. This means you will have optimized your child's energy level and increased learning opportunities for more durable social learning. Here are some tips for increasing your fun factor with your child.

When your child seems withdrawn, uninterested, unresponsive, or bored, increase their energy and motivation as follows:

- Stay in your child's spotlight, narrate your actions, and be face to face. Exaggerate your fun responses and gestures with big smiles, laughter, silly faces, tickles, funny noises, and bigger voices with more emotion: draw attention to your face.
- Play games such as peek-a-boo, hide and seek, find the hidden object, pattycake, finger play, or build a fort in your living room.
- Determine your child's favorite rhythmic song or physical game such as, Ring around the Rosy, When You're Happy and You Know It, the Chase Me Game, or rough housing. Use picture choice cards to help your child make the choice of song or activity.
- Occasionally surprise your child with a variation of routine such as new sound effects, new verse, or new step in the routine or game.

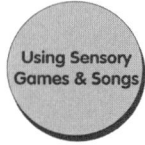

Using Sensory Games & Songs

- Frequently pause or freeze sensory routines to prompt your child to signal what they want next.
- Once you get the signal (verbal or nonverbal), continue the game, and then pause again, waiting for another signal.
- Make sure there is back and forth communication between you and your child. Rather than simply entertaining your child, encourage them to stay connected by responding to your prompts, pauses, and communication efforts.

Avoid getting your child over aroused:
- Pay attention to your child's arousal level.
- Make the play softer, gentler, quieter as soon as you notice your child getting overly aroused.
- Sing calmer songs that calm your child down.
- Freeze the play to take deep breaths or use positive imagery.
- Redirect the play before your child shuts down or dysregulates.
- Once your child has calmed down, don't be afraid to increase your enthusiasm and optimize your child's energy level again.

Face to Face and Joint Attention During Snack Time

Most children learn from imitation and modeling the words, expressions, and actions of their parents and teachers. This helps them feel emotionally connected. Children on the autism spectrum are less inclined to imitate what others do, perhaps because they are not paying attention to others, or perhaps because they aren't motivated to engage socially with people. In prior scenarios you have learned how to turn up the volume of your narrated interactions to get in your child's attention spotlight and help shift their gaze from objects to people and back again. This joint attention is important to promoting your child's language, social, and cognitive development.

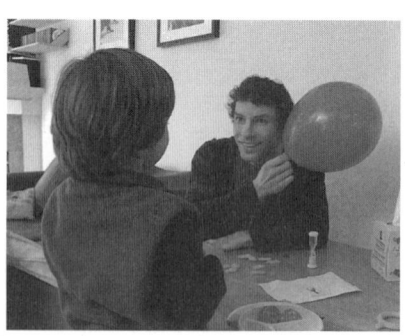

You have learned that parents can enhance their children's joint attention by using exaggerated facial expressions, getting close to their child's face, and waiting for a verbal or nonverbal response. In the next scenario, Hudson is having a snack and his father sits across the table from him with a balloon. Hudson's father gets his son to give him eye contact and to make a verbal request before giving him what he wants. Then he pretends the balloon is an airplane. Think about what else this father is doing to get in Hudson's spotlight and what social behaviors he is teaching him.

Father: This balloon is like a big floating airplane.
Hudson: This is a big floating airplane.
Father: Yeah, it's going to land right here...
Hudson: (grabbing balloon)
Father: Oh you want the balloon? Yes? (looks Hudson in face and smiles).
Hudson: Yes (not looking at his father).
Father: Can you look at me with your eyes? Hudson can you look at me with your eyes, look at my eyes.
Hudson: I want the balloon please (glances very briefly at father).
Father: Thank you for looking at me and asking so nicely (gives him balloon). Coming in for landing...swish.
Hudson: Swish.
Father: Swish.
Hudson: Swish.
Father: He's going up, up, up in the sky now. Maybe he's taking off. He's taking off from the airport. There he goes. (*narrates Hudson's actions*).
Hudson: There he goes. He's going to airport.
Father: It must be fun to be an airport pilot.
Hudson: There he goes.
Father: There he goes, the kitty cat cracker. (picks up a cracker that looks like a cat)
Father/Cat: Hi Hudson. I'm a kitty cat I want to go for an airplane ride. Can I ride your airplane? (*pretend play*).
Father: You want to put the kitty cat on top of the airplane. She wants to go for a ride (puts cat there). She wants something to eat. MEOW!

Considerations

Hudson's father does a great job of getting in his son's attention spotlight by using imaginary ideas with one of his favorite objects (the balloon is a floating airplane and cookie kitty cat wants a ride). He knows that Hudson wants the balloon, so he uses it as a motivator to get Hudson to look at him. Since Hudson has difficulty with eye-contact, his father sets a small goal and gives Hudson the balloon after brief eye-contact. It would be easy for Hudson to disengage and withdraw into his own nonsocial world during snack time, but the father's approach to bring in one of Hudson's likes (the balloon) to the play as well as do something imaginary or unexpected makes it hard for Hudson to disengage. Think about what fun, unexpected, or silly things you do during your social interactions that will keep you in your child's spotlight.

Think about what fun, unexpected, or silly things you do during your social interactions that will keep you in your child's spotlight.

As mentioned earlier, one of this father's goals is to get more eye contact from Hudson. However, some children may find this eye contact too overwhelming. If your child is not ready for eye-contact, your social goal may be something different such as sharing the snack kitty crackers, or requesting a particular snack. Choosing the most developmentally appropriate social goal for your child is important when setting up these social coaching play practices.

Prompting Sharing, Helping, Verbal Responses and Asking

"Prompting" means suggesting or supporting your child to engage in a desired behavior. The prompt could be asking your child to help you, so that they practice the action of helping, or physically prompting and guiding your child's hand through the desired action of sharing something, or modeling by suggesting the words or gestures for your child to imitate. If your child complies with your prompt by imitating you, then you praise his friendly actions or words. If your child does not comply, you let it go, as the prompt is a suggestion, not a command that must be obeyed. Your goal is still to be child-directed. Be patient and remember the prompt will help your child learn a social response that could be used another time. Eventually, you can fade out the prompt as your child initiates this social action on their own. In the next scenario, let's see how Hudson's father prompts and models sharing, helping, and asking behaviors in his interactions with his son. Think about what this approach helps his son learn.

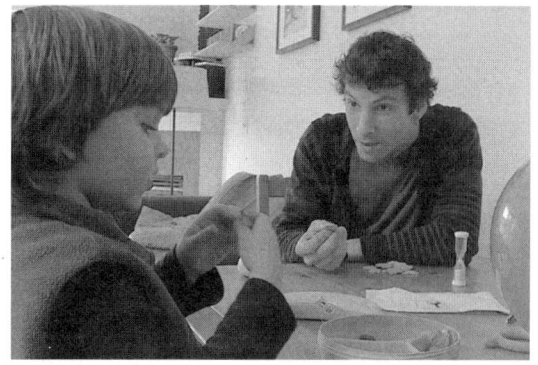

Father: Can I have one more raisin please Hudson? (*prompting sharing.*)

Hudson: (gives him a raisin)

Father: Thank you so much. You are being so generous with sharing your raisins. You are giving me all the raisins I want. (*praises sharing and models social skills of saying thank you*) Since you are being so friendly with me, I will be friendly with you. Would you like a kitty cracker? (*models sharing.*)

Hudson: (reaches for cracker)

Father: Would you like a kitty cracker? Yes or no? (*prompts verbal response*)

Hudson: Yes.

Father: Say: "yes please." (*prompts adding another word.*)

Hudson: Yes please.

Father: There you go. Great speaking! Would you like two kitty crackers? (holds cracker up to his face.)

Hudson: Two kitty crackers.

Father: Okay here you go (gives him crackers) (*models sharing*).

Hudson: (takes crackers and puts them together)

Father: Two kitty crackers. They are like kitty cat friends. Are they kissing? Are they giving each other a nice hug? Are they playing? I think they might be giving each other tickles, tickle, tickle, tickle. Time to go in the mouth, yum yum yum.

I'm going to eat another one too (models eating a cracker). I'm going to eat some banana, Hudson, and I might need some help. Can you help me peel this banana please? (*prompting helping behavior.*)

Hudson: (no response)

Father: Are you focused on your kitty cat? (*drops his prompt for help with the banana and refocuses on Hudson's interests*)

Father: (stands up his kitty crackers) He's standing up... he's standing up on the table. There is a line of kitty cats. Jump one, two, three, four. That's a lot of kitties. Are you counting kitty cats?

Hudson: (takes cracker from his father without asking)

Father: Hey you took it away from me. That makes me a little bit sad. Can you ask me? Can you ask nicely? (*prompting asking*)

Hudson: I want a kitty cat.

Father: Okay since you asked, here you go. I'll give you the kitty cats. (*rewards desired asking behavior*)

Hudson: You asked. (echolalic)

Father: Now I have three and you have three, so we are both happy. Meow, meow, meow. I need your help, will you help me open this banana please? (*prompts helping again*)

Hudson: Will you help me open this banana please? (echolalic)

Father: You are so good at opening and peeling bananas, all right...you are going to give me the peel back too, thank you. (*praises helping and models social skill thank you*)

Hudson: (peels the banana and hands his dad part of peel)

Father: Thank you, thanks for the peel. Now you're going to give me the banana too. Now I am feeling pretty lazy! You are so helpful!

Considerations

This father effectively gets into his son's spotlight by praising his sharing of the raisins and by offering Hudson a kitty cracker. In terms of the ABC of child learning he uses the kitty crackers as his motivating antecedent to prompt (B) a verbal response (yes) and then for (B) asking for them (I want kitty cat) and then the consequence being that he gets 2 kitty cats. He makes these kitty cats even more interesting by being silly and turning them into kitty cat crackers that are kissing, hugging, tickling each other, and saying meow. He continues to model the social skills he wants Hudson to imitate and prompts Hudson by asking him for help with opening the banana. Did you notice that Hudson doesn't respond to this prompt, probably because he is distracted by the kitty cats? The father doesn't force his son's compliance, rather he follows his lead engaging in the kitty cat game by standing up the cats and counting them. When Hudson takes a cracker from him, he gives him the words to ask (I want kitty cat), and when Hudson responds by asking, his father praises and gives him more crackers. The father tries again to prompt helping, and this time Hudson complies and is thanked and praised.

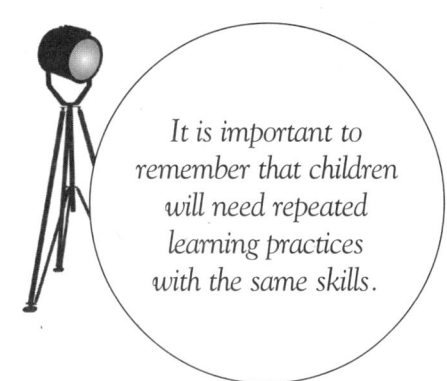

It is important to remember that children will need repeated learning practices with the same skills.

It is important to remember that children will need repeated learning practices with the same skills. As this snack interaction continues Hudson's father continues to prompt Hudson to help and interact with him.

Father: Will you also help me throw the banana peel in the garbage? (*prompts helping*) You are so good at throwing the banana peel in the garbage—you can even throw it in the compost. Press the button and open the compost. (*praises*)

Hudson: (puts banana peels in compost)

Father: Very helpful Hudson, press the button and open the compost. There you go, perfect. Thank you so much Hudson, give me five (*praising compliance to instruction*).

Hudson: (sits back down)
Father: Now do you need help opening your banana? I can help you too. (*models helping*) You helped me and I'll help you back. Can you open it all by yourself do you think? Can you help me open this Hudson... grrh, I'm trying, I'm not strong enough...see if you can do it for me.
Hudson: (peels banana)
Father: Oh, you are so strong! Grrh...you pulled the top off and there it goes, whee, you did it!

Consideration

The father gives Hudson another learning opportunity to learn how to help by asking him to throw the banana peel in the compost. He praises and reinforces his son's compliance to his request, contributing to his understanding that responding to his father's request and helping him is important. Next, as Hudson peels his own banana, the father offers to help him, modeling how to offer help to another. Then when Hudson continues to try on his own, his father praises his independent efforts. All of this positive social interaction and praise from his father helps Hudson to feel confident, independent, and eager to keep interacting with his father, who has become his favorite playmate. In addition, it helps Hudson learn what it means to help someone and how to offer help to another.

Managing Children's Anxiety and Promoting Independence

In the next scenario, notice how the same father responds when Hudson accidently tips the bubble bottle over. Notice how the father helps Hudson stay emotionally regulated, teaches him how to ask for help, and supports his independent behavior.

Father: Hudson, we're going to do two more minutes of bubbles okay? Two more minutes. (*gives warning*)
Hudson: I lost it (wand lost in bubbles and container falls over spilling bubble material. Hudson looks distressed and starts flapping his hands.).

Father: You lost it. Oops. That's okay. We'll get a rag and clean it up okay (gets rag) Here you go Hudson, want to wipe it up? You can use the rag.
Hudson: (wipes area)
Father: Thank you. You are helping to clean up! (*reinforces helping behavior*)
Hudson: Spilled.
Father: You can say. It's okay. It spilled, but it's okay. No big deal. (*prompts calming language*)
Hudson: No big deal.
Father: No big deal. We'll just clean it up.
Hudson: No big deal.
Father: Here's the rag to clean the floor, please. Thank you for your help. Hudson you have been very helpful.
Hudson: I lost it. (looking in bubbles for missing wand).
Father: Do you want me to help to get the bubble wand out? Can you reach in there and get it out with your finger? (*offers choice and if he wants help*)
Hudson: (tries to get it out himself) I need help.
Father: Nice asking. (*waits as he continues trying*) Did you get it?
Hudson: I need help to get it.
Father: Will you look at me and ask for help? (*prompts target asking behavior and eye contact*)
Hudson: I need help. (not looking)
Father: With your eyes.
Hudson: I need help please. (glancing up briefly, but then gets the bubble wand himself)
Father: You got it, and did it all yourself! All by yourself good job Hudson! Okay now we're going to do two more minutes, okay? (sets timer)

Considerations

This father helps his son manage his anxiety about the bubble spill by modeling a calm reaction to the spilled bubbles. He turns the distress and frustration into a learning opportunity for Hudson to practice being helpful and to use his self-talk language to stay calm by saying, "it's okay, no big deal." Once things are cleaned up, the father asks Hudson if he wants help getting the bubble wand out of the bottle, "do you want help" As this is what caused the spill in the first place, it would have been tempting to get the wand out for Hudson. Instead, the father turns this into another learning opportunity for Hudson to learn to ask for help. Even when Hudson echoes, "I need help," his father waits to see if he can do this on his own. In the end, Hudson completes the task independently, and his father acknowledges his success, contributing to Hudson's sense of independence and confidence.

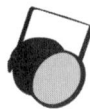

Think about how you teach your child to ask for help during daily activities such as mealtimes, getting dressed, bath time, or using a challenging toy or game. Also think about how you can encourage their beginning independence by doing some of these tasks on their own, with your support and scaffolding.

Coaching to Foster Independence in Everyday Activities

The principles of getting into your child's attention spotlight, narrating actions, modeling, prompting, following your child's lead, imitating, and praising social skills can also be used during regular caregiving routines. Think about coaching social interactions during these routines as another learning opportunity and chance for your child to connect with you and for you to encourage social language. You can use these social prompts to promote your child's independence. Does this take more time? Absolutely! It is easier and faster to take your child's shoes off, bathe them, get them ready for bed, or clean up for them; however, doing this as a joint activity will be helping your child learn to be independent. It will also foster an understanding

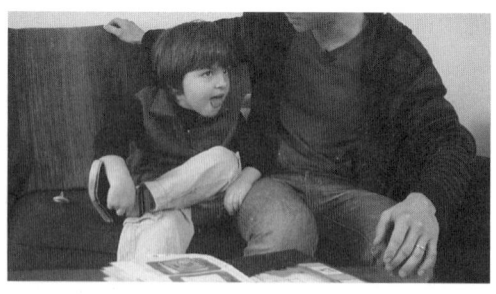

of how to follow directions, listen, help and take turns. In the next scenario, watch how the father uses coaching methods during the daily routine of Hudson taking off his shoes.

Father: Sit down. Here we go. Can you open your straps? Can you open the straps, Hudson? (*prompting desired activity.*) You can do it all by yourself.
Hudson: (undoing Velcro)
Father: There's one strap and another strap, you got it. Take this one off! Oh you're going to do the straps first. (*describing actions and being child directed.*) There you go. You can pull it back there. There you go, you got your shoe off... nice work. One strap, and you are opening the other strap, you are using your hand to pull it off, that is great.
Hudson: (shoe falls off)
Father: You did it... yippee! (*encouragement, praise.*)

Considerations

Hudson's father used patience, coaching, encouragement, and descriptive commenting to help his son learn to take off his shoes. This took more time and patience than doing it for him, but with repeated experience, Hudson will soon learn to take off his shoes independently, fostering his self-confidence and self-care skills!

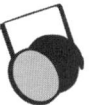

A child without ASD seems to find pleasure in moving from dependence to independence. For example, they want to dress themselves, put on their own shoes, eat with utensils, and "do it all-by-self" like their older siblings or parents. They spend time observing their parents, sibling, and peers and imitating them, and they feel reinforced by the social responses of others to their efforts. However, children with ASD don't seem to have the same urge to be independent or do things for themselves, nor are they necessarily motivated to be like others around them. Therefore, they are not imitating others and they miss out on the many ABC learning opportunities that naturally occur for children who are motivated and reinforced by learning to do things independently. While parents may be tempted to place fewer demands or expectations on children with ASD, this approach will delay their learning of independent skills. Instead, use the ABC's to help teach target independence behaviors by setting up motivating antecedents and behavior goals, modeling and prompting the target independent behavior, and reinforcing its occurrence. At the same time, make sure your child is not being rewarded or reinforced for unwanted behaviors and communication, and set up opportunities to teach them replacement behaviors or "positive opposite" behaviors.

Social Coaching During Mealtimes

Mealtimes are a great opportunity to use social coaching. In the next scenario notice how the father gets into his son's attention spotlight, sparks his interest and sets up fun learning opportunities so he can model and practice how to greet someone and say goodbye in social interactions.

Father: Okay, do you want a whole banana or a little piece? A little piece of banana, or whole banana? (holds up half a banana on one side of his head and whole on the other side and makes a funny face.) *(prompts choice response)*

Hudson: Whole banana.

Father: Whole banana! That is a lot of banana. Ring, ring, ring, but I want to use it for a telephone first, do you want to do phone banana or do you want to eat the banana? Ring, ring, ring.

Hudson: Eat the banana.

Father: All right here you go, banana for you, I will eat the half banana. *(reinforces response)*

Hudson: (puts banana phone to his ear)

Father: Oh, you are talking on the phone too.

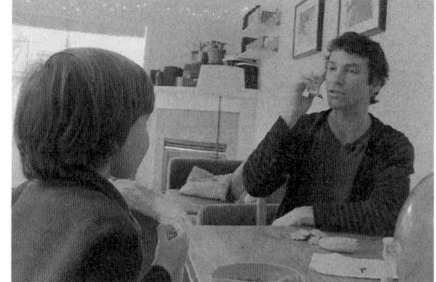

	Ring ring. I only have half a phone here.
Hudson:	ring ring
Father:	Hello, who's there, what's your name? (*prompts greeting*)
Hudson:	ring ring
Father:	What's your name? Is your name Hudson?
Hudson:	ring ring
Father:	You can say "Hi my name is..." (*prompts actual words*)
Hudson:	Hi, my name is Hudson. (child imitates)
Father:	Ah my name is Papa.
Hudson:	My name is Papa. (child imitates)
Father:	Yeah, I like talking to you on the phone. All right, see you later. Can you say: "Bye bye, Papa?" (*prompts saying goodbye*)
Hudson:	Bye bye, Papa.
Father:	(waves) Bye bye, Hudson. Okay, hang up. Click, hang up the phone. It was fun to talk with you on the phone, Hudson.

Considerations

This father does a great job of getting into his son's attention spotlight and prompting and encouraging his son's conversational skills by pretending his banana is a telephone. He encourages eye contact by putting the desired object (banana) next to his face. He prompts Hudson's use of language and turns this snack time into a fun make-believe social game. Here we see that Hudson has immediate echolalia, that is, he repeats what his father says immediately after hearing him. For example, when the father says, "My name is Papa," Hudson imitates this but is not really understanding the meaning of what he is saying; that is, his communication is not quite intentional yet. Hudson is at the beginning stages of learning how to introduce himself and how to say goodbye. Throughout this conversation the father models communication skills by using expressive language, smiles, gestures and excitement about what they are doing.

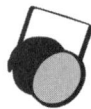You can think of your child being on a *continuum of intentional communication*. Some children are not yet using gestures or sounds to initiate intentional communication. For these children, parents will focus on helping the child learn to use a gesture, visual prompts, or sound to express their needs or wants. Hudson uses communication mainly in a transactional way; to get what he wants such as, to blow the bubbles, have the balloon, or to be spun again. At the other end of the continuum are children like Amelia who communicate to get information, such as when she asked what Truman's favorite color was, or whether she used the word please. In this case she is asking questions to get information about another person, to get feedback, and in some cases commenting simply to be sociable.

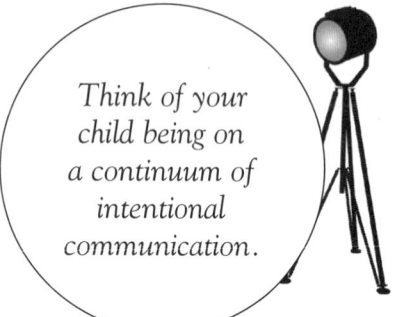

Think of your child being on a continuum of intentional communication.

Using Visual Prompts to Help Children Know How to Participate in Social Interactions

Because children on the autism spectrum are delayed in spontaneous gestures and nonverbal communication, it can be helpful to make pictures of key nonverbal gestures and words such as: waving *bye-bye* and saying *hi, all finished, sorry, please,* or *pointing*. As we discussed in Chapter Two, the meanings of the pictures are taught by pairing them with the actual gesture, word, or social skill behavior that has been targeted for learning. These pictures can be used to help children remember and know what to gesture or say in social situations such as on the playground, playing with another child, or during mealtimes. Perhaps the child always plays alone on the playground and doesn't know how

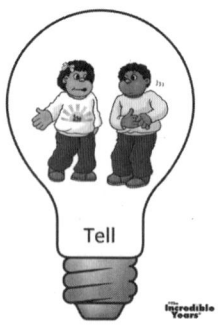
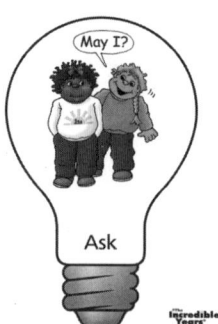
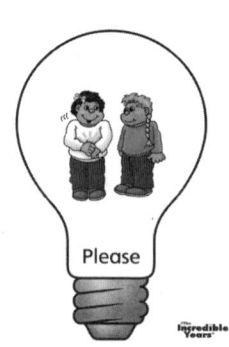

to initiate play with another child. They might be provided with some visual options of what to do in these unstructured social play times such as asking, "May I play with you," saying "hello," or waving.

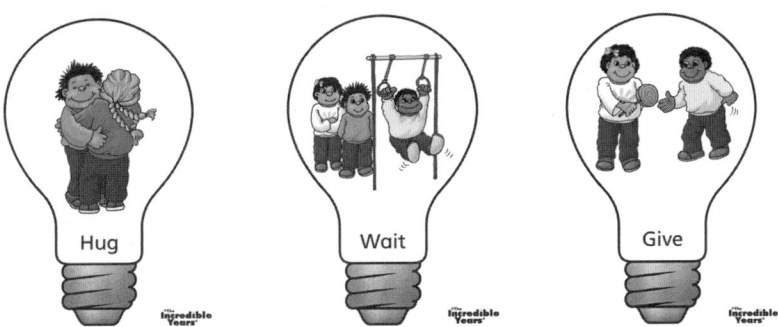

Communication pictures will be tailored to your child's play stage, social skills, and communication goals. For example, you might have pictures of asking, sharing, giving, helping, waiting, saying sorry, and complimenting. You can use these picture options to support your teaching when you model, prompt, and teach your child one of these social skills. For example, in the play scenarios we have seen with Amelia, Hudson, and Kalani, the parents could show the share or give picture card whenever the child shared, or the helping or giving pictures when they helped their sibling or parent by giving them something, or, the waiting picture when they waited their turn. Eventually the child will understand the connection between the social behavior and the picture. At that point, the pictures can be used as a prompt in situations where the child is uncertain about what to do.

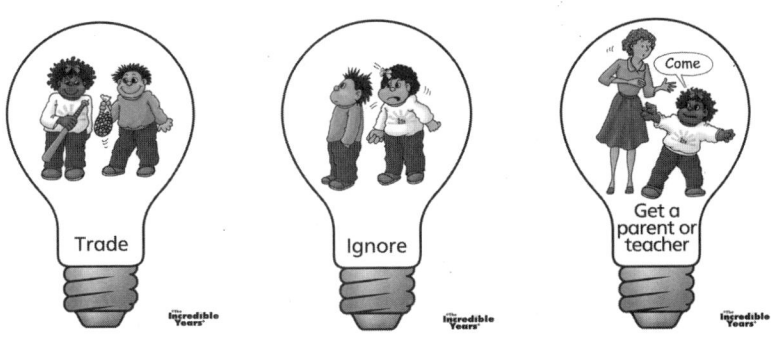

For these visual social prompts to be successful, teachers and parents will need to use them in conjunction with verbal social coaching, modeling of the behaviors, enthusiastic support, and praise in their child-directed play times. Here are a few examples of these social pictures from our *Incredible Years Child Dinosaur Program*. For children who can't read, the best pictures are those like hug, share, wait, give, and ask for help from parent or teacher because the picture depicts the behavior action.

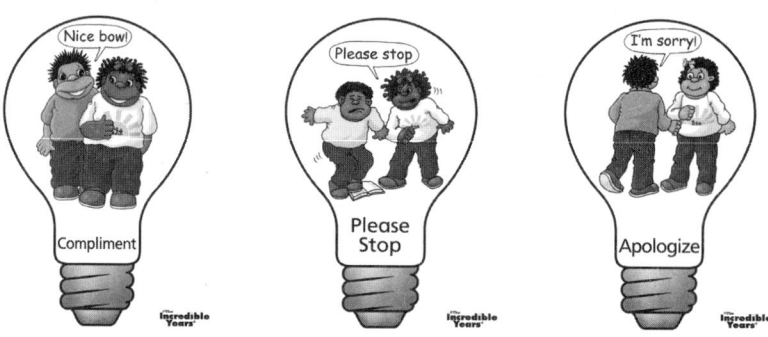

If children can read, then you could use apologize, compliment, ask, and please images. Start by using one or two pictures to depict the target social skill you are working on. Remember, you can always take photographs of times your child is waving, giving a thumbs up, sharing, asking, or hugging to depict the social behavior you are promoting,

Parent Reflections on Social Coaching

Mother: *I wanted to try to improve Amelia's social interactions. She really wants to interact. It's just that sometimes she just didn't do it appropriately. She couldn't pick up social cues, didn't know body space, so I hoped that the social coaching would help. She knows what the social behaviors like asking for a turn and trading mean but coming up with them in the moment is really hard for her. Sometimes for a child on the spectrum, they really have to memorize their options and learn the rules for what to do in a situation.*

When I coach Amelia socially, I primarily do it one-on-one. When my son is there, it's a little challenging because Truman is 21 months old, and Amelia's almost four. So I've got to manage the issues that a typical 21-month-old has with not really fully understanding sharing and the three-and-a-half-year-old who is still trying to gain the skills needed to ask for a turn or to trade or share. However, I've seen that Truman is learning a lot of these words already even though he doesn't have the language to express them. It's interesting. She'll say trade, and he knows to hand her something. I can see that Truman already understands some social interactions in a way that it is not intuitive to Amelia.

Father: *In regard to social coaching, there's been some mixed results. Like, when there's actually other kids around, and I'm trying to get him to take a turn or wait a minute, there is too much going on, and he can't process the interactions. But when I've done role-plays with him alone, it's been a lot easier. In the situation with other kids, it's like, he's usually already upset before it comes up. When I've done practice with him, he's seemed engaged and interested in it. He's not as emotionally involved, so it's not such a big deal. So he's willing to practice it. I think we need a lot more one-on-one practice before he'll be able to do this with another child.*

To Sum Up...

We have talked about using the ABCs to get in your child's attention spotlight and to able to set up social learning practice opportunities. You have learned to engage your child in play through songs, sensory physical routines, and social coaching where you model, prompt, imitate, and reinforce targeted social behaviors. You have started to widen your child's social spotlight to be more aware of you or siblings in the social interactions. In some cases, you have begun to help your child develop beginning empathy skills. At first your child will need a great deal of support to learn these social skills. Explicit visual prompts or cues can be beneficial reminders. Sometimes you may need to use physical prompts as well as visual cues for your child to fully understand what it means to give, help, share, or take turns. For example, physically taking your child's hand with the toy in it and offering the toy to you or a sibling will help your child understand what it means to give or share.

Eventually you will be able to fade out these prompts, so the child learns to take turns or share without your help. You saw from the scenarios in this chapter how physical sensory and fun pretend games can give your child an opportunity to show you how they can take turns and socially interact with you. In so doing your child will have discovered that his favorite activity is his social time and engagement with you.

Describing, modeling, prompting, and praising children's friendly behaviors is a powerful way to strengthen children's social skills. The following is a list of social skills that you can model and comment on when your child is playing with you or a friend or sibling. These are also social behaviors that can be used as the target behavior in an ABC learning opportunity. Combine picture and physical prompts with gestures and reduce the number of words according to your child's language level. Use this checklist to target the specific social skills that are your goals and write down the nonverbal and verbal communication approaches you will use. Start by working on only 1-2 social skills at a time.

Teachers and Parents Social Skills Coaching Checklist

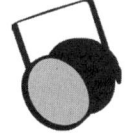

Describing, modeling, prompting, and praising children's friendly behaviors is a powerful way to strengthen children's social skills. The following is a list of social skills that you can model and comment on when your child is playing with you or a friend or sibling. These are also social behaviors that can be used as the target behavior in an ABC learning opportunity. Combine picture and physical prompts with gestures and reduce the number of words according to your child's language level. Use this checklist to target the specific social skills that are your goals and write down the nonverbal and verbal communication approaches you will use. Start by working on only 1-2 social skills at a time.

Social/Friendship Skills	Goals
_____ helping	
_____ sharing	
_____ teamwork	
_____ using a friendly voice (quiet, polite)	
_____ eye contact	
_____ listening to what a friend says	
_____ taking turns	
_____ asking	
_____ trading	
_____ waiting	
_____ responding to a friend's suggestion	
_____ gesturing (e.g., pointing)	
_____ smiling at peer	
_____ using soft, gentle touch	
_____ asking or gesturing to use something a friend has	
_____ cooperating	
_____ including another in play	

Prompting
- "Your friend is asking for a block. Can you give him that block? " (Praise child if s/he tries to help and/or point to yellow block, or put block in child's hand and give to other child)
- "Oops. You can say 'I am sorry' to your friend."

Modeling Friendly Behavior
- Parents and teachers can model asking, waiting, taking turns, helping, and complimenting, so children know what these social skills look like. For example, "I'm your friend (pat your chest) and share my block with you." (give block to child & show Sharing picture cue card.)

CHAPTER 5

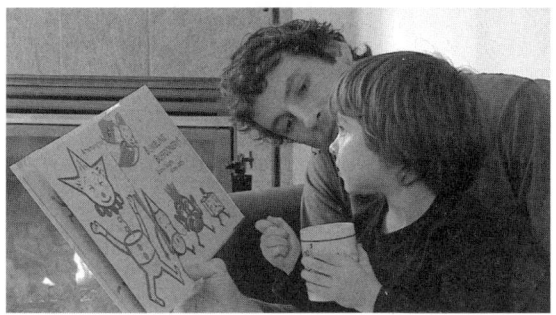

Emotion Coaching Promotes Emotional Literacy– Spotlight Your Child's Feelings

INTRODUCTION

In Chapter Four we talked about using the ABC model with social coaching to support, practice, and reinforce children's social interactions. Because children on the autism spectrum can be more preoccupied with objects than people, they need to be motivated to observe and interact with others. This spotlighted *"observational learning"* encourages them to observe, model and socially engage with others. In turn, these social experiences provide them with powerful practice learning opportunities.

In this chapter, we will discuss the importance of drawing children's attention to their own and other's feelings by using *emotion coaching*. This approach helps children develop feelings literacy; that is, a vocabulary for expressing their emotions to you and others. This is especially helpful for children with autism who can be delayed in emotion language and their ability to read nonverbal facial signals that typically convey emotion. Sometimes these children are described as withdrawn, flat and without affect or feelings. However, it is not that they don't have feelings, but rather that they don't know how to express their feelings or read emotion facial cues or gestures in others. They may withdraw due to confusion and anxiety. Moreover, since many of these children avoid eye-contact and do not look at others when communicating, they miss important cues that people typically use to read the emotions of those around them. For example, they might not see or register facial expressions such as smiles, frowns, or drawn or raised eyebrows.

Social Emotional Coaching

This chapter will build on all the nonverbal and verbal communication skills you have already learned, such as the importance of hand gestures and facial expressions, smiles and exaggerated positive tone of voice. You will target emotion words to model and spotlight the emotion words you want your child to learn. We will also discuss how to use visual feeling prompts to give your child more cues to understand their own feelings and the context for those feelings. Eventually, when your child can recognize and share their own feelings verbally or nonverbally, you can begin to help them recognize feelings in others, the beginning stage of empathy.

Modeling, Naming and Prompting Emotion Language

Emotion coaching starts when you name your child's emotions whenever you see them nonverbally expressing an emotion, such as when they seem happy, excited, content, confident, surprised, curious, proud, brave, calm, patient, frustrated, sad, lonely, disappointed, embarrassed, anxious, tense, fearful, or angry. Labeling feelings at the time you observe your child's emotional reactions or facial expressions helps your child link the feeling word with their internal emotional state and become more self-aware. You can also model feelings words and facial expressions by gesturing and naming your own feelings with words and

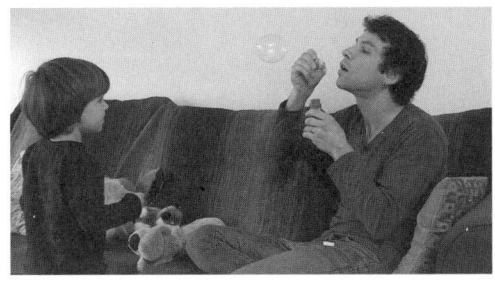

linking them to your child's experience during play. For example, saying with enthusiasm and a big smile, " I am so happy playing with you," or with a curious face, "I am so curious to see where the next block goes," or with a frown and hands up in air saying, "Oops, I'm sad that it broke," or with a frustrated face saying, "That is frustrating when the pieces won't go together". The number of specific feeling words targeted in emotion coaching will depend on your child's language stage. Remember also that what you give attention to will be repeated by your child, so try to give more attention to positive emotions than unpleasant emotions.

Once children have developed a feeling vocabulary, they can learn to recognize their own feelings and share them verbally or nonverbally with others. Ultimately, they will be able to recognize feeling gestures and words in others and respond sensitively to others' feelings. Supporting your child's emotional communication will contribute to your child's eventual ability to more easily regulate their own emotional and behavioral responses; that is, to develop emotional self-regulation skills.

Be sure to have a balance of positive and uncomfortable feeling words, and give at least as much, or more, focus to your child's learning about positive feeling states.

In the next scenario, notice all the ways Hudson's father models and prompts his son's expression and understanding of emotions.

Hudson: (bouncing)
Father: You look excited, Hudson, are you feeling excited? Say "I'm excited." *(prompts use of feeling word)*
Hudson: (does not respond but continues to bounce.)
Father: Are you having fun? I'm having fun. I like to blow bubbles. I like to blow bubbles with you Hudson. *(models feeling language)* Okay should I blow a big one? *(prompts request)*

Hudson: Blow a big one.
Father: Are you feeling nervous or are you feeling excited? (*prompts feeling response*)
Hudson: I'm feeling excited.
Father: You're excited! Your body is bouncing. You like bubbles. (blows more bubbles)
Hudson: Smiles and tries to pop bubbles
Father: You also look happy. I see a happy smile.
Hudson: (flapping)
Father: There it goes up in the air. Oh it's going to fall on your head, boop. There's a little one right by your foot. (waits for Hudson to look at him and ask before blowing)
Hudson: Hudson (looks at his father) and says: "More bubbles"
Father I'm feeling pretty happy right now. I'm proud of you for using your words and looking at me with your eyes to ask for bubbles. (*models feeling language*) What do you think, should we do it again?
Hudson: So do it again (jumps up and down).
Father: How should I do it this time? (*prompts verbal request*)
Hudson: Blow a bunch of bubbles.
Father: A bunch of bubbles okay. Are you flapping your arms because you are excited? You can say, "I flap my arms when I am excited." (*prompts feeling words*)
Hudson: I flap my arms when I'm excited.
Father: Yeah if anyone ever asks you can just tell them you are happy. (blows another bubble).

Considerations

Hudson's father uses one of his son's favorite activities (bubble blowing) to get in his son's attention spotlight and teach him feeling words such as excited, happy, and proud. He puts the bubbles close to his own face to encourage eye to eye contact and communication. He models expression of feelings himself by saying with a big smile, "I'm feeling pretty happy right now. I'm proud of you for using your words." Hudson's father also describes Hudson's physical feeling cues: "You are excited. I see you bouncing." Or, "You can say, 'I flap when I'm excited,'" and "I see your happy smile." He prompts his son to repeat the feeling words: "Are you excited or nervous?" Hudson answers by accurately identifying his excited feeling.

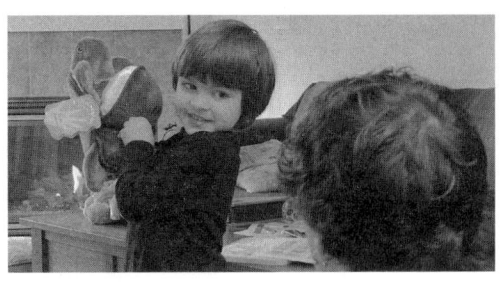

In this short scenario the father repeats the feeling word "excited" seven times and the word "happy" four times. This repetition will enhance Hudson's learning of the meaning of these feelings. When you are interacting with your child, look for opportunities to name your child's emotion and to model and label your own positive feelings about being with your child. For example: "You look excited about getting your favorite snack." Or, "I'm feeling happy that we are having snack together."

Using Visual Prompts to Teach Your Child Emotion Words

Using feeling picture prompts along with spoken words and gestures will give your child more cues to understand the feeling and the context or reason for the feeling (for example, being sad because it is time to stop spinning). In the next scenario think about how the Hudson's father uses laminated feeling pictures cue cards to teach his son some emotion language. Think about what else Hudson is learning.

Hudson: (shows his father a picture of sad face)
Father: How does he feel?
Hudson: Sad.
Father: He feels sad. Looks like he's crying. (father makes a sad face). Here's my sad face. I think you are sad when you have to stop spinning.
Hudson: (pulls another picture)
Father: What's he doing?
Hudson: What's he doing?
Father: He's pushing the...
Hudson: He's pushing the...
Father: What's that? (points to the wall in the picture)

Hudson: He's pushing the…what's that?
Father: (turns to touch wall) What's this here?
Hudson: He's pushing the wall.
Father: He's pushing the wall. That's right. It's called wall push-ups. Maybe if you feel angry or sad you can push the wall and feel calm again.
Hudson: (shows him a picture of calm face)
Father: Yes! You found the calm face. This says "calm". Can I see your calm face?
Hudson: This is my calm face.
Father: Yes, you seem calm now. This is my calm face.

Considerations

Hudson's father has a selection of laminated feeling pictures he uses to teach his son feeling words. In the scenario above, he is following Hudson's interest in looking at and talking about the feeling pictures he has chosen. When Hudson is looking at the sad feeling picture, the father adds information by showing his own sad face. He also adds context by naming a situation that makes Hudson sad. When Hudson selects a new picture of the wall push-up, the father follows his lead, and talks about how wall push-ups can help him calm down when he is angry or sad. When naming negative or uncomfortable feelings, it is important to offer a coping strategy that the child can use to feel better.

Hudson's father has worked with him on feeling language over many weeks. He has gradually added new feeling word pictures to his feeling book as Hudson has practiced and learned new words (e.g., starting with happy, mad, sad, and then adding frustrated, nervous, and excited, patient and brave).

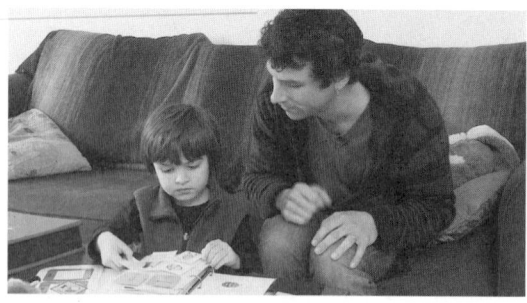

When Hudson exhibits one of these feelings, his father shows him the feeling picture, naming it and saying, "you feel excited when you flap your arms and are playing with bubbles" or, "you are frustrated when spinning stops". He connects the feeling word and picture with a possible reason for the feeling and the body cues or facial gestures that go with the feeling. This is important because it will help a child link an experience with a particular feeling and understand its meaning.

Once your child has learned the name for each of the feelings, you can prompt them to share their feelings by pointing to the picture of the feeling and naming the word. This is the beginning of being able to communicate feelings to others. Recognizing and communicating feelings eventually leads to self-regulation and empathy for the feelings of others.

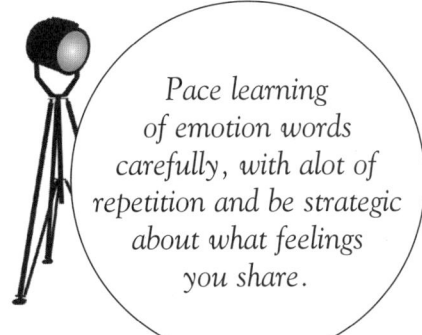

Pace learning of emotion words carefully, with alot of repetition and be strategic about what feelings you share.

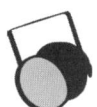

Think about what feeling words you model when you are communicating with your child and what specific feeling words you want your child to learn. Be sure to have a balance of positive and uncomfortable feeling words, and give at least as much, or more, focus to your child's learning about positive feeling states. Remember that the average number of feeling words expressed by a neurotypical 3-4 year old child is 3 words, although they will likely understand more feeling words than they can speak. So, pace this learning of emotion words carefully and slowly with lots of repetition.

Some Tips for Using and Making Feeling Picture Prompts to Help Your Child Understand Feelings

Start by identifying two feeling emotion words to teach your child. Pick one positive and one negative/uncomfortable feeling such as happy and sad, fearful and brave, or frustrated and calm. Find a picture to represent each feeling. Remember, you can use picture line drawing communication symbols (PCS) of feelings and many other free line drawing printables found online by Boardmaker (Mayer-Johnson) or other companies. Or, you can make your own set of feeling pictures by cutting pictures from magazines or using real pictures of your child and other family members showing each feeling face. For example, to show happy, you could take a picture of your child smiling while eating ice cream, going down the slide at the park, or playing with a favorite toy.

Social Emotional Coaching

Put the word of the feeling on the picture. Initially it is best to use close-up pictures of your child's face that show an exaggerated facial expression—for example a big smile, open excited mouth, scrunched up angry face. You want to have obvious facial cues for your child to notice.

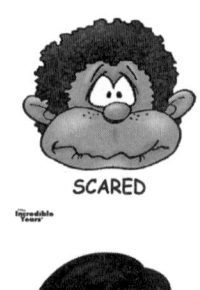
SCARED

When you show your child the visual card, name the emotion and link with the experience: "Kalani is happy when he is on the teeter-totter." "Amelia is sad when she falls down on the scooter. Hugging mom makes her feel better," Or, "Hudson is mad when he has to stop spinning. He takes a deep breath to calm down." When labeling an uncomfortable feeling, name the feeling and then add a coping response to indicate a way to manage the feeling, or to reassure the child the feeling will eventually change.

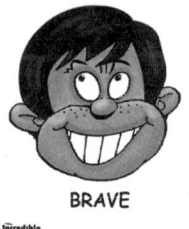
BRAVE

When you show your child the visual card, name the emotion and link with the experience.

When you show these pictures to your child, be sure to mirror the expression of the feeling on your own face. As your child learns new emotions, you can gradually add more feelings to your child's emotion picture board. Eventually your child will be able to point to a picture of a feeling on the feeling board to show you their feeling. With time, repetition, and ongoing modeling, your child will be able to name his feeling with a word without the feeling cue cards. Ultimately your child will learn to recognize feelings in others.

Spotlight Feeling Activities

Feeling book: It can be helpful to make a feeling book with drawings or photographs of different feelings and examples from the child's life. Positive feelings can be pictured with the positive event: *"Jolie is happy when she eats grapes." " Nico is proud because he has learned to ride a bike." " Hudson is excited when he blows bubbles with his father."* Uncomfortable or negative feelings should be paired with a coping or "feel-better" strategy. *"Alex is sad when he falls down. Getting a bandaid & kiss from mom makes him feel better"* or *"Menta is mad when she has to stop spinning.*

She takes a deep breath to calm down." "Amelia is anxious at school but feels better when she asks a friend to play with the doll house." The key is to link the emotion word to an experience.

Feeling key chain or board: Make small (3x3) pictures of feeling faces such as those shown here, laminate them and put them on a key ring or portable Velcro board. This can be taken with you and used to help your child communicate and share their feelings in any setting.

Mirrors: Use mirror and take turns making feeling faces while looking in the mirror. This allows your child to see their own face when making a feeling expression.

Feeling Dice: Put a different feeling face on six sides of a square cardboard box. Take turns tossing the box and then label and imitate the feeling face that comes up on top of the box. If your child has more language they can share a time they felt that way.

Feeling bingo: There are many feeling bingo games available for purchase, or you can make your own bingo cards and board. Play traditional bingo, or just use the cards for feeling exploration. Some children will enjoy matching the cards to the bingo sheets, others will like sorting the cards, or just looking at and talking about the pictures and times they felt that way. You can also play a matching game by turning over the feeling cards and finding the match with another one of the same emotion. When you find a match you can say the name of the feeling and show the face.

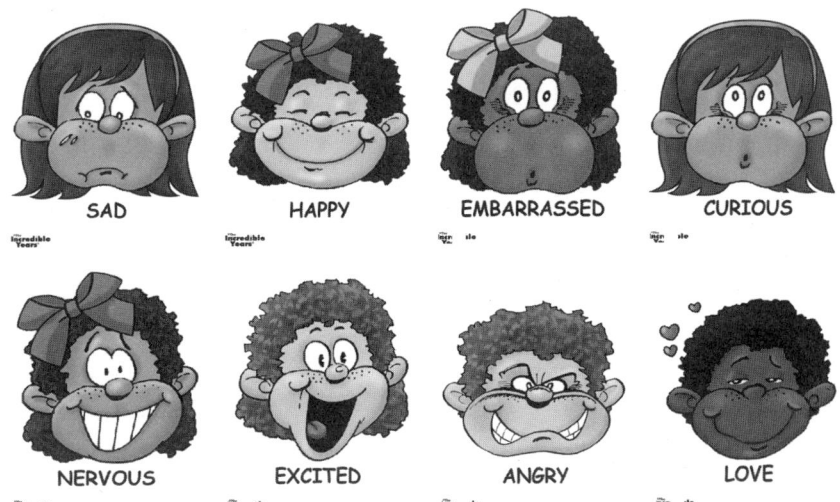

Reading to Build Emotional Literacy

Another way to begin to build your child's feeling literacy is through books. While it is typical to read with your child sitting in your lap, sitting with your child facing you will allow you to make eye contact and to model feeling facial expressions and gestures while you are reading. To enhance your child's emotion awareness, label the feelings of characters in the books, mimic the emotions with your own face, point out feeling cues in the illustrations (tears, grimaces, smiles), and link the emotions of the characters to your child's own experiences. Continue to remain child-directed, narrating what your child is looking at and allowing your child time to show you what is interesting in the book and to respond to your questions or comments. Provide opportunities for your child to fill in a partial prompt or mimic your language. Sometimes adding a sound effect or action can make the story more interesting for your child. In the next scenario watch all the strategies the father uses to keep his son's attention and how he makes reading this book a shared social experience.

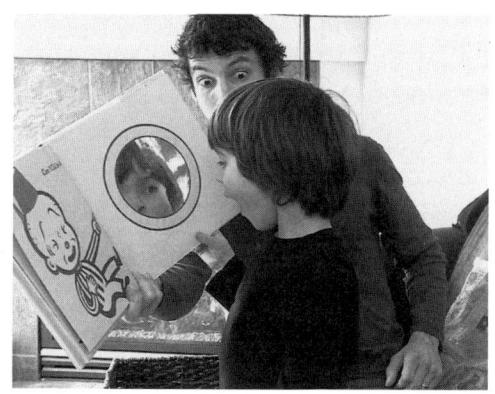

Father: There is an exclamation point, big one.
Hudson: There's exclamation point.
Father: (pointing at picture in book). What does this license plate say? What are those letters?
Hudson: What are those letters?
Father: That's a...(partial prompt)
Hudson: S
Father: S, What's that one?
Hudson: I
Father: I
Hudson: L
Father: L

Hudson: E and another E.
Father: Another E. SILLEE and that spells sillee.
Hudson: That spells sillee.
Father: Here comes Willy really silly.
Hudson: Here comes Willy really silly.
Father: Hey he's got a big smile, look... I think he's happy – what's he doing with his mouth? (big smile on his face)
Hudson: He's licking.
Father: Licking. He's sticking out his tongue, yeah (sticks out his tongue). I'm being silly. Can you be silly too?
Hudson: A parade of sillies.
Father: (tries to look at him but Hudson is gazing off) They all have funny hats on... do you have a favorite hat?
Hudson: (gazes away)
Father: I like the triangle hat. Oh, at look the monkey, Is he mad now or is he happy? How's he feeling?
Hudson: He's happy.
Father: Yeah, he feels happy. I see a smile.
Hudson: Happy
Father: Now he's relaxed just hanging out, funny faces wink and smile...I'm going to show you this face okay? I'm going to move you for a sec so you can look at my face (moves Hudson so he can get eye contact). This face! (sticks his tongue out) What kind of face is that? That's a silly face.
Hudson: I want to see the mirror.
Father: Oh, the mirror okay you want to look in the mirror... you remembered the mirror, that's right.
Hudson: The mirror (turns the pages).
Father: There's Hudson's face. (shows him mirror in book).
Hudson: (smiles at his own face)
Father: You are smiling. You look happy. Are you going to make a silly face? Can you make a silly face?
Hudson: (opens his mouth looking at mirror)
Father: (imitates Hudson's face.) That's pretty silly. Okay look at me, Hudson. Look at me. I'm going to make

>   a silly face, okay? (sticks out his tongue and blows
>   bubbles and makes noises).
> **Hudson:** (takes book and looks in mirror making funny noises)
> **Father:** (imitates Hudson's voice while they both look in mirror)

Considerations

While they read together, this father teaches his son what it means to look and feel silly. It is interesting that Hudson knows his letters and can spell Silly, but it is unlikely that he understands the meaning of this feeling word until their joint social interaction reading experience. During the reading, the father moves so he can get more face-to-face interaction. This allows his son to see him when he exaggerates his silly feeling gestures and facial expressions to engage his son's interest and to increase Hudson's understanding of the silly feeling. The father remains child-directed in his approach, turning to the mirror when Hudson asks to see that.

Remember the E-CARE reading strategies we discussed in Chapter Three and Four to promote your child's pre-academic words and understanding of social skills. The same approach can be used to teach your child emotion words when you read. Think about how you can focus your discussion of books, rhymes, songs, and pictures on the feelings for the characters. For example, talking about how Humpty Dumpty felt when he fell and broke into pieces and then how he felt when he was put together again. Or, how the Itsy Bitsy Spider felt: first when the rain washed him away, and then when the sun came out. You can use your feeling picture cards with the books and rhymes and have your child point to the feeling picture representing how the characters felt.

Combining Emotion Coaching with Physical Sensory Routines

Notice how Amelia's mother uses a physical sensory game, imitation, and coaching to motivate her daughter's learning of feeling vocabulary. Think about what else Amelia is learning in this social interaction.

>   **Amelia:** (throws her head in pillow)
>   **Mother:** You can say "I'm feeling a little shy, but I'm going to
>   be playful soon."

Amelia: (throws head in pillow again)
Mother: (laughing and gets eye contact.) That's so silly. Where are you going? (imitates Amelia, also throwing her head in pillow). I feel shy. I feel so shy, hello.
Amelia: (throws head down again in pillow)
Mother: (imitates Amelia) I'm shy, but I'm going to come out and play.
Amelia: (throws head repeatedly)
Mother: Wow that's silly. Are you feeling silly now? (imitates her putting her head in pillow)
Amelia: I'm not shy any more, I'm silly.
Mother: You are being silly now? (Laughing)
Amelia: (throws head some more)
Mother: That's silly.

Considerations

As you may recall Amelia is frequently shy and anxious around other children and people. With others she withdraws and says very little. In this scenario the mother teaches Amelia emotion words while engaged in a fun physical sensory pillow reciprocal game. By imitating what Amelia is doing, the mother enters her spotlight and makes it more likely that Amelia will engage and learn from her. Notice that Amelia's mother does label Amelia's shy feeling but gives at least as much attention to her positive silly state. This helps Amelia understand the feeling word shy and then how her feelings can change when she is silly. Amelia's mother spotlights her silly and fun emotions. If Amelia's mother had only labeled the shy feeling, Amelia might have stayed longer in her shy and withdrawn state and would not have had the chance to experience the fun silly emotion.

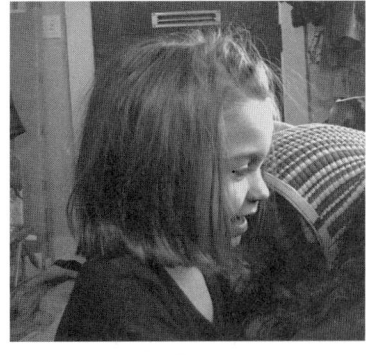

Combining positive emotion coaching with preferred physical sensory activities can help strengthen children's understanding of positive feeling states. If your child frequently seems fearful, frustrated,

Pay attention to which feelings you are teaching and labeling.

or avoidant, it is important to also notice and name their feelings at times when they are feeling happy, confident, curious, brave, content, or patient. Pay attention to which feelings you are teaching and labeling. It is important for your child to have words for both positive and negative feelings, so you will teach and validate all feelings. However, remember that your child may stay stuck in negative emotion states if you focus most of your attention on those states. Give even more attention to neutral, calm, patient and positive feeling states.

Responding to Children's Unpleasant Emotions

In the next scenario, we see another example of a mother using emotion coaching to help her son identify and then cope with an unpleasant feeling. Kalani is playing with a tub of water.

Kalani: Yum, dum, dum. (stirring water with wooden spoon)
Mother: Are you going to cook something with your spoon? We can stir it up, (laughs) stir it up, I am happy cooking with you.
Mother: (Kalani puts toe in water and jerks out again.) Is it cold?
Kalani: No.(shakes his head and looks startled).
Mother: Cold water – splash.
Kalani: In water.
Mother: You want to go in the water? Okay it's going to be cold on your feet. Ready (she helps him in the tub, and he slips a little).– Whoa and slippery! Was it slippery? Too slippery? A little bit scary?
Kalani: Yea, a little.
Mother: Was that a little bit scary? Cold? It's cold slippery water.
Kalani: Whoa.
Mother: Oh it's cold, but you are brave. You're in the water!
Kalani: Cold.
Mother: Kalani is standing in the cold water! You're brave.
Kalani: More water.
Mother: More water please.

Kalani: More water.
Mother: It looks like you are having fun. You like the cold water!
Kalani: More water.
Mother: There's more—more water—you just want to get in there, let's see. How does it feel? It was scary and now it's fun!
Kalani: (squeals in delight)
Mother: (hugs Kalani) A hug! A hug!

Considerations

In this scenario Kalani is a bit afraid of putting his feet in the water because it is too cold or slippery. His mother teaches him the word "scared" and validates his anxious feelings. She also encourages him to try new things and to manage his trepidation about getting in the water. She provides physical support so that he feels secure to try something new. As he gets used to the water and starts to enjoy himself, she labels that he is having fun and he is brave. This interaction provides Kalani with the vocabulary to understand his scared feelings and to experience that these feelings can change to fun when he is brave and takes a risk.

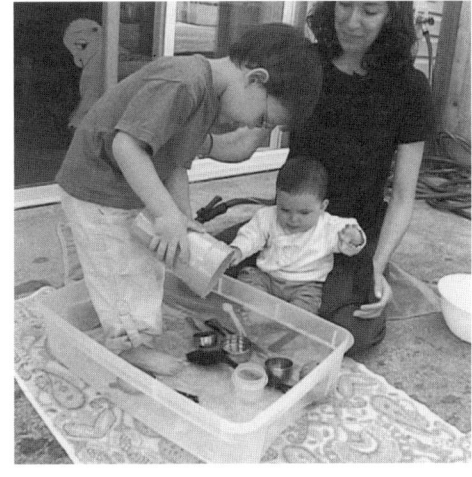

Research shows that a child's brain grows and is stimulated by things they are interested in. So, if your child likes paints, big blocks, or water play, they'll be most receptive to learning new emotions when they are engaged in these preferred activities. In this scenario the mother helps Kalani learn about feelings while he's having fun with water play.

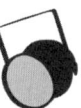

It is not necessary to have fancy toys. In fact, simpler unstructured toys, such as blocks, are probably preferable because they allow the child to use their own imagination and creativity. Also, many household objects such as cereal boxes, pots and pans, and a bucket of water can be wonderful toys for young children. Some old-fashioned toys are still the best fun such as building blocks, playing dress up with parents' old clothes and shoes, playdough, sand and water, building a fort out of the living room furniture, or playing with a doll house and family with a baby.

Helping Children Learn that Unpleasant Emotions Change

Coaching children's dysregulated emotions is tricky because giving excessive attention to negative emotions can make your child more angry, frustrated, scared, or sad. However, if done skillfully, coaching unpleasant emotions can strengthen your relationship and make your child feel validated and understood. It can also promote coping strategies and the recognition that these unpleasant feelings change with time. It is important to pair your comments about uncomfortable feelings with positive coping statements and predictions. In the next scenario, watch how the mother uses emotion coaching in regard to her child's worries.

Coaching unpleasant emotions can strengthen your relationship and make your child feel validated and understood.

Amelia has a small scratch on her finger.
Amelia: Oh no, oh no, oh no. (waving her finger vigorously and talking in a whining voice)
Mother: Is your finger still bothering you?
Amelia: Yeah. It hurts. It hurts (loud and dramatic voice).
Mother: It looks like that hurts. (*validating Ameila's experience but using a calm voice*) Do you want me to get a Band-Aid?
Amelia: Put some medicine on it and wash it.
Mother: I think that you are worried about your owie. Let me get a Band-Aid. I'll be right back. (leaves to get Band-Aid) Oh look what I have? A Band-Aid for your owie.
Amelia: Holds out finger and is still whimpering, but not as loudly.
Mother: We can help the hurt feel better with a Band-Aid. Oh, I need some help to open it. Can you help? (*offers distracting activity*)

Amelia:	(opens Band-Aid and stops whimpering)
Mother:	Nice pulling it apart for me all by yourself, thank you. You seem calmer! (names feeling)
Amelia:	It hurts.
Mother:	Oh, your owie hurts. Let's make it feel better. First I'll kiss it, (kisses finger) then I'll put a band aid on it.
Mother:	Do you feel better?
Amelia:	Yeah.
Mother:	All better. You are not hurt now. You're calm and okay.

Considerations

This mother expresses the feelings that she thinks her daughter might be having while at the same time letting her know she is cared for and will feel better. She labels and validates Amelia's emotions: hurt and worried. At the same time, she models self-regulation by talking in a calm voice and letting Amelia know she is cared for. She provides reassurance her the bandaid will help. By giving Amelia the task to pull apart the Band Aid, she supports her independent action and then praises her for doing this by herself. This mother has assessed that Amelia is not seriously hurt, but that the "owie" is a serious worry for Amelia. She validates and nurtures her daughter's distressed feelings without feeding into and increasing the worry. She provides comfort and a distracting activity with the fun Band-Aid. By the end of this the interaction, Amelia is calm, and her mother points out this new, calm feeling state.

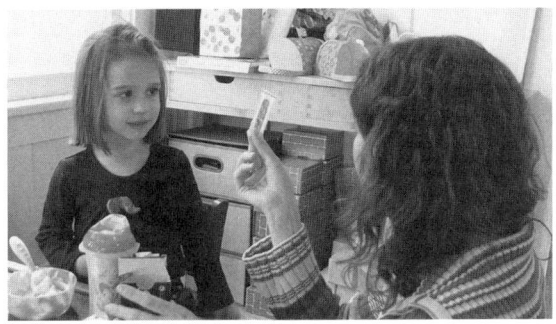

Linking Helping Social Behavior to Feelings

In the next scenario, Amelia's mother uses pretend play game to help Amelia understand more about emotions. Think about the importance of linking a feeling to a helpful social response especially for children on the autism spectrum.

Playing a game with a squirrel action figure, acorn pieces, and a tree stump

Amelia: Oh no mama! (an acorn has just fallen off the tree stump).

Sneaky Squirrel: (mother as squirrel) Oh no, my acorn fell out of my tree stump. That makes me sad! I need help! Help somebody. Help my acorn. I can't quite get it. It keeps falling.

Amelia: Is he sad?

Mother: Yes, I think he's sad that his acorn fell. I think he would feel better if he could get it back on the tree. Do you need help squirrel?

Amelia: Do you need help squirrel?

Sneaky Squirrel: Yes I do! This purple acorn fell, and I'm sad. Are you big and strong to help me and be my friend?

Amelia: I'm sad.

Sneaky Squirrel: You're sad, oh no. We are both sad. Are you okay? (strokes Amelia gently.)

Amelia: Yeah.

Sneaky Squirrel: Would you like to come and play with me? I'll be nice to you. Here you can help me put my acorn in my tree.

Amelia: (helps)

Sneaky Squirrel: Thank you, you helped me, now I feel so much better I have my acorn back. I'm happy now. Are you happy now too?

Amelia: I feel happy too.

Considerations

This mother skillfully sets up a scenario where her game character Sneaky Squirrel is sad because his acorn keeps falling, and he can't get it back in the tree. Amelia shows empathy and concern and asks her mother if the squirrel is sad. This indicates that the mother has been successful in teaching her daughter to think of other people's feelings. The mother models and prompts Amelia in how to ask squirrel if he

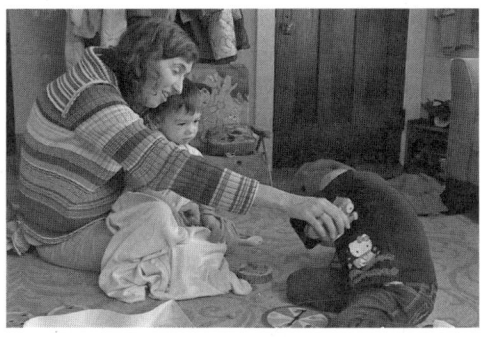

needs help. Amelia also copies and mirrors squirrel's feeling state of being sad. This allows squirrel to model helping and caring behavior and to invite Amelia to help her put her acorns in her tree. In the end, Squirrel helps Amelia discover that feelings can change because of her help. The modeling and prompting on the part of the mother with squirrel make this a powerful social and emotion learning experience. In the next Chapter Six, we will talk more about how to use puppets and toy characters to enhance children's social and emotional skills.

Parent Reflections on Emotion Coaching

Mother: The emotion coaching, both for myself and for Amelia, has gone really well. It's always a work in progress with any child, but especially with a child on the autism spectrum.

We worked a lot on just identifying emotions. I've been giving her the words to say. So if she got sad, I'll say, "Oh, I see you feel sad, but it's gonna be better soon. You're hurt because you fell, and I'm helping you rub it. We're cleaning it. We're gonna put a Band-Aid on it. And it's gonna be better."

I give her words, "I feel sad because I fell down." You know? She's very good at repeating, as kids on the autism spectrum are. Then, she says, "I feel sad 'cause I fell down." Just in the last couple weeks started to be able to say things without me prompting her. So that's been really big.

Father: I've tried a lot of emotion coaching because that's a main difficulty in dealing with his emotions and emotional regulation.

A big part of that is reading books with him. He likes reading and so it helps to focus on the characters in the books. We've gotten a lot of really good books that talk about emotions. Even books that are not about feelings have characters with expressions on their faces. So, he can now identify quite a few facial expressions and emotions. I try to link these to talking about the feelings that he's having.

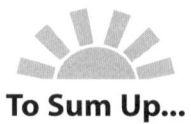
To Sum Up…

While young children with autism often have difficulties understanding feelings in themselves and others, they are capable of making enormous gains in this area. This can happen when parents model feeling language themselves and spotlight their child's feelings by labeling the feelings their child is experiencing. Parents can help their child understand more about feelings by pointing out the physical cues and context that go along with different feelings. To promote self-regulation parents can provide reassurance and coping strategies to help children manage uncomfortable or dysregulated feelings. Books, games, and visual feeling prompts can also be a helpful way for children to learn feelings language. Emotional self-awareness will eventually lead to the development of understanding and empathy for the feelings of others.

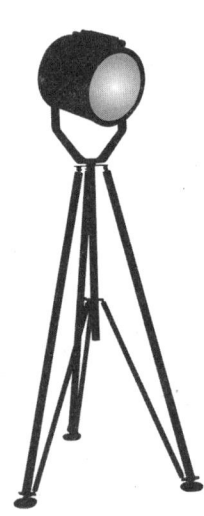

SPOTLIGHTING
Emotion Coaching

- Try to think about what your child might be feeling and wanting.
- Describe your child's feelings (don't ask what they are feeling because they are unlikely to have the words to tell you).
- Validate all feelings, but make sure to label your child's positive feelings more often than negative feelings.
- When naming uncomfortable feelings such as frustration or anger, point out and praise the coping strategy your child is using: "You look frustrated, but you are staying calm and trying again."
- Cuddle and soothe your child when they are hurt or frightened. Stay calm yourself to provide extra reassurance.
- For children who are non verbal, use visual prompts of feeling faces to teach feelings. Keep your language simple and repeat words often. Prompt your child to use the picture cards to show you how they are feeling.
- Use the one-up principle to provide explanations of the context for feelings. Tailor these phrases to your child's language level.

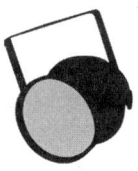

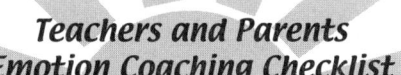
Teachers and Parents Emotion Coaching Checklist

Describing children's feelings is a powerful way to strengthen their emotion literacy. Once children have emotion language, they can better regulate their own emotions because they can tell you how they feel. From the following list of emotions choose a few that you could comment on when interacting with your child. Combine the verbal emotion words with your facial expressions and use of picture emotions. Slowly add more feeling words and be sure to have a balance of more positive than uncomfortable feeling words. When using uncomfortable emotions combine with a coping emotion word.

Feelings/Emotion Literacy		Goals
____ happy	____ brave	
____ frustrated	____ disappointed	
____ calm	____ fearful	
____ proud	____ loving	
____ excited	____ tired	
____ pleased	____ energetic	
____ sad		
____ helpful		
____ worried		
____ confident		
____ patient		
____ having fun		
____ jealous		
____ forgiving		
____ caring		
____ proud		
____ curious		
____ angry		
____ mad		
____ interested		
____ embarrassed		

Modeling Feeling Talk and Sharing Feelings
- "I am proud of you for solving that problem." (Show Proud picture.)
- "I am really having fun playing with you." (Show Happy picture.)
- "I was nervous it would fall down, but you were patient, and your plan worked." (Show Nervous picture.)
- "Your friend is so happy that you shared with her."

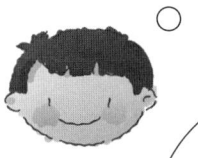

"friendly dog, you happy"

"You look proud of that drawing."

"You seem confident when reading that story."

"You are so patient. Even though it fell down twice, you just keep trying to see how you can make it taller. You must feel pleased with yourself for being so calm and trying hard."

"You are forgiving of your friend because you know it was a mistake."

"I am having fun with you and am excited about your discoveries."

 Spotlight your child's feelings!

CHAPTER 6

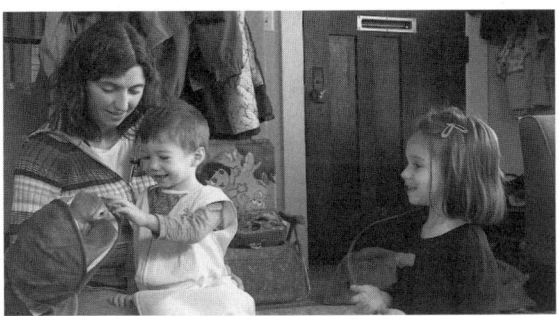

Using Pretend Play to Spotlight Empathy and Social Skills

Introduction
For young children on the autism spectrum, the world of pretend and imaginary play does not emerge naturally; it needs to be encouraged and strengthened. Such children may be very adept at playing with puzzles, knowing shapes, letters, numbers and even reading, and may be good at understanding concrete facts. However, using ideas that come from their imagination, rather than ideas that are factual or based on real-life objects is more difficult for them. In this chapter we will discuss how you can encourage your child's imaginary play skills. Studies have shown that when young children develop pretend play,

their language abilities and social skills also increase. Pretend play with you helps you and your child engage in a shared social communication experience. In addition, pretending helps your child learn what others are feeling and thinking. When encouraged by parents and teachers, imaginary play provides powerful opportunities for enhancing children's language, social skills, emotional regulation, and ability to make sense of real life events.

In prior chapters we saw Hudson's father using pretend play with Kitty Cat crackers as if they were alive and a banana as a symbolic substitute for a phone to enhance his son's social communication. We also saw Amelia's mother communicate through the Sneaky Squirrel toy to prompt her daughter's helping behavior and to help her see the connection between friendly actions and good feelings. These parents got in their children's attention spotlight with joint pretend play experiences and engaged their children's social conversation skills. Let's think about some other benefits of using imaginary objects, characters, or puppets with children. We know that young children talk more easily with a puppet than with adults, perhaps because puppets resonate with their emerging fantasy and imaginary world stage of cognitive development, that is, Piaget's pre-operational second stage of thinking (ages 2-7 years). This is when children think at a symbolic level but are not yet using logical cognitive operations. Fantasy and reality are easily confused, and they are able to make one thing stand for something else. Almost anything can be alive and have feelings. Although children on the spectrum are said to be delayed in pretend play, they seem particularly attracted to and engaged with puppets, perhaps because they already have a preference for objects over people. Or, perhaps because puppets have less complex facial gestures and seem more predictable and less confusing than people. If you choose your puppet's language and actions strategically, puppets can be a great way for you to get in your child's attention pretend spotlight and model and prompt specifically targeted social and emotional skills. Here are some possible puppet scenarios:

Puppets can be a great way to get in your child's attention pretend spotlight and model and prompt targeted social and emotional skills.

Puppet Models and Prompts Your Child's Social Skills

- **Friendly Greeting to Others.** Your puppet can model how to greet someone by saying, "Hi, I am Tiny Turtle. What is your name?" When your child answers with their name, your puppet can thank them for being so friendly. Use a puppet with a moving mouth and incorporate greeting gestures such as waving hello or good-bye.

- **Showing Interest in Another.** Your puppet can model being interested in your child by asking, "What do you like to do?" or, "What is your favorite game?" When your child shares their interests, the puppet can reciprocate by sharing their own interests. You can even prompt your child to ask your puppet what they like to do? For example, whisper to your child, "You can say, 'Tiny Turtle what do you like?'" Remember to tailor these interactions to your child's language developmental level. Your puppet's language should follow the "one-up" rule for number of words. If your child is not yet responding to questions from others, then your puppet should imitate your child's sounds, words, and gestures.

  > *If your child is not yet responding to questions from others, then your puppet should imitate your child's sounds, words, and gestures.*

- **Asking for Help.** Your puppet can prompt your child's targeted social behavior by asking for help with something. For example, your puppet says, "I can't find the puzzle piece (or blue lego) that fits, can you help?" When your child helps your puppet, the puppet can say thank you or compliment them for helping and friendly behavior. For example, your puppet says, "that was so friendly. You found that. I feel happy." For a child with less language, the puppet might hold up a block, gesture or point to another block, and ask "help please" while trying to stack the blocks. If your child responds by helping, the puppet could say, "Thank you! Happy!" and gesture by patting themselves on chest. Connecting the puppet's feeling to the social behavior helps your child understand the relationship between a behavior action and someone else's feelings, a first step towards building empathy.

- **Sharing.** Your puppet can model how to share by offering a block, toy, marker, or food item to the child. For example, puppet says, "you want cracker" and holds it out to child. When your child takes the cracker, you can prompt a thank you by whispering and saying, "Say, thank you." If your child responds, praise them for being friendly by saying, "Good thank you!" For children with more language, the puppet can also label the friendly behavior: "Would you like some banana? I will be friendly and share it with you!" This helps the child connect the label for the friendly behavior to the action.

- **Waiting, asking, and sharing.** Your puppet can model waiting for a turn and sharing. For example, while your child is playing, the puppet can say, "I am waiting for turn with green playdough." When your child shares the playdough (you may need to prompt this), you can praise them for sharing. Next look for opportunities to praise your child for waiting for a turn. "Now the puppet is playing, and you are waiting!" Interactions like these provide chances to practice waiting, asking, and sharing. For example, you can prompt your child to ask the puppet, "Can I have some yellow playdough?" Praise your child by saying: "That was friendly asking!" When the puppet shares the playdough, you can say, "Good sharing, puppet. Your friend asked and you shared the playdough." Or, you might teach the idea of asking to trade instead of waiting and sharing. In this case the puppet can say, " Can I trade my car for your truck?" If your child agrees and hands your puppet the truck, you can say, " You are being friendly sharing and trading with each other!" The number of words would be reduced for children with less language and perhaps combined with a visual prompt of waiting or sharing or asking.

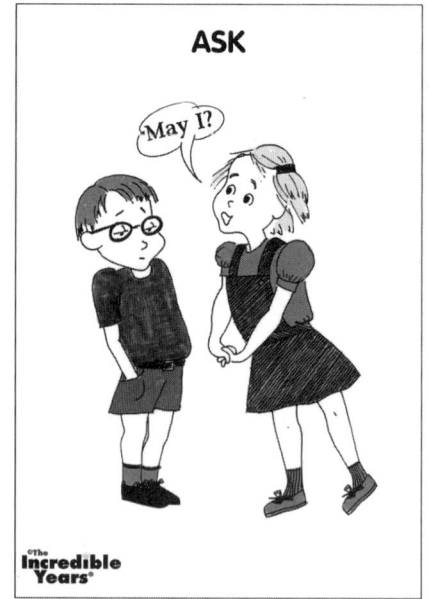

- **Reversing Roles.** After your puppet has modeled one of the social skills scenarios described above, you might reverse roles and prompt your child to use their own puppet or favorite stuffed animal to introduce themselves, ask a question, or share their interest or a toy. You might say, "Can your puppet tell my puppet what he likes to play with?" Some children might find it easier to talk through their puppet. However, this is a much more complex skill than responding to your puppet.

Puppet Models or Names Emotions and Prompts Beginning Empathy

- **Naming Child's Emotions and Prompting Empathy:** Your puppet can label your child's emotions during play times, focusing on the feeling words that you have targeted for them to learn. For example: "You look excited. Your body is jumping!" "You look happy to be spinning. I see a smile." Or, for less verbal children: "Kalani happy, smiling!" "Hudson excited, jumping!" Your puppet can offer empathy and label feelings when your child is struggling with a task: "You look frustrated. Can I help?" or, "You look confused, but you are trying hard."

- **Modeling Emotion Words:** Your puppet can model his own feelings, such as saying, "I am excited to play with you" or, "I am sad my tower fell down." Then you can prompt your child to respond: "I am happy to play too." You can also encourage an empathic response; "The puppet is sad. You can ask him if you can help." When your child offers help, your puppet can say, "Thank you! I am happy now that you are helping, thank you."

- **Showing Connection Between Social Behavior and Feeling:** When your child offers to help your puppet or share with them, your puppet can say, "I feel happy now". You can respond to your child by saying, "That was very friendly. You look proud and your puppet friend looks happy because you helped them."

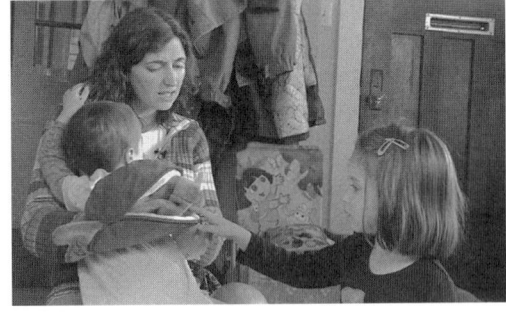

Tailoring Your Puppet's Language

The amount of language your puppet will use follows the same one-up language rules you have for your own verbal language. If your child speaks in single words, then your puppet can speak with 2-word phrases, keeping it simple and repetitive. Keep your puppet's language consistent with the goals you have for your child with respect to the kinds of descriptive commenting you are using. For example, your puppet may name objects, positions, actions, or some pre-academic concepts such as shapes, colors, some social skills, or emotion language. If your child has no language and is using visual prompts, your puppet can use these same visual prompts. For example, your puppet can show a picture of a toy they want, or show a picture of a feeling they have and then name it when they show the visual. If your child is learning physical prompts, your puppet can use their arms to point at something they want, clap with delight, give a high five, point to themselves when it is their turn, or push their hands down when all done. In essence, your puppet is using the same nonverbal or verbal language modeling and prompting that you use when playing with your child.

Parent Role

When using a puppet, you will continue with all the same gestures and enthusiastic tone of voice, sounds, and songs that you usually use to get you into your child's spotlight. Amazing how your puppet has learned the same songs you know! Or, perhaps your puppet can teach you both a new song! It is helpful to use a silly/different voice for your puppet character and then go out of puppet role and use your own voice to praise your child and your puppet character for their friendly behaviors. When you use a puppet, it is as if you are playing with two children, one is your child and the other the puppet. The puppet has good social skills and is modeling the skills you want your child to learn. You can even whisper prompts to your puppet as you would do for your child. For example, whisper to your puppet, "You can say, 'please can I have book?'" Your puppet amazingly always seems to copy your suggestion, modeling

Your puppet amazingly always seems to copy your suggestion, modeling for your child how to respond to a prompt.

for your child how to respond to a prompt. When you prompt your child, it is important not to insist on a response. Just look for another opportunity for your puppet to model or prompt the targeted skill you are working on.

Using the Wally's Detective Books for Solving Problems at Home or at School

When reading books to children who have good receptive language, you can also include puppets or your child's favorite stuffed animal in your pretend interactions. Your puppet can express their emotions about a character, ask your child questions, offer to take a turn turning the page or 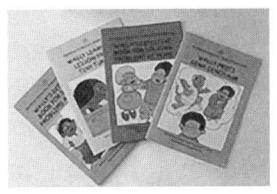 reading words, or act out something such as sharing an idea. Many children's books have scenarios that lend themselves to this kind of problem-solving practice. The Wally detective books from the Incredible Years® Child Dinosaur Program are designed to facilitate social problem solving practice between children and their parents or teachers. There are two books that contain many common interactions or problem scenarios that children encounter. For example, book one, *Wally's Detective Book for Solving Problems at School*, consists of 28 difficult situations that Wally and his friends encounter at school such as being left out by peers, being teased and bullied by other kids, being poked, feeling unpopular, losing at a game, forgetting to do homework, having trouble with writing, and not feeling liked by a teacher. Book two, *Wally's Detective Book for Solving Problems at Home* consists of 22 situations Wally encounters at home. Examples include: being scared to stay overnight at a friend's house, sibling difficulties with sharing, parents fighting, losing a belonging, and feeling discouraged that something is too hard. The parent or teacher uses 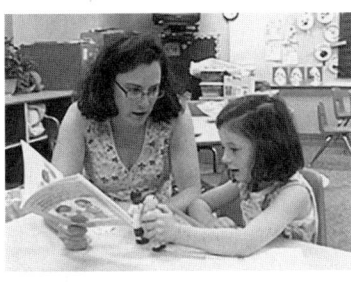 the book by reading the child one of the scenarios and then talking about possible solutions. After discussing a few solutions, the adult and child act out the scenario with puppets. The adult and child may also look to the back of the book to see the solution Wally chose for the problem and possibly act out that solution. These books can be purchased through the *Incredible Years* website: incredibleyears.com. They are most appropriate for children who have good receptive and expressive language, similar to Amelia.

Next are some scenarios where Amelia and Hudson's parents use pretend play and puppets to teach their children social behaviors and promote their empathy and awareness of other perspectives.

Using Pretend Play to Teach Helping Behavior
In the next scenario, notice the way Amelia's mother uses pretend play to engage her daughter in social interactions and to prompt her learning about helping others. Amelia and her mother are playing with balls

Amelia: Where are you going to put it?
Mother: I could pretend it's an apple (pretends to eat ball), kind of yummy, want to try some?
Amelia: No. You eat it.
Mother: (laughing) Is it tasty?
Amelia: Yes.
Mother: Hmm, I like it.
Amelia: I don't because it's always, always…because it's a lemon.
Mother: Oh it's lemon, and you don't like lemons. I like lemons because I like sour. I like red strawberries. Do you like my red strawberry? (tastes it and hands on to Amelia).
Amelia: (tastes strawberry colored wooden ball) This is a strawberry.
Mother: I would love some strawberry. Do you have strawberries? It would be so friendly if you gave me a strawberry? I'm so hungry.(*prompts sharing*)
Amelia: Looks at mom but does not give her the strawberry ball.
Mother: Can you help me get some strawberries? Or, can I have an apple. (*prompts sharing*)
Amelia: You can have an apple.
Mother: Okay, thank you for sharing that apple. I wanted a strawberry, but the apple is good too. Did you want to keep the strawberry? I can wait for a bite.
Amelia: (goes to her doll house and offers the strawberry to her Barbie doll)

Mother: I think someone is taking all my food and bringing it to the Barbie dolls. Are they eating all my food? Are you being friendly and giving Barbie some food? Is Barbie eating all the food?

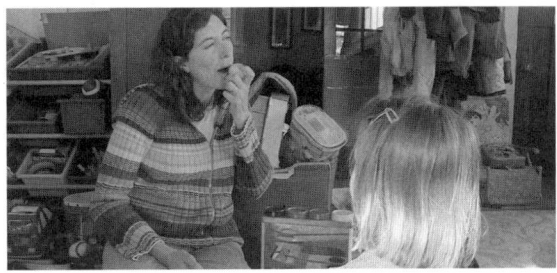

Amelia: (brings food to mother)
Mother: Oh you are so friendly and so nice. I waited and you shared with me. I get to eat all the food. Thank you so much for being helpful and friendly. (*praises friendly behavior*)
Amelia: Mom can I have those back...because I pretend...can I have those...now can I have it?
Mother: Sure, thanks for asking. I will share them with you because you asked to nicely! Here, you've got them all. (*reinforces Amelia's asking*)
Amelia: (picks up yellow ball) I can pretend this is lemon.
Mother: Lemon, oh you like the sour lemon.
Amelia: I can pretend this is a lollipop.
Mother: What a great idea, I love lollipops...yum, yum.

Considerations

Through pretend play, this mother is able to prompt Amelia to think about another person's needs and to reinforce the social skills of asking, sharing, and waiting. She is patient and calm when Amelia does not share at first. When her daughter finally responds to her request for food, she praises her friendly sharing and reinforces her by quickly returning the food when she politely asks to have it back. At the end we see that Amelia is beginning to join her mother in the pretend scenario by first pretending she has a lemon and then a lollipop, a new word not previously modeled or mentioned. Because her mother joins in her spotlight, Amelia is open to new learning. We see that eventually this imaginary play triggered Amelia's ability to share her own imaginary world with the imaginary lollipop idea. As this pretend play continues, notice how the mother continues to teach Amelia some other social skills.

Using Pretend Play to Model and Teach Friendship Skills

Mother: Very good pretending. I'm feeling really hungry. I'd love some strawberry, grape, or lemon. Can I have a turn? Is it my turn? (*gestures to self, prompts sharing behavior*)

Amelia: Not yet.

Mother: I will have to wait. Waiting is hard.(*models waiting*) Can I trade you? Do you want to trade? (*models another social strategy*)

Amelia: Yeah.

Mother: Oh good. Trading is friendly. Want to trade my cue ball for a strawberry? (*models trade solution to problem*)

Amelia: Not yet.

Mother: Not yet. Sounds like you are not ready to share? Okay I'll wait. I'll wait patiently. I'm going to wait my turn (*models waiting behavior*).

Amelia: (sings) If somebody wants a turn, you give it to somebody or if they say no, wait one minute, you don't have it...

Mother: Did you make that up?

Amelia: Yes. (goes to get long leaf to twirl)

Mother: I love that song! You said "if somebody wants a turn you can wait a minute, or you can ask for a turn, or you can trade, right?" Is that another thing we could do? I'm waiting for my turn. I'd love to trade you (offers another ball).(*models trading*)

Amelia: (takes mother's ball and gives her the ball)

Mother: Thanks for trading. That's so friendly and that makes me feel so happy. I think you feel happy too because you traded with me and are a good friend. (*praises social skill and connects it to feeling*)

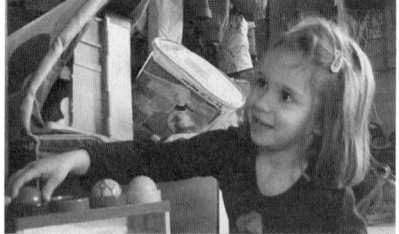

Considerations

This time Amelia's mother models how to respond when one's request for a turn is denied. In this case the mother models how to wait patiently. She also introduces a new social skill: to offer to trade one object for another. When Amelia responds to the trade solution, the mother praises her friendly behavior and connects the friendly action to her own feelings. In this way she is helping Amelia understand how sharing, taking turns, or trading can result in both people feeling happy. Thus, we see how valuable it can be to combine social coaching with emotion coaching.

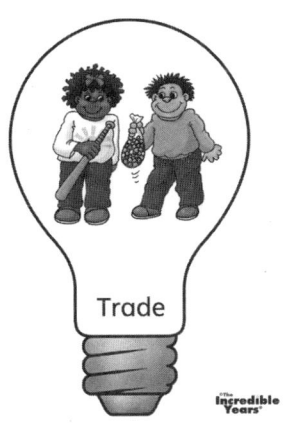

Increasing Your Child's Symbolic Play Skills

In this scenario we see that Amelia has a fairly high level of symbolic pretend play. She is treating the wooden balls as if they are fruits even though they don't look at all like fruit.

This imaginary idea comes originally from the mother who models something unexpected and pretends that a wooden ball is an apple to eat! This prompt immediately engages Amelia who imitates this idea and goes on to make the balls into strawberries and feed them to her Barbie dolls. This allows the mother to build on this joint attention to prompt Amelia's other social skills of sharing, asking, and trading.

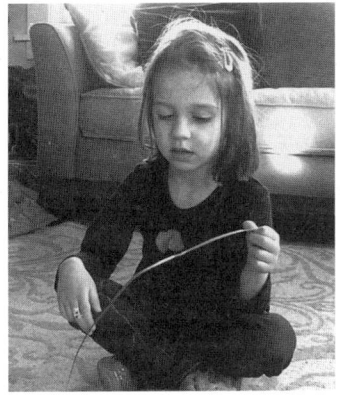

Here are a few steps to introducing symbolic play with objects and toys.

- Start with functional play where the toys or objects represent realistic-looking or conventional objects and are used in the "right" way. This is the first step of symbolic play. This could include a toy phone, tea set with cups and teapot, doctor kit, doll house with family dolls, beds, bathroom, and kitchen, or self-care items such as brush, tooth brush and mirror. With these realistic objects you can act out conventional daily activities such as getting ready for bed, talking on the phone, having a meal, going to the doctor, or bathing a baby. For example, you model having a phone call on the toy phone and then give the toy phone to your child and prompt, imitate, narrate, and coach your child to make their own call.

- Next, incorporate a doll or your child's favorite stuff animal or puppet into the pretend action. For example, your puppet can pretend to talk on the phone with you, show how they get ready for bed or for school, sit at the table for a meal, help set the table, or sit on the potty chair. Remember to stay in your puppet or doll character role and that you are no longer the parent. Adopt a name and voice. Your child also can be prompted to feed your puppet with a spoon or give them a drink, brush their teeth, or put their baby doll to bed using their daily routine of bath, story, song and kiss. For example, your puppet can say, " I need help brushing my teeth." Keep these scenarios fun and creative. As these dolls, stuffed animals, and puppets become more real, they will help to animate your child's imaginary play and practice self-care routines.

- As you are directing and acting out these actions and dramas with your props and dolls or puppets, your child will be developing more ideas about pretend actions and eventually will initiate some ideas themself. You will be able to pull back from modeling the actions with the dolls and follow your child's lead by imitating what they do. We saw this in the scenario above where Amelia's mother first modeled the idea that balls were fruit and then Amelia came up with her own idea of a ball being a lollipop. Her mother responded enthusiastically, thus reinforcing Amelia's imagination and pretend play.

- The next type of pretend or symbolic play is where the object is treated like something else. For example, Amelia's balls were fruits and Hudson's father used the banana as a phone. With this type of imagination, your child can turn almost any object into any other object. When this happens, it is a huge step for children with ASD because their pretend play thoughts are no longer bound by the limits of the actual objects. Their mental world is becoming more abstract. At this point props don't have to be so realistic, because any object can become a cookie, baby bottle, cup, or rocket ship. Or, your child may even pretend to be a puppy and walk on all fours. In this final stage of symbolic play your child will begin to make up stories from their imagination and act them out, pretending to be someone else.

- After learning to use one object to represent another object, the next step of imaginary play is to incorporate invisible objects. For example, a tea pot no longer has to have real water in it, but you and your child both pretend to pour and sip tea. Or, your child could feed a baby with an invisible bottle or pretend to talk to an imaginary friend. Experiment with introducing the idea of an invisible object, but if your child does not understand or rejects the idea, move back to imaginary play with real objects. Children with ASD like realistic objects much better and forcing them to engage with invisible objects could reduce their engagement. Still helping your child learn about invisible objects is helpful because it increases creativity and is useful for times you don't have props. Moreover, other children do incorporate invisible objects and people into their play, and some practice will help your child to understand when it occurs in their play with peers. As with every other skill in this book, understanding invisible imaginary objects is a developmental skill, so if your child rejects this play at first, follow their lead, but then reintroduce the idea at a later time. You may be surprised at how your child responds differently a few weeks or months later.

The process of learning about pretend play is a gradual developmental process for all children, and it is linked to language development. While your child may be delayed in this area and not be able to pretend at first, with your coaching and modeling simple pretend play, they can learn to pretend. For example, when your child is playing with playdough, suggest they are cooking cookies, ask for a bite of their playdough cookie, and pretend to eat it. Have your puppet bear pretend to be hungry and ask to eat something or perhaps lick your child's face. Have your doll or figurine pretend to be a kitty cat or airplane pilot. If your child likes cars, trains, airplanes, dinosaurs, or action figures, start pretending with these favorite objects.

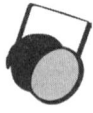

Think about acting out a short sequence of pretend actions or scenes with your child before starting any new event such as visiting a dentist, going to a birthday party or restaurant, first airplane ride or swimming experience, or the arrival of a new baby. These pretend play routines will help children learn and prepare for the new social routine, including how to respond and make sense of the experience.

In the next examples we will provide scripts of how to use puppets and pretend play to promote children's imaginations, understand how others feel, practice social skills, and learn how to solve problems.

Using Pretend Puppet Play to Promote Social Skills

As noted earlier, puppets are another effective way to encourage children's imaginary play. In fact, children on the autism spectrum often love interacting with puppets more than with people. You can set up common friendship scenarios with your child's favorite puppet to help your child learn to think of others' feelings and practice friendly social responses. Notice in the next scenario how the father engages his son with the Tiny Turtle puppet. Think about what Hudson is learning.

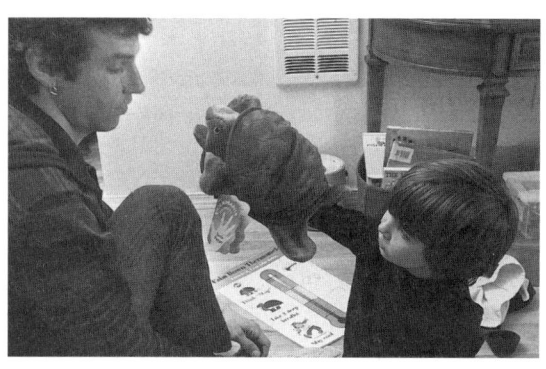

Father: (using turtle puppet, talks as puppet) Hi Hudson! My name is Tiny Turtle. Can I give you a tickle? Tickle, tickle, tickle. I am very slow. Turtles move very slow.

Tiny: (Father in role as turtle.) So, when I'm feeling sad or worried, I can go inside my turtle shell.

Hudson:	I go inside my turtle shell.
Tiny:	In my shell I say, "I can be calm. I can do it,"
Hudson:	I can do it. (pulls the puppet off his father's hand).
Father:	Oh you see it's my hand. Look, it's a puppet. I can make the turtle move. I can make him say... (puts puppet back on)
Tiny:	Hi Hudson I want a hug. Will you give me a hug?
Hudson:	(hugs him)
Tiny:	Oh thank you Hudson that's a nice hug. I feel happy when you hug me. Can I have a couple of kisses on my cheek?
Hudson:	(kisses him)
Tiny:	Oh thank you. I feel loved.
Father:	Hudson, that is very friendly. You are so nice to this turtle giving hugs and kisses. Whoa you took my hand out...do you want to try it? Do you want to try to put your hand inside?
Hudson:	I want to try it (puts on turtle puppet).
Father:	Okay you can make him talk, if you put your hand in there, you can say, you can give yourself a funny voice, say "hi."
Hudson:	Hi.
Father:	Hi, I'm Tiny turtle.
Hudson:	Hi, I'm Tiny turtle.
Father:	Oh, hi Tiny turtle. It's friendly that you said hello. Do you want a kiss? (kisses Tiny). I'll shake your hand (shakes Tiny's hand)—Give me five Tiny turtle. Tiny turtle give me five.
Hudson:	(gives him five with his puppet)
Father:	You are so friendly.

Considerations

By using the puppet, the father engages Hudson in a social interaction. The turtle puppet models how to introduce oneself by saying, "Hi Hudson. I am Tiny Turtle." He also models a calm-down strategy: going in his shell to calm down when he is sad or worried and saying: "I can do it. I can be calm." When Tiny asks for a hug and kisses, Hudson cooperates and is reinforced with Tiny's praise and a thank you for being so friendly. Once this father has captured Hudson's attention with Tiny Turtle, Hudson wants to use the puppet himself. This leads to the father coaching him in how to introduce himself. This dialog with the puppet has motivated Hudson to pay attention to someone else (the puppet), respond to a greeting, show affection, and introduce himself. These are skills that he does not yet show spontaneously in his everyday interactions.

Using Puppets to Promote Empathy

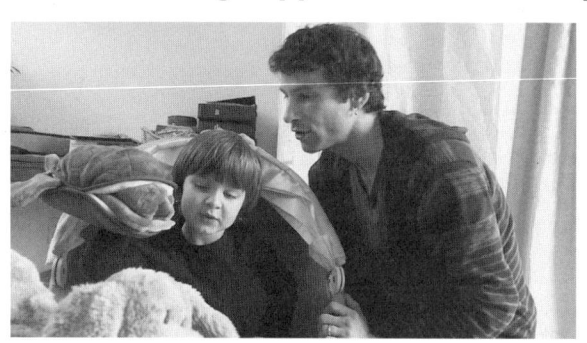

Young children can become quite attached to their stuffed animals and puppets. Hudson has become so interested in the Tiny Turtle puppet that he wants to take him into his spinning egg. This is a good sign of his caring and empathy for another, albeit a puppet. Notice as his father builds on this theme to further his son's empathy by asking him to consider how Tiny Turtle is feeling while they are spinning. Think about what this father is helping his son to learn.

Hudson is in his egg, ready to spin.

Father: If you say stop, I'll stop you really quick. Then we'll go again. Are you ready? Is Tiny ready?
Hudson: Ready. (spinning with Tiny on his lap)
Father: Tell me when you want me to stop. I think Tiny the turtle might want to stop.
Tiny: (father in role) This is Tiny Turtle. I want to stop.
Father: (stops spinning) Okay the turtle wanted to stop.
Hudson: Go.
Father: The turtle wanted to stop because he's getting dizzy.
Tiny: I'm getting dizzy oh…
Hudson: Go.
Tiny: I'm getting too dizzy and scared…
Hudson: Go go go go! (more insistent)

Father: Ask the turtle if it is okay. Can you ask Tiny Turtle? Say: 'Can we go, please?'
Hudson: Can we go please?
Tiny: Thanks for asking me. Well okay one more time, but then I'm going to be too dizzy.(they spin again)
Tiny: I'm getting pretty dizzy now I think I'd like to stop.
Father: (stops spinning) Okay Tiny Turtle. Hudson, the turtle wanted to stop because turtles get dizzy pretty quickly… They aren't used to spinning around fast. Turtles walk pretty slowly.
Hudson: (looking at turtle) I like spinning.
Father: Great that you looked at Tiny to tell him that. Can you ask him if he wants to spin with you?
Hudson: I want to spin and hold it.
Father: You want to spin and hold the turtle.
Hudson: I want to spin and hold the turtle.
Tiny: Thank you for asking me. I will feel safe if you hold me. I will spin with you.

Considerations

Hudson's father is working on helping his son to consider Tiny Turtle's feelings. He narrates how the turtle feels and also has Tiny directly share his feelings. Hudson is highly motivated to spin, but he is also fascinated with the turtle. The competing wishes: to spin and to be with Tiny (who is scared to spin) force him to verbally communicate and interact with the turtle and with his father. Stopping the spinning allows the father to promote joint social interaction, language development, and beginning empathy skills for considering the turtle puppet's feelings.

Think about how you could use a puppet to help your child think about the puppet's feelings and to be able to understand why the puppet might have these feelings.

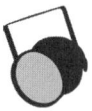

Using Puppets to Promote Empathy

Next, Amelia's mother uses a baby dinosaur puppet to help her daughter understand shy feelings and how to cope with them. She has developed this puppet scenario because she knows that her daughter is anxious at school and has difficulty initiating interactions with other children.

Baby Dina: (baby dinosaur puppet) I'm kind of shy. I am afraid to come out. I'm scared.
Amelia: Why's he scared?
Baby Dina: I feel shy.
Amelia: You don't feel shy.
Baby Dina: I do, I am going to hide in here.
Mother: Oh, little dinosaur. It's okay we're friendly. You can come out. (points at Amelia) Try to tell him that it's safe to come out. (*prompts Amelia's helping response*)
Amelia: We're friendly. You can try and come out.
Mother: That was so nice of you to say those things to make him feel safe.
Baby Dina: Are you sure? (Amelia pats him) Okay, oh wow, you are so friendly.
Amelia: Is he shy now?
Mother: Could you ask him? (*prompts him asking puppet*)
Amelia: Are you shy now?
Baby Dina: Thanks for asking. I feel a little bit braver because you told me you were friendly, and it was okay to come out.
Amelia: Who's talking?
Baby Dina: I am, I am feeling a little shy.
Amelia: (grabs baby Dina's face)
Baby Dina: Oh, that scares me.
Amelia: (laughs and grabs him again)
Mother: Gentle with him. He's afraid to come out. Gentle hands. It's okay little dinosaur. It's okay little dinosaur (strokes him gently) to come out and play. I think he will come out if you are gentle, and you are a good friend with him. (*intentional communication*)

Baby Dina: I really want to come out and play with you Amelia. I am so hungry. Oh, do you have some food for me? I could be nice and friendly.
Amelia: (gives baby Dina an orange) Here's an orange.
Baby Dina: (takes orange) Oh thank you for sharing. I love oranges.
Mother: That was nice helping him feel better when he was hungry.
Amelia: Is he shy?
Baby Dina: I feel brave now because you are so friendly, and you are helping me come out. Are you a really nice little girl?
Amelia: Yes.
Baby Dina: I feel better now because you are so friendly.
Amelia: Ah my finger hurts.
Baby Dina: I'll give you a kiss, are you okay?
Amelia: Mama my finger hurts.
Mother: Does it really? (kisses finger) Kiss and feel better.

Now notice what happens a little bit later that afternoon and how the mother reminds her daughter of the expected friendly responses.

Vignette 5 continued
Amelia: Where's the dinosaur?
Mother: Well maybe we can invite him for snack. That would be so nice.
Amelia: Is the dinosaur shy?
Mother: He was feeling shy, but I think you made him feel brave because you were so friendly and said "come out it's okay." Shy feelings can turn to brave feelings when you meet friendly people.

Considerations

Amelia has good language skills but is delayed in social skills and is reluctant to interact with other children at preschool. The mother uses a baby dinosaur puppet to express feelings of being shy about interacting with others. She prompts her daughter with the words to help the puppet feel safe to come out and play. Later Amelia is curious about whether the dinosaur feels shy. When the baby Dina puppet says she is feeling braver, Amelia responds with an aggressive action. The mother responds to this by modeling and prompting gentle friendly behavior. Amelia responds with friendly behavior and shares oranges with baby Dina. Her mother reinforces her for this friendly helping behavior. Later in the morning when Amelia still is worried about baby dinosaur's shyness, the mother reminds her of how she helped him feel brave. She also points out that shy feelings can turn into brave feelings. This puppet scenario is set up to help Amelia learn to interact with others in appropriate ways and to recognize that shy feelings can change. Notice that while this play provides an opportunity to label and identify with Amelia (and Tiny's) shy feelings, there is also a focus on coping with shyness and on the alternate feeling, brave. If Amelia's mother had only shared Tiny's shy feelings, Amelia would not learn ways to feel brave.

Using Puppets to Promote Empathy & Friendship Skills

Notice how the same mother uses a different puppet to help Amelia learn about being gentle and helping someone who is hurt.

Mother: Hi turtle. Come on out.
Amelia: Is he being gentle?
Mother: He is being gentle. He is so nice.
Amelia: Pats turtle's head.
Tiny Turtle: Thanks for being so gentle with me. I'm feeling a little sad.
Amelia: Why is he being a little sad?
Tiny Turtle: Thank you for asking. I hurt my arm.

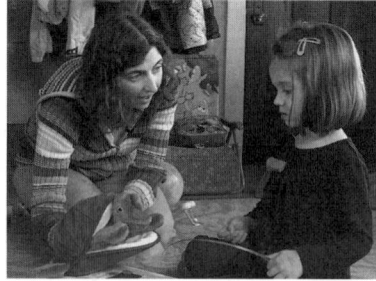

Amelia:	Why is he being a little sad?
Tiny Turtle:	I feel sad because I hurt my arm. Can you kiss it for me and be a good friend?
Amelia:	(touches arm) I put some bastion (medicated ointment) on it.
Tiny Turtle:	Oh, you are such a good friend, thanks for doing that for me. I see you have an owie too.
Amelia:	(looks at her finger)
Tiny Turtle:	Do you feel better?
Amelia:	Yup.
Tiny Turtle:	Oh you have a band aid on it, and you got a kiss. Oh I'll kiss it too (kisses her finger). Does that make you feel so happy and good?
Amelia:	Yeah.
Tiny Turtle:	That's great. I feel happy too because you helped me when I got hurt.

Considerations

So far in this scenario the mother helps her daughter understand the importance of being gentle. The puppet shares a feeling. He is sad because he hurt his arm. Amelia is encouraged to show empathy by giving a kiss and helping take care of his hurt. Tiny Turtle praises her friendly responses. Then Tiny notices Amelia

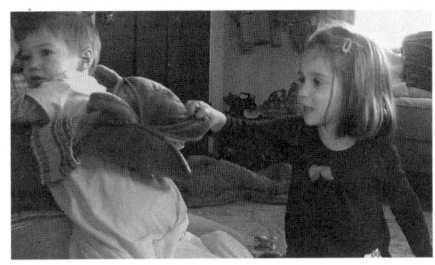

has a hurt finger and asks if he can kiss it better. He checks on her feelings. Amelia agrees she is feeling better and Tiny Turtle says he feels better because she helped him when he was hurt. Here the mother helps Amelia understand how helping someone can lead to happy feeling for both people. Now watch how the mother responds when Amelia grabs the turtle.

Mother, Amelia, and younger brother Truman are sitting on the floor with Tiny Turtle.

Amelia:	(roughly grabs turtle)
Tiny Turtle:	(ignores Amelia and gives attention to Truman.) Hi Truman.

Truman:	(pats Tiny Turtle)
Tiny Turtle:	Oh, you are gentle with me. That is so nice. That makes me feel safe.
Amelia:	(leans forward to touch Tiny Turtle's mouth)
Tiny Turtle:	Hi, did you want to see my mouth? I have a red mouth. You can be gentle. If you ask me, I'll show you my flippers.
Amelia:	(touches Tiny Turtle's face)
Tiny Turtle:	You are being gentle.
Mother:	You are being gentle. Can you ask before you touch him?
Amelia:	(leans forward to touch)
Mother:	(moves Tiny Turtle back so he can't be touched) You can say, "May I touch your tongue?"
Amelia:	(doesn't say anything but tries to grab Tiny Turtle again)
Mother:	(*ignores and gives attention to brother*) Truman do you want to touch? Say, "touch please."
Truman:	(reaches to touch Tiny's body)
Mother:	Say touch please. Oh you are being so gentle. That was so nice being gentle.
Amelia:	(reaches to give gentle touch like Truman did)
Mother:	Are you feeling gentle?
Amelia:	Yes.
Mother:	Okay gentle, gentle pat.
Amelia:	(grabs Tiny Turtle again)
Tiny Turtle:	Ouch! I don't like that. (*then ignores and turns to Truman*). Hi.
Amelia:	Is he sad?
Tiny Turtle:	I'm a little scared, when you yank at me it makes me feel scared.
Amelia:	I will be gentle.

Considerations

Amelia often becomes over stimulated and rough in situations where she is uncertain, such as meeting someone new. When Amelia grabs the puppet, the mother calmly ignores and instead gives attention to

Truman's gentle behavior. This gives Amelia a chance to re-regulate her emotions and also to learn that if she grabs, she will not get the puppet's or her mother's attention. This interaction continues several times. In addition to ignoring, the mother emphasizes that the grabbing hurts ("ouch!") and makes the puppet scared, while the gentle behavior helps him feel safe. She reminds Amelia of how to be gentle. As Amelia calms down and experiments with being gentle, the puppet begins to interact with her again. Amelia is learning how her actions affect others and how to regulate her dysregulated feelings.

When playing with your child with puppets, it is important not to give attention to aggressive behaviors in their pretend play interactions. Instead, use this as an opportunity for the puppet to tell the child about the feelings these nonfriendly actions cause. Don't be surprised if your child sometimes hits your puppet or acts aggressively; this is common. The important thing is avoid giving attention (your own or the puppet's) to inappropriate behavior. The puppet may briefly react by telling your child how he feels: "Ouch, that hurts" but then focus on prompting your child to use a friendly behavior: "Could you pat his head gently?" Give attention to friendly and gentle reactions. If your child repeatedly acts aggressively, they may be too dysregulated to continue at that moment. You can say, "Tiny doesn't feel safe. He's going to take a break, and we can play again later." It's important to follow up soon with another chance for your child to play with the puppet more gently. Overtime, they will learn that if they want the puppet to stay and play, they will need to be gentle. Eventually this social skill can be transferred to gentle play interactions with other children.

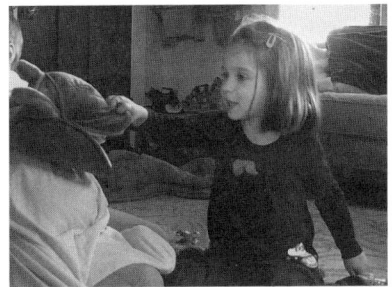

Parent Reflections—Using Pretend Play

Hudson's Father: *Hudson likes to pretend play with stuffed animals, and it started with a big bunny rabbit he got from his Uncle Danny. Pretend play and imaginative play has been really delayed I think, for his age, which I*

suppose is normal for somebody on the autism spectrum. It has been really exciting to see him start doing those things recently. And at the beginning, he was imitating me or my wife. I think it helped him out just to see us modeling that. Now he sometimes starts an imaginary idea on his own.

Amelia's Mother: *We use pretend a lot in our house. That's actually one of her preferred activities. So I use it, even to draw her out with playing with others. Because sometimes she wants to use pretend to play by herself. She loves to pretend she's different people, different names, different ages, different birthdays. So we take pretend and use it a lot for social coaching. If someone wants a turn what can you do? Such and such fell down, they're sad. Can we ask if they're okay? Things like that.*

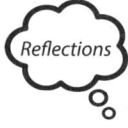

Hudson's Father: *I guess what I've done is practice taking turns and then say, "that's very friendly." Or I've done it a few times with the voice of the animal saying "oh, I feel happy because you let me take a turn, it was very friendly of you." And then I'll step back and say "that was very friendly of you, letting the animal take the turn." I still get the voices mixed up sometimes. I think Hudson listens more when I'm using the funny voices.*

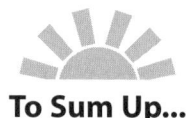

To Sum Up...

You may be nervous at first if you haven't done much puppet or pretend play before. But when you see the joy on your child's face and how much they enjoy this playful interaction, you will quickly be entranced by how your puppet or toy character can help you enter into your child's attention spotlight. As you model, prompt, and reinforce targeted social and emotional skills, be sure to adjust the language your puppet uses to your child's receptive language level. Pretend play starts with pretending to do real life actions. For example, drinking from a toy cup, talking into a toy phone, or cooking on a toy stove. Your child will be copying things they have seen you do, using real objects or realistic looking toys. As pretend play develops, the child may feed his toy bear a pretend meal or get him ready for bed. Gradually the objects in pretend play can become more imaginary. For example, we saw Amelia imagine the hard colored balls were food that could be fed to others or Hudson pretend that a banana was a phone. In the final and more challenging stage of symbolic play, your child can make up stories from his imagination and act them out. Sometimes your child may pretend to be someone else such 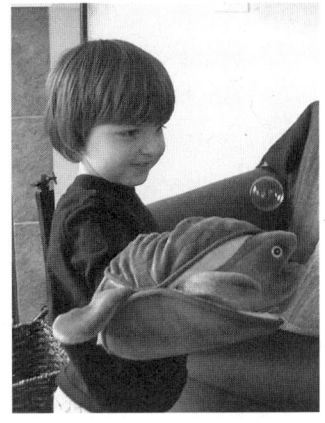 as a doctor, parent, or animal. Don't worry if your child is not able to pretend at first. You can start this sequence by pretending yourself. Amelia likely wouldn't have turned the balls into fruits if she hadn't seen her mother do this first, and Hudson's father initiated the idea of a pretend banana phone call. Doing the unexpected helps your child become more flexible and try new things. This makes the play even more fun.

Remember to follow your child's lead, imitate what your child does, keep the puppet scenarios simple and have fun. Do not have your puppet model inappropriate behavior. Keep it positive.

SPOTLIGHT
Getting in Your Child's Spotlight with Pretend Play

- Start pretend play with realistic toys such as a toy phone, dolls and doll clothes, dress up clothes, puppets, cars, trains, planes, dinosaurs, pretend food, a doll house, or a toy kitchen with stove, refrigerator, and pots and pans. When your child is able to pretend with these realistic objects, then you can progress to pretend play where objects can be anything.
- Use puppets and dolls, family figurines, or lego characters to model and prompt social skills such as helping, sharing, trading, taking turns, and asking.

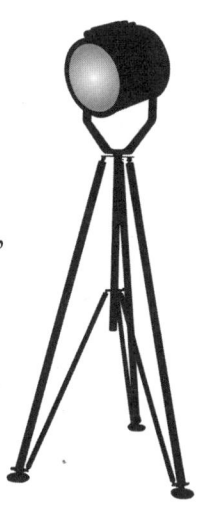

Pretend & Puppet Play

- Puppet and figurine communication methods should mirror what you use with your child. For example, the puppet uses the "one up" rule for language, imitates, is repetitive, uses gestures, and plays at a slightly higher level than your child's language and play level. Keep the scripts short at first.
- Use doll houses and family figurines to set up every day scenes from daily life such as bedtime routine of bath, teeth, pyjamas and story, getting up in the morning, having a meal, or having a friend over to play. Narrate these everyday scenes using the "one up" rule.
- Use puppets, dolls and toy characters to model emotional language and prompt your child's beginning empathy skills.
- Use puppets, dolls, figurines, and toy characters to teach self-regulation skills such as taking deep breaths and thinking of their happy place.
- Use puppets, dolls, family figurines, and toy characters to set up problem solving scenarios where you act out solutions.
- Act out with puppets pretend scenes from favorite story books or movies. For example the Wally Problem solving books can be used to set up play scenarios and then to act out solutions with puppets or dolls.
- Once your child has learned how to engage in pretend play, let your child come up with their own ideas for the script.

CHAPTER 7

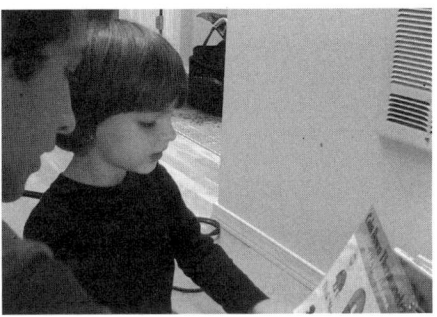

Spotlighting Your Children's Emotional Self-Regulation Skills

Introduction

A major developmental task for preschool children is to learn to manage and regulate their emotional responses (e.g., anxiety, anger, frustration, sadness, embarrassment) to arousing situations. This is sometimes referred to as learning *emotional regulation skills*. In earlier chapters we discussed ways to build children's ability to recognize and express emotions. Emotional awareness of one's feelings and the ability to express these emotions is a foundational step to eventual emotion regulation and developing empathy for the feelings of others.

Just as there is wide variation in when children learn to crawl, walk, talk, read, or become toilet trained, the development of emotional regulation and empathy is a gradual process that develops at different rates in different children. This is especially true for children on the autism spectrum and those with language delays. The processes underlying the ability to regulate emotions include neurological maturation, temperament, developmental and language level, and parental and teacher support. While you cannot change a child's neurological system or developmental status, you can help your child learn to regulate their emotions by providing consistent support, limits, and predictable routines. This will be discussed in the next chapter. In addition, you can use emotion coaching to model, prompt, and give attention to feelings, and you can teach your child some self-calming strategies. Because many children with autism are visual thinkers and learn to love pretend play, it is effective to use books, puppets, imaginary stories, games, songs, and coaching to build their self-regulation skills. In this chapter you will see examples of parents using pretend scenarios such as imaginary visualizations or imagery, simple coping self-talk, visual prompts, breathing, and physical sensory routines to support their children's emotion regulation. These scenarios will give you ideas for pretend play scenarios you can use to support your child's self-regulation skills.

Teaching Beginning Self-Regulation Skills—Breathing

In the next scenario notice how Hudson's father promotes emotion literacy and uses a visual prompt to help his son learn a breathing method for staying calm when angry. Think about why this visual prompt might be helpful in teaching a child how to self-regulate.

Father: (showing picture of an angry child face) How do you think he feels?

Hudson: Angry.

Father: Angry or frustrated. That's right. He goes grrr. (shows mad grimace on his face)

Hudson: (shows a picture of person smelling a flower and blowing out a candle—this is a visual signal to take a deep breath by breathing in and breathing out)

Spotlighting Your Children's Emotional Self-Regulation Skills 223

Father: Oh! We know what to do with that one right?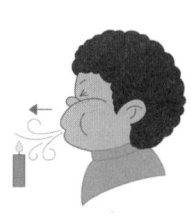
Hudson: We know how to do that one.
Father: What to try it? Smell the flower. Want to smell the flower with me? (*models breathing in*). Blow out the candle (*models blowing out*).
Hudson: (takes breaths and blows out)
Father: That's right. Sometimes if you feel angry or frustrated, you can practice smelling the flower and blowing out the candle. You want to try it again? (*models taking in deep breaths and blowing out*)?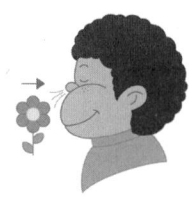
Hudson: (selects a picture of deep breathing))
Father: And that one says take a deep breath, that's like smelling the flower but bigger, (takes deep breath) if I want to feel calm, it helps me to feel calm again.

Considerations

We can see that Hudson has learned the feeling word for *angry* and the father expands on that idea by introducing another related feeling word: *frustrated*. He then models and encourages Hudson to practice taking deep breaths while visualizing smelling a flower and blowing out a candle. This fun visual prompt and visualization helps children learn how to take a deep breath (breathing in through nose and out through mouth). Deep breathing is an excellent self-regulation strategy because it automatically triggers the body to relax and become calmer. It is also a simple strategy that even very young children can learn to do effectively. The father links this breathing activity to the feelings of anger and frustration. When Hudson looks at another picture, his father repeats the breathing strategy, models taking a deep breath, and explains he uses this breathing himself because it helps him stay calm.

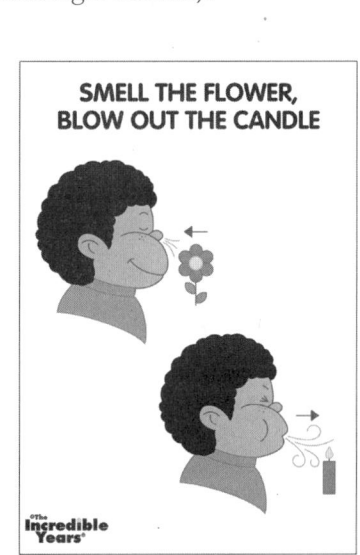

After your child understands the meanings of several feeling words, you can begin to teach simple self-regulation strategies. It is key that this teaching occurs at a time when both you and your child are calm. Your child will need to practice the strategy (in this case deep breathing) many times before using it for actual self-regulation in a conflict situation. You can practice with puppets, model using the strategy yourself, talk about characters in books or videos, or use other imaginary play scenarios to set up breathing practices.

Eventually, you will be able to prompt your child (verbally or with a visual prompt) to use the regulation strategy to calm down when they are actually upset. The timing of your prompt is important; try to offer the prompt right as your child begins to become upset. This is when they will be mostly likely to be able to process your prompt and use the self-regulation strategy. Don't wait until your child has escalated into a full melt-down. At this point they will be too dysregulated to process any outside information. Be patient with this process. It will take time and repeated practice for your child to really use the self-regulation strategies to manage their real-life emotions.

> *Offer the prompt right as your child begins to become upset, when they will be most likely able to use the self-regulation strategy*

Remember one of the first steps in teaching your child any new behavior is to get into their attention spotlight. Once you have their attention, you can introduce the visual prompt and model the desired behavior for your child. For example, when you are playing with your child, you or your puppet can pretend to be frustrated with the blocks, a puzzle, or a drawing. Then model a self-regulation strategy for your child by saying, "I am going to calm down by taking deep breaths to smell the flower and blow out the candle." After modeling this breathing and showing the picture, you or your puppet can say, "Okay I feel calm, I will try again." Have the visual calm down picture readily accessible to show your child as you model the breathing skill. If your child shows interest, you can ask your child to practice with you and praise them for being so calm. To make the learning more fun and concrete, you can use props: a real or silk flower to smell and a flashlight or candle to blow out. If your child enjoys smelling the flower and blowing out the flashlight, you can use the anticipation of smelling and blowing as the antecedent motivator (A) to prompt the breathing practice (B) and the reward (C), seeing the flashlight go out. In the scenario below we will see how this father used the egg spinner as a motivator (A) for helping Hudson practice this breathing.

A second calm-down strategy you can teach your child is a muscle relaxation exercise. Help your child learn to tense and relax each muscle by repeatedly clenching the muscles in each body part and then letting go (feet, legs, stomach, hands, arms, shoulders, face). Talk with your child about how it feels to be tense (stiff, hard, tight) and how it feels to be relaxed (soft, floppy, wiggly). This exercise can be combined with the deep breathing so that your child learns to recognize their tense body, use the deep breathing exercise, and then notice the relaxed feeling. It may help to have your child squeeze (tense) a stress/relaxation ball and then let it go (relax).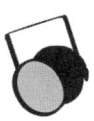

Using the Calm Down Thermometer Visual Poster to Teach Calm Down Breathing

In the previous scenario Hudson's father is teaching his son a fun imaginary visualization to practice deep breathing. In the next scenario, he uses a calm down thermometer picture poster to help his son learn another way to calm down. Hudson is intrigued by the arrow and Velcro on the poster, and so is motivated to practice and stay engaged in the activity with his father. Notice all the strategies the father uses to stay in Hudson's spotlight and keep him engaged in the calm down practice.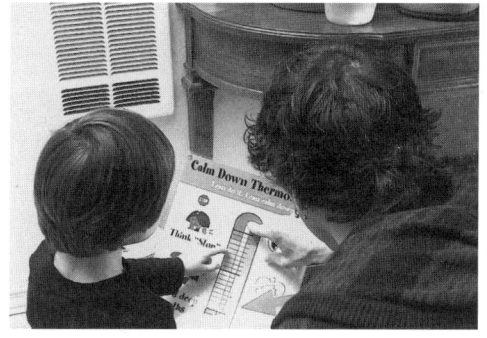

    Father: (sitting on floor and shows poster) This is a thermometer. It's the Calm Down Thermometer.
    Hudson: It says "stop." (points at stop sign)
    Father: "Stop," That's when you are in the red and you feel really mad. You are really angry. If you want to yell or break things you are way up here. (points at mad face and top of thermometer)
    Hudson: (points) The orange (red and orange are the colors that represent the top of the thermometer).

Father: That's when you say "stop," you think "stop."
Hudson: You can do the yellow.
Father: Yes, yellow is down, getting calmer. What do you do to get to yellow? You take 3 deep... (*partial prompt*)
Hudson: Breaths.
Father: That's right! Three deep breaths.
Father: There is also an arrow you can move down so if you take deep breaths, you can move it from red to yellow.
Hudson: (moving arrow on poster to red) Top.
Father: If you are feeling really mad you can put the arrow up here, you can say, "Papa I'm mad." (makes a mad face)
Hudson: Papa I'm mad.
Father: Then you say, "I'm going to stop." (gestures stop with his hand)
Hudson: I'm going to stop.
Father: (points to turtle on poster) And the turtle, this is what the turtle does; look he is opening his mouth and he's taking deep breaths – he's going (takes a deep breath) three times.
Hudson: Yellow now (arms flapping).
Father: Yes, he takes a deep breath and then the arrow comes down to yellow. Can you move it there?
Hudson: (takes the arrow and moves it to yellow).
Father: Now he's getting calmer. Can you take another breath and move it down more, to blue?
Hudson: To blue (moves arrow).
Father: Now he's calm and happy. Hudson looks calm and happy too.
Hudson: Calm and happy

Considerations

It is clear that this thermometer picture poster engages Hudson, and he is keen to use the arrow and move it up and down the thermometer. As he plays with the arrow the father effectively describes the pictures and prompts Hudson to practice taking deep breaths, using his words to tell his feelings and to think of something happy. At the end he helps him understand the word for his current feeling of being calm.

Try using a picture of a thermometer with your child to explain how to calm down with breathing and get into "cool blue". Make this interactive with an arrow and Velcro so that your child can move the arrow to show how emotions change. Or, to make it even more fun, you can take a real thermometer and put it in cold water and take deep breaths as you watch the thermometer line or numbers go down.

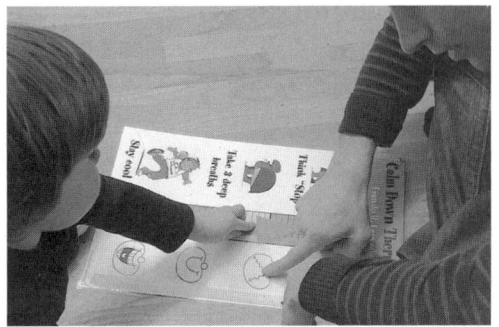

Remember other family members can model how to use the calm down thermometer and breathing to stay calm. Keep this poster on your refrigerator and anyone in the family can go over and move the arrow when they feel the need to take deep breaths. Narrate your actions when you do this: "I'm feeling a little angry right now. I need to take some deep breaths to calm down."

Visualizations: Using a Happy Thought or Memory Visualization to Calm Down

Hudson and his father continue to look at the thermometer together. Hudson's father introduces the idea of using a calm or happy thought or memory visualization to calm down. This is another calm-down strategy for children who are able to understand enough language to listen to a description of a scene and picture it in their minds.

Father: (pointing to the turtle picture). And maybe the turtle's thinking about some place he likes, like the ocean. He's thinking about standing on the beach and watching the waves of the ocean. The turtle loves the ocean, and he feels happy when he thinks of the ocean. When he thinks about the ocean, the arrow goes down even further. (moves arrow down)

Hudson: (puts arrow back at top on red)

Father: (does not correct Hudson's arrow placement, but instead follows his lead). The red one has a face like this – what is this face? Is he happy or mad? (points to picture of face on poster)

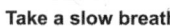
Take a slow breath

Hudson: Mad.
Father: He's mad...He needs help to calm down. When you are mad, you can think about bubbles. Bubbles make you happy. (Father points to Hudson's bubble feeling picture card. Hudson reaches for the arrow).
Father: You want the arrow.
Hudson: The arrow.
Father: Let's think about bubbles. Do bubbles make you happy? Show me where the arrow is when you are happy with bubbles (hands him the arrow).
Hudson: (looking at thermometer with his arrow)
Father: Do you feel calm?
Hudson: In the red.
Father: Are you feeling mad right now Hudson? Or are you feeling calm?
Hudson: Calm.
Father: You are feeling calm, pretty calm. That means you are down here in blue…. Yeah you do seem pretty calm. (points to bottom of thermometer)

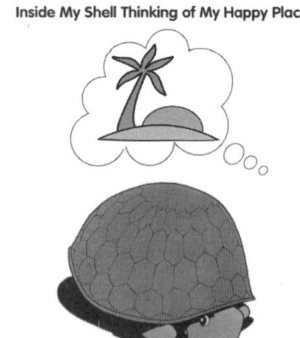

Hudson's father introduces the strategy of thinking about a happy thought or calming memory visualization. This positive visualization strategy is more challenging for young children than deep breathing because it involves an internal cognitive process. Hudson's father first shares the Turtle's happy thought and memory and then shares a happy thought for Hudson. Hudson continues to be engaged in this activity but is likely not yet understanding the connection between the happy thought or visualization of blowing bubbles and his own feelings. The father uses the picture cue card to help Hudson connect the concept of thinking of one of his favorite activities and calming down. He stays in Hudson's spotlight by engaging him with the arrow and is not bothered when Hudson puts the arrow in places that don't match the feeling that they are discussing. With repeated exposure to the idea of a happy thought

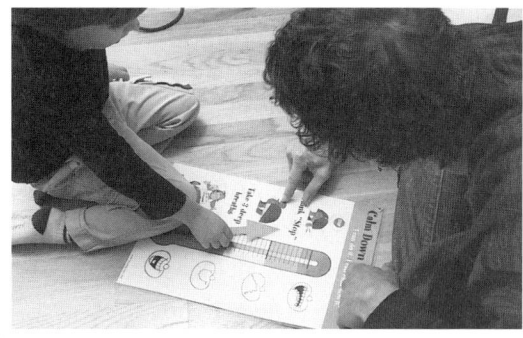

or memory visualization, Hudson will eventually be able to make this connection.

The relaxation thermometer combines several different calm-down devices (the turtle, the feeling faces, and the thermometer). For some children talking about the feeling faces, thermometer, and turtle pictures may be too complex for one discussion. Pace your discussion to your child's level. First talk about the faces and practice making those faces as you move the arrow on the thermometer and calm down. Another time discuss the Tiny Turtle ideas and practice with a turtle puppet. When your child can use the Turtle idea to calm down, then link that with the thermometer. Similarly, putting a real thermometer in hot or cold water might be too abstract for some children on the spectrum. You would only want to do this after you have taught them to understand the visual calm down thermometer poster. Keep this discussion simple and fun and gradually add new aspects of the poster as your child shows interest. For children without much language, use gestures and practice breathing or muscle relaxation steps. Keep the number of words simple: "smell" and "blow" or "tense" and "relax" your hands.

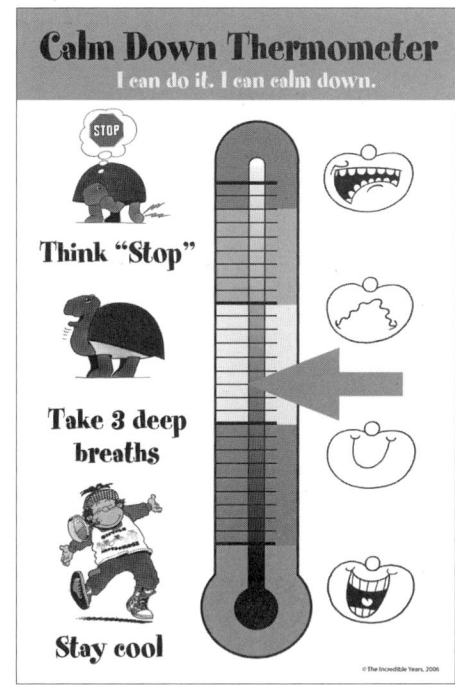

Using Puppets to Help Your child Learn Self-Regulation Skills

As we discussed in Chapter Six, using puppets can help you get into your child's attention spotlight. In the next scenario, think about how Amelia's mother uses the Tiny Turtle puppet to model calm down strategies with her daughter.

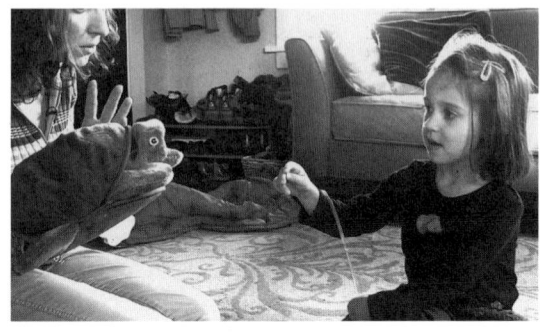

Think about what Amelia is learning. Notice how Amelia responds differently than Hudson to the use of positive visualization.

Amelia:	Are you shy turtle?
Tiny Turtle:	(mother in role as turtle) I'm not feeling shy right now, but my engine is hot...I feel mad! I'm going in the red. I need to stop, take a deep breath (takes a breath), and go in my turtle shell. I am going to count 1...2..3...4, and I take a deep breath in my turtle shell (breathing). Can you do that with me?
Amelia:	Yeah, you go first.
Tiny Turtle:	Let's to it together. Let's go into our shells and breath. (Amelia and Tiny practice together).
Tiny Turtle:	I'm feeling better. I'm calm now. You know, another thing I do when I'm upset is to think of something that I love doing like, like going on the swing. That makes me feel happy and calm again. I'm going to try that. I'm thinking about swinging back and forth! How do you think I feel when I think about swinging?
Amelia:	Happy?
Tiny Turtle:	Yes, happy and calm! What makes you happy? What could you think about to feel happy?
Amelia:	What makes me happy?

Mother:	Are you happy on the swing or the trampoline?
Amelia:	The swing.
Tiny Turtle:	So, you could think about the swing just like me. Do you like to go high?
Amelia:	Yes, I like to go high.
Mother:	Wait, I need to go get your baby bother. He's awake. (comes back with baby brother who is crying)
Amelia:	(asking about her brother who is crying) Is he in his turtle shell?
Mother:	Is he in his turtle shell? That is a very good question. I think Truman might need to go in his turtle shell. Is he taking a deep breath?
Amelia:	(takes turtle puppet and acts part) I am in my turtle shell taking a deep breath.
Mother:	Taking a deep breath and maybe thinking of your favorite place like the swing or the trampoline, (baby cries). It's okay Truman, I know sweetheart. I know. You are in your shell. You are in your turtle shell like the little turtle (rocks him) taking deep breaths.
Amelia:	Are we taking deep breaths?
Mother:	We can try. Let's show turtle and Truman how to do it. Turtle, smell the flowers and blow out the candles. Amelia, do you want to help turtle do it? Truman this is how we do it. Show him you are such a big girl you know how to do it. I know you can show him.
Amelia:	(takes a deep breath, using the turtle).

Considerations

Amelia really likes Tiny Turtle, so her mother effectively uses him as a model for how to take deep breaths as well as how to think of his favorite place. Amelia has a better understanding of these concepts than Hudson and is able to participate in a conversation about

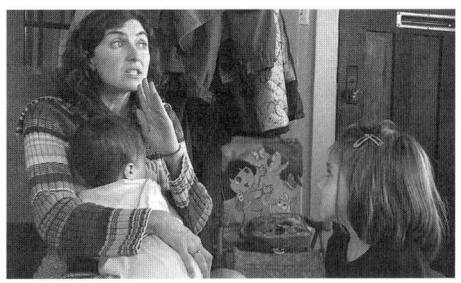

the connection between swinging and being happy. Since swinging is one of Amelia's favorite activities, her mother chose swinging for the turtle's happy place.

Amelia notices her brother's distress and asks if he is in his turtle shell. This awareness of others is part of Amelia's newly emerging empathy. Amelia's mother encourages Amelia to teach Truman and Tiny Turtle these calm down breathing steps. This provides Amelia with additional practice opportunities as well as the chance to feel competent and helpful in her role as a big sister.

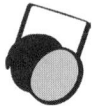

Try using a puppet to practice teaching your child self-regulation skills such as taking deep breaths, thinking of a happy place, telling yourself "I can calm down," counting down, taking a break and relaxing. Incorporate visual prompts such as the Smell the Flower picture, Calm Down thermometer, Tiny Turtle pictures, or count down from ten picture, or Take a Break pictures. (See sample scripts below that you might try. Be sure to adjust the amount of language you or your puppet use according to your child's language level.

Staying Patient and Modeling Self-Regulation Skills

Parenting is stressful at times for most parents, but research indicates that parenting a child with developmental disabilities, such as autism, results in significantly elevated depression and anxiety symptoms and disorders. Struggling to get support services, relentless worry about the future, and financial strain all can seem overwhelming at times. Try to curb your negative thoughts, use positive imagery, take deep breaths, get enough sleep, and develop support systems to stay calm. If you model taking your own deep breaths by smelling the flowers and blowing out the candles, or verbalize a happy thought, or share that you are thinking of a positive image while you move the arrow down on your thermometer poster, you will strengthen your child's emotion regulation skills. In the next chapter, we will talk further about

Try to curb your negative thoughts, use positive imagery, take deep breaths, get enough sleep, and develop support systems to stay calm.

self-reinforcement and self-care for parents and teachers, another important strategy for reducing your stress.

Using Visual Prompts for Self-Regulation

Pictures can be used to represent different self-regulation skills such as taking deep breaths, thinking of a happy place, using the calm down thermometer, using the countdown method, going into a turtle shell, or taking a break. All of these calm down strategies can be practiced with children by showing the pictures while they are helped to do guided practice with the breathing skill. Moreover, you and your puppet can model the self-regulation skill and encourage your child to practice. Once the self-regulation skill is learned, these visuals can be used to prompt a child to use these strategies when they begin to get frustrated or angry or sad. See pictures in this text of sample calm-down strategies using some of our puppets. Of course, you can make some of your own pictures, for example, of your child practicing smelling the flower/blowing out the candle, using the thermometer, or taking a break by running

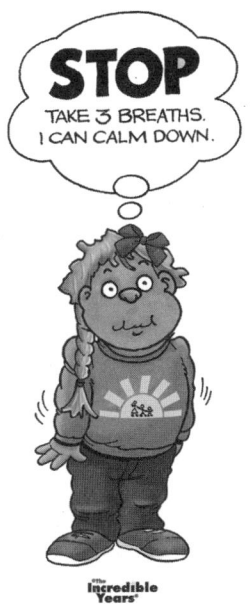

around the coffee table, or jumping on the trampoline. You could also take a picture of your child with the Tiny Turtle puppet taking deep breaths or showing the Stop sign. You could make a book of your child's happy and relaxing places. Read this often and encourage them to remember these calming times when they are beginning to dysregulate.

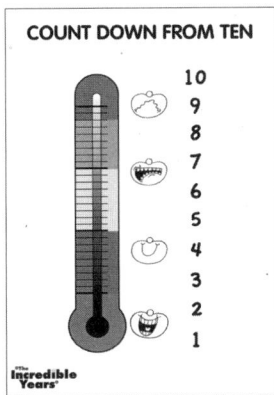
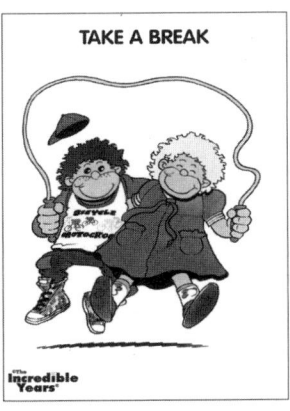
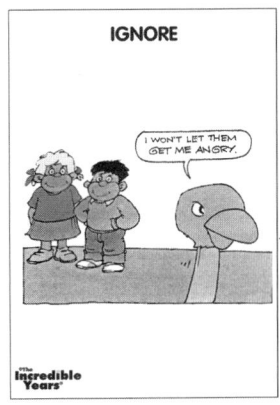

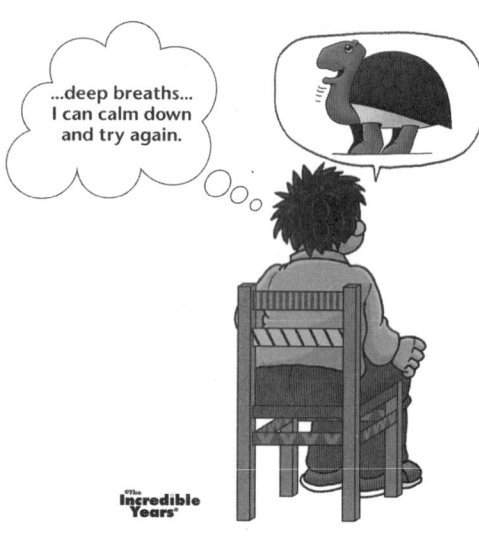

Sample Scenarios for Teaching Your Child Self-Regulation Skills

Here are a few scripts for ideas of how to use the Calm Down Thermometer poster and Tiny Turtle puppet. Each of these scenarios would be done in a short session and repeated at different times when your child seems relaxed and interested in some puppet play. Adjust your language according to your child's language stage. Try to keep these scenarios simple, fun, and imaginative; follow your child's lead; and use gestures along with the visuals. Remember to mirror the puppet's feelings on your own face and sit face-to-face with your child.

Tiny Turtle Explains how the Calm Down Thermometer Works

Your Tiny Turtle puppet introduces the Calm Down Thermometer and explains how it works. For example, *"Hi, I am Tiny Turtle. I want to tell you about this amazing feeling thermometer that can measure your feelings."* Your turtle puppet can tell your child that he is feeling sad, mad, worried, frustrated, happy, calm, relaxed, or proud. While Tiny is telling a story about his feelings, point to the place on the thermometer that shows Tiny's feeling. (Red for hot for angry versus blue for cool or calm.) You can also ask your child to point to the color on the thermometer or move the arrow to the place that represents Tiny's feeling. When your child points to the place on the thermometer, you can add to the fun by asking them to show you that feeling face.

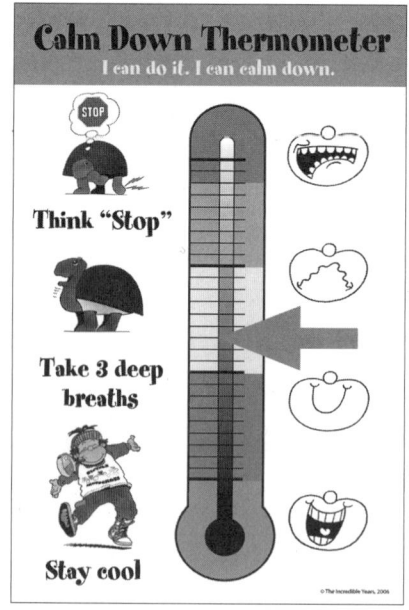

Spotlighting Your Children's Emotional Self-Regulation Skills 235

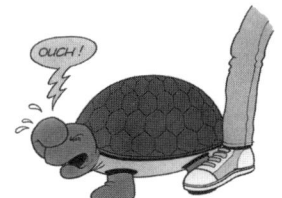

- Tiny Turtle tells your child a story about a time he was mad, hurt, or upset. Add a simple explanation for the feeling: "someone stepped on me," "my mommy said no more screen time," "someone called me a mean name." Then Tiny explains how he took three deep breaths to get back into blue. For example, *"One time someone made fun of me because I am so slow. I was up here in red, feeling mad. I took three deep breaths and practiced smelling a flower and blowing out a candle. Then I came down into blue and felt calm."*
- Ask your child to practice taking deep breaths with Tiny Turtle and let him or her move the thermometer arrow down from red to green.
- Tiny Turtle asks your child to tell a time he or she felt angry or sad or excited or safe. (Use a variety of comfortable and uncomfortable feeling words.) For example, Tiny asks, "Have you ever had someone make fun of you? How did that feel?" When your child shares a situation, help him/her move the arrow to how he/she was feeling and them move the arrow down as deep breathing is practiced.

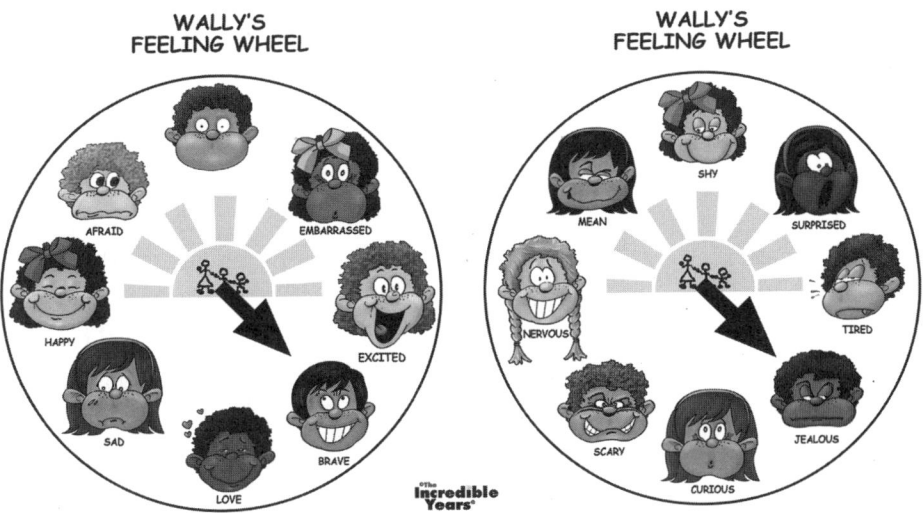

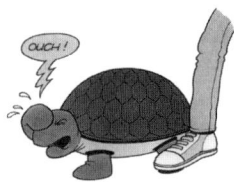

1

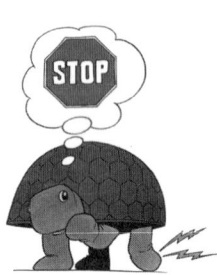

2 Think STOP

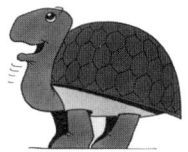

3 Take a slow breath

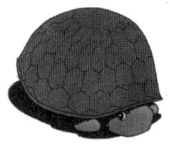

4 Withdrawing into shell

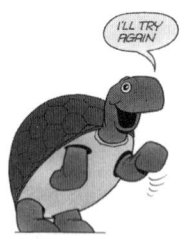

5

- Using the Calm Down Thermometer, Tiny Turtle asks your child what feelings the faces on the thermometer represent. For example, *"See these feeling faces on this thermometer, what feelings do you think they are?"* When your child names a feeling, praise their understanding and ask them to show you that feeling face. You can mirror the feeling face back at them.
- You could also use the feeling spinning wheel. When the arrow stops on an uncomfortable feeling, you (or the puppet) could talk about a time you felt that way and then practice how you can take deep breaths and think of your happy place to stay calm.

Tiny Turtle Explains How to Calm Down

- Tiny Turtle explains how he recognizes an uncomfortable feeling, says "stop," and goes into his turtle shell to take deep breaths. For example, *"One time someone stepped on my foot, and I was mad, but I said "stop" and went in my turtle shell and took deep breaths like this. Then I felt better."* Ask your child to practice this with Tiny Turtle and either imagine they have a magic turtle shell or suggest they put their head under their shirt.
- Tiny Turtle explains how he uses his happy place visualizations when he is in his shell to help him calm down. For example, *"When I am nervous, I take deep breaths and think about a time I learned to ride my bike. I was proud of myself. Thinking about that makes me feel better."* Or, *"When I am afraid or sad, I think of my teddy bear and that helps me feel safe."* Or, *"Sometimes I think about being in the water at the beach."* After Tiny has explained his happy or safe places, he can ask your child where their happy place is and how your child can use this when to feel better and calm down. This exercise can help your child develop some positive imagery of things to think about when in their shell.
- Tiny Turtle explains what he says to himself when he is in his shell. For example, *"When I am in my shell, I say to myself:*

I can do it. I can calm down and try again." Ask your child to repeat these words with Tiny and do it together.
- Tiny Turtle asks your child when they could use their Turtle Power. Then Tiny asks your child to show you how they use Turtle Power. For example, *"What makes you angry? So, you are up here in red on the thermometer. How can you get yourself down here in green? Can you use your turtle power to calm down?"* Praise your child for showing you or Tiny how to take deep breaths, think of their happy place, or use positive self-talk.
- Make a calm down area with your child. You might call this the turtle cave or cozy corner. Make the area inviting perhaps with a blanket over a card table, adding a pillow, Tiny Turtle puppet, and relaxation thermometer. You and your child can work together to decorate the area in a way that will help your child calm down. Going to the cozy corner can be another self-regulation strategy for your child to use when they are beginning to feel upset.

Remember when using Tiny Turtle, follow your child's lead and ideas and praise their willingness to practice taking deep breaths, use happy place memories, and do muscle relaxation exercises or positive self-talk. Make these play scenarios fun, imaginative, and interactive. For children with limited language use less language, simple words, a slow pace, more gestures of breathing, and repeat key words often. Avoid complex stories and just have fun with the puppet breathing in his shell and saying, "I can do it".

Parent Reflections—Promoting Children's Emotion Regulation

Father: *One of the pieces of advice that seemed helpful is practicing calming strategies, like breathing, when Hudson's not upset. Because, at the point when he's upset, even when he's not in the red on the thermometer, even when he's maybe just a little bit upset, halfway there, he's still not really willing to practice taking deep breaths.*

I feel like some of the things that have helped with self-regulation are giving him a lot of encouragement that he's okay, or he's gonna be okay, and he can calm down.

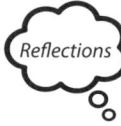

Mother: *I've tried to model how to calm down myself, because obviously, when you have two children, one and three, you're gonna get a little frustrated at times, and so there've been moments where I'll say, "mama's frustrated, I need to take some deep breaths." And so, I'll even model smelling the flowers, blowing out the candles.*

Father: *I have started modeling some emotions, like I have started taking more deep breaths, and I try to remember my yoga classes, and how much the focus is on the breath there. And if I'm really tired, then I'll try to just take a break, and see if he'll do something on his own. Or even sometimes recently I've just laid down in bed, and he's actually come in with me.*

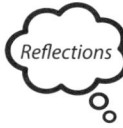

Mother: *We talk about the different things that she could do when she's angry. I think once I actually caught her in her turtle shell. I don't know if she was really, really angry or if she was just starting to get angry, but I caught her in her turtle shell, and I right away praised, saying, "I see you're in your turtle shell, you're making yourself calm down all by yourself, that's great!" So, really defining it, describing it, talking about how to regulate it, kind of putting it all together really helps her learning.*

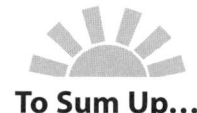

To Sum Up...

All of this teaching and practice occurs at times when your child is emotionally regulated. Once your child knows an emotion regulation strategy or two, you can prompt them to use the strategy when you see the first warning signs that your child is becoming tense and frustrated. As long as they are not too dysregulated, you might be able to intervene with a prompt to take deep breaths, go to the calm down thermometer, use turtle power to move the arrow, or show you one of the emotion or self-regulation visuals. However, don't be surprised if your child rejects this suggestion and becomes oppositional. As children enter a dysregulation cycle, they quickly become too dysregulated to respond. Your intervention and coaching may even make the tantrum worse or provide attention that reinforces your child's tantrum. So, if you try a self-regulation prompt and it does not work, it is best to ignore, while monitoring and making sure your child is safe. Through your ongoing social and emotional coaching and your self-regulation teaching, you will be helping build your child's positive self-image and ability to self-regulate. You will be helping your child perceive themself as someone who can be successful at handling emotions. You can predict your child's success by saying things like, "you are staying strong with your breathing."

Of course, if your child is behaving in a way that is harmful to himself 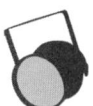 or to someone else, this behavior cannot be ignored. You may need to physically move your child away if he has hurt another child or move the other child away and then try an ignore combined with a distraction. In Chapter Nine we will talk more about managing misbehaviors.

SPOTLIGHTING
Building Children's Self-Regulation Skills

- Coach and praise your child's self-regulation skills such as staying calm, being patient, trying again when frustrated, waiting a turn, and using words or gestures when frustrated.
- Support your child when they are frustrated but recognize when they are too upset to listen and need space and time to calm down.
- Encourage your child's practice of calm down steps with puppets, books, calming thermometer, and games.
- Model and prompt your child to use feeling words, feeling pictures, or puppets to express their needs and feelings (e.g., "Show me the card with the face of how you are feeling.").
- Help your child learn ways to self-regulate such as using a special stuffed animal or blanket, taking deep breaths, telling themself they can calm down, waiting, or solving a problem.

- Teach the Tiny Turtle calm down steps.
- Use picture prompts to cue your child to wait, take deep breaths, or take a break.
- Model self-regulation skills yourself, such as taking deep breaths, positive self- talk, or taking a break.

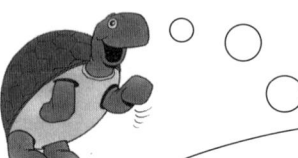

Parent Prompt Examples:

"You can think of your happy place."

"Can you pretend to use Tiny's secret shell to take deep breaths & calm down?"

"You did a good job using your words to talk about your problem. That's what friends do."

"That is so strong to use your waiting muscles."
"Let's check the Calm Down Thermometer and get into the blue zone."

CHAPTER 8

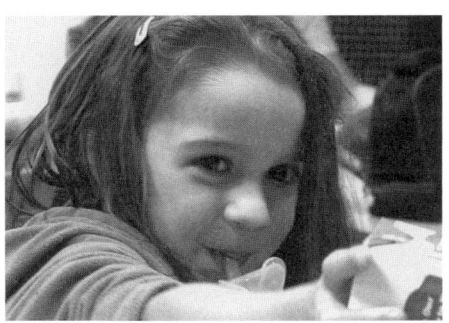

Using Praise and Rewards to Motivate Children

Introduction
The task of teaching a new behavior to a child on the autism spectrum is often difficult and slow. Patient and consistent child-directed play and well-paced descriptive commenting, social and emotional coaching will support their learning. In addition, praise and encouragement and, sometimes, a tangible reward can be a crucial part of strengthening and maintaining a child's targeted social behaviors. Because children on the autism spectrum often seem disinterested in pleasing, imitating, or connecting with others, parents and teachers may think they are unaware of and unmotivated by expressions of pleasure, approval, or praise. It is true that praise, encouragement, and rewards that motivate most children may

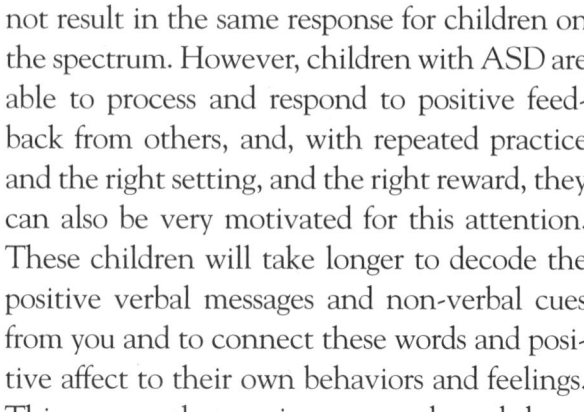

Praise cannot be subtle or vague; it must be put in your child's spotlight in an attractive, exciting, and engaging way.

not result in the same response for children on the spectrum. However, children with ASD are able to process and respond to positive feedback from others, and, with repeated practice and the right setting, and the right reward, they can also be very motivated for this attention. These children will take longer to decode the positive verbal messages and non-verbal cues from you and to connect these words and positive affect to their own behaviors and feelings. This means that praise cannot be subtle or vague; rather it must be put in your child's spotlight in an attractive, exciting, and engaging way. Just as these children need to learn to participate in, and enjoy social interactions with others, they also need repeated practice and positive experiences to learn to enjoy receiving and giving praise to

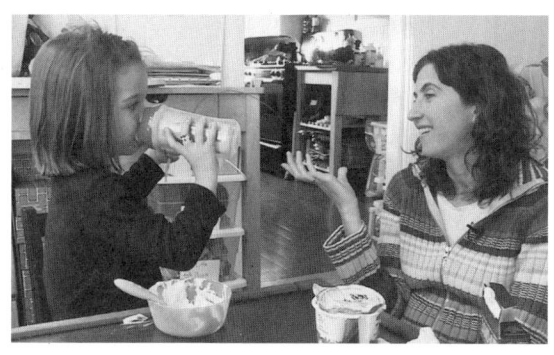

others. In this chapter we discuss how to praise and reward children using many of the same coaching strategies that were used to teach other communication language and social skills.

In the next scenario, watch how Amelia's mother praises her daughter. Think about what makes her praise approach effective.

Face-to-face praise

Amelia: I need some cherry yogurt.

Anna: Nice asking. Let me see if I have cherry yogurt, I might just have raspberry. Raspberry or strawberry, Amelia? Which one would you like?

Amelia: Strawberry (looking down).

Anna: Which one? (moves her face closer to Amelia's face)

Amelia: Strawberry (looking up at her mother).

Anna: (moves closer with a smile) Thank you for looking at me when you are talking. Strawberry it is!

Amelia: (smiles)

Considerations

Amelia's mother is very specific about the behavior she is praising and does it with a warm tone, and with a smile and face to face with eye contact. She pairs her praise with one of Ameila's favorite foods; pairing the tangible reward of yogurt with her praise. When children on the spectrum are learning to receive and enjoy praise, it can be useful to pair the praise with another positive consequence like a preferred activity, food, or desired object. At first, the child may be more motivated by the object or activity, but gradually, if the activity is paired with enthusiastic praise, or a warm non-verbal gesture such as a hug, kiss, or tickle, the child will gradually learn to appreciate and be motivated by the positive interaction.

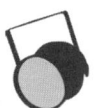

Make a list of the target social or emotion regulation skills or independent behaviors you want to praise and encourage in your child. Some examples might include tying shoe laces or doing up buttons, using a spoon to eat, using the toilet, cooperating with washing in the bath, using a picture prompt or word to indicate a preference or request, responding to your request, initiating a conversation, greeting someone with a hello or saying good bye, washing hands, or getting dressed for school. From your list, pick one or two skills at a time to target with your praise. Before your child does the targeted behavior, or even starts or approximates that behavior, give warm and enthusiastic praise. Clap your hands, or whistle, or use a thumbs up to add impact to your praise. Show that you are anticipating your child's success.

Praising Gentle Behavior—
Labeled Praise

In the next scenario we see Charlie, a 6-year-old boy who often handles his cat too roughly. He doesn't seem to understand that his behaviors can hurt his cat. Previously his parents have scolded him and removed the cat when he behaves this way. In the next scenario, they have decided to teach Charlie to treat the cat

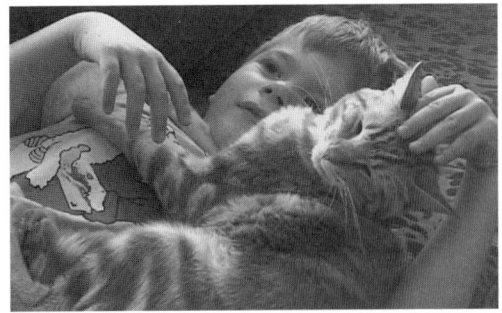

appropriately by turning their attention spotlight around so that he gets their attention and praise for being gentle with the cat. Notice how they use social and emotional coaching as well as praise to encourage the social behavior they want to see more of.

Charlie: (lying on couch with cat, patting cat slightly too hard, but not aggressively)

Father: Hey Charlie, you being gentle? Charlie? Charlie? Be gentle with Simba. (Charlie's pats become more gentle). That's a good boy. That cat loves you. You're being gentle.

Charlie: (hugs cat with a tight squeeze and the cat growls).

Father: Hey Charlie, That bothers Simba. I don't want to hear Simba make any noise. Show me how you can be gentle with soft pats.

Charlie: Okay. (pats more softly)

Father: Thank you. That's so good. Thank you for taking care of Simba. I am going to pat you gently so you know how it feels. (pats lightly)

Mother: And Charlie, you know what? Simba looks pretty happy with you right there, so you must be doing a good job.

Charlie: Yeah, I am.

Father: You're being good and gentle.

Charlie: Mm-hmm.

Mother: Nice, soft touches.

Charlie: I am not being mean anymore.

Mother: You're not being mean. You're being gentle. When you're gentle, do you know what that means?

Charlie: What?

Mother: That means—what does Simba want to do?

Charlie: Stay.

Mother: Yeah. Simba likes to stay with you when you're being gentle.

Charlie: When I'm mean, Simba has to run.

Mother: Simba has to run away from you when you're being mean. That's right. But you're being nice and gentle right now. Which takes a lot of work, doesn't it?

Charlie: Can you guys go play?
Mother: Oh, you want us to go away? How come?
Charlie: Because I want to have fun with Simba.
Mother: Okay. Well, you're being nice and gentle, so I think that's a fair thing, to let you have your fun. All right. I love you. Look at that Charlie, Simba's still staying with you because you're being nice and gentle. Thank you. You love your Simba.
Charlie: And Simba sits. I gotta pet him.
Mother: You know what? You're petting him, making him feel real comfortable.
Charlie: And he shakes.
Mother: He shakes? I think he likes to shake his head by himself. Don't you?
Charlie: Yeah.
Mother: Yeah? Do you think it's more comfortable for him when he shakes it or when you shake it?
Charlie: He shakes it.
Mother: Yeah. I think that's a good idea. See now his eyes are all closed? And he's relaxing, because you're being so gentle. And he likes it.

Considerations

These parents are teaching their son what it means to be gentle. They do this by giving him repeated labeled praise for his soft, gentle touches: *"Simba's still staying with you because you're being nice and gentle. Nice soft touches."* His father pats Charlie gently so he will understand what gentle means while his mother helps him understand the connection between his gentle touch and Simba's happiness and willingness to stay with him. She says, "Simba's relaxing because you are being gentle. And he likes it." She helps Charlie understand when he is "mean" his cat runs away. This is the beginning of helping Charlie develop some empathy for his cat and understanding that his gentle behavior results in more positive consequences for himself. It is also important that these parents are both working with Charlie on the same goal. Their consistent message will double the impact of their praise.

Sometimes parents praise using vague statements that are nonspecific and unlabeled. For example, "good job" or "well done" or "great." While these statements do convey a positive message, they are impersonal and they do not describe the behavior you are trying to praise. It is more effective to give praise that clearly labels the particular behavior you like at the time it occurs. For example, Charlie's parents immediately describe him being gentle at the very time he is patting his cat in soft ways. This helps him understand what it means to be gentle. They also help him make the connection between this gentle behavior and his cat's comfort. This is repeated several times by both parents. The number of words you will use in your praise statement will vary according to your child's language stage. For a child with very little language, you may use the words "soft" and "gentle" repeatedly at times when your child is experiencing that combined with physically modeling being gentle when touching your child. In addition, your positive tone of voice and smile will help your child understand you like this behavior.

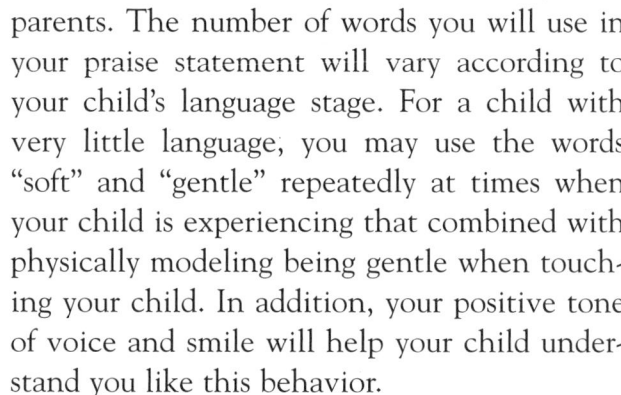

It is more effective to give praise that clearly labels the particular behavior you like at the time it occurs.

Rewarding Self-Regulation Practice with a Sensory Activity

In addition to enthusiastically praising and giving focused attention to your child's chosen target behaviors, you can also use tangible rewards such as stickers, hand stamps, small candies, fruit, or crackers. Another powerful motivator is the sensory activities your child enjoys. These can be used along with your praise as a reward for practicing a social skill, following a direction, or using a self-regulation strategy. In the next scenario, notice the way Hudson's father uses his son's favorite egg spin activity to reward him for practicing his calm down breathing strategy.

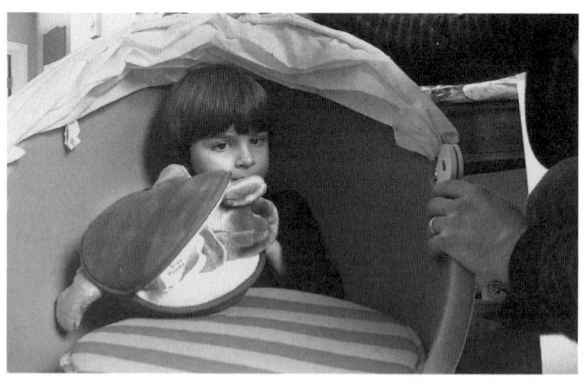

Father: (spinning Hudson in his egg spinner) Whee, Hudson while you are in your "take a break" chair, you can practice your deep breaths. You can "smell the flower and blow out the candle." Like this: (*models taking deep breaths*).

Father: (stops the spinning and opens the cover to see Hudson's face) Let's do one smell the flower and blow out the candle, and then we will spin some more. Okay, we'll do it together. Ready? (takes deep breaths.)

Hudson: (takes a breath)

Father: Good practice! One more breath. (Father takes deep breaths and Hudson watches) Okay! More spin. Wheee…

Father: (spins again) Okay, I'm going to count to 10 then I am all done spinning. One… two…

Father: (stops spinning) Stop! Okay let's do one more deep breath, and then I'll spin one last time. Okay? Ready –are you breathing deep? Through your nose go… (deep breaths and blows out. Hudson imitates breath) Good practice, Hudson! Good breathing!

Father: Here comes the final spin. It's going to be the fastest one this time. Wow, it is pretty exciting. Spinning is fun.

Hudson: It is exciting.

Father: It is like you are at the amusement park.

Hudson: Exciting.

Father: Pretty exciting.

Considerations

Hudson's father has previously taught his son about using deep breathing, and now he motivates Hudson to practice this new breathing skill using the ABC learning sequence. First, he starts with the motivating antecedent, egg spinning chair, (A) and uses this to motivate and coach his son to practice breathing (B: behavior). This is followed by another egg spinning reward (C: consequence). Each time the father stops the egg spin, he gets face to face contact with Hudson and models and coaches him to practice the breathing method before he gets the reward of his father's praise and another spin. This approach accentuates the fun of social interaction and provides repeated learning opportunities. This father also labels his son's excited emotion to enhance his emotion literacy. At first, Hudson may be more motivated by the spinning than by his father's praise. However, if the praise and rewarding spinning experience are repeatedly paired, Hudson will begin to internalize the good feelings that result and will associate them with the social interaction as well as the spinning. Overtime, he will be reinforced and motivated by the father's praise.

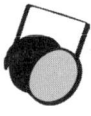

Think about and write down what sensory physical routines you could use to reward your child for your target behavior goal. Effective rewards are things that your child desires or likes such as food, comfort objects, interesting sounds, and sensory movements, and games. Remember to pair these rewarding activities with your praise and enthusiasm when your child engages in the target behavior.

Motivating Children

In the next scenario notice how Hudson's father uses rewards to help his son become toilet trained. Think about what makes this approach effective.

Father: (stops spinning Hudson and opens up cover of egg to get face to face) One more spin and then it's time to do a dry pants check. Are you ready for a spin and then dry pants?

Hudson: Spin!

Father: Spin and then dry pants check. Here we go—spin! And now stop. Okay, time for dry pants check and then another spin.

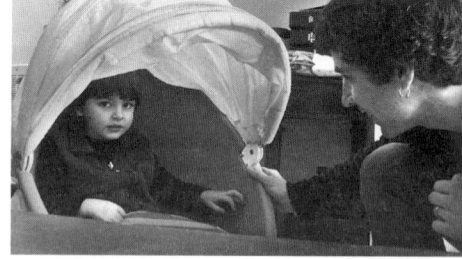

Hudson: No dry pants check. Spin!

Father: Yes, first dry pants and then spin. (*ignores Hudson's mild protest and calmly reaches to check his pants*). Dry pants check, let's open this up and I'll look at your pants. (Hudson let's his father check pants). Thank you for letting me look! (*labeled praise*). You are cooperating Hudson! Let's look at your pants. Are they dry?

Hudson: Are they dry?

Father: Yes! They are dry. Hudson, thanks for helping with the dry pants check. You helped AND you are dry. Wow! Now you get to spin.

Considerations

Hudson's father is working on helping Hudson learn to use the toilet. Hudson has been reluctant to cooperate with toileting routines in the past, so his father has broken this process into very small steps. In the scenario above, he focuses on a small cooperative behavior: checking for dry pants. All that is required of Hudson is that he let his father check his pants. Notice that his father gave a warning prior to initiating the dry pants check: "One more spin and then it's time to do a dry pants check. Are you ready for a spin and then dry pants?" This helps Hudson prepare for the transition. Then he uses a first/then sequence to help motivate Hudson to cooperate. "Yes, first dry pants and then spin." Hudson is not immediately cooperative, but his father ignores the mild protest and calmly follows through with the dry pants check. This is important. Hudson is not ready yet to proactively cooperate with this request, but his passive cooperation in allowing his father to check is a step in the right direction. His father enthusiastically praises this cooperative behavior and thanks him. Then he rewards Hudson with another spin. Gradually Hudson will learn to participate more willingly and cooperatively with this checking routine.

Motivating Children: (continued)

Later, after Hudson has finished spinning and is wandering around the living room, his father engages him in trying to use the toilet. You will see that he is using Skittles (small candies) as a reward for sitting on the potty. This is a system that he has already explained and practiced with Hudson on multiple occasions.

Father: Okay Hudson. Now it's potty time. Time to go pee pee in the potty.
Hudson: Not potty time.
Father: You get two Skittles, remember? Two Skittles. (small candy)
Hudson: (refusing reward) No two Skittles.
Father: (shows Hudson the Skittles) When go pee pee, you can choose what color to get.
Hudson: (turns away)
Father: Want a green and red one? Green and red Skittle (moves in front of Hudson and shows him the candy again).
Hudson: Green and red skittle. (reaches for them).
Father: Yes, first pee pee in the potty, then green and red Skittle. That's right Hudson! (takes Hudson's hand and gently leads him towards the bathroom).
Hudson: Green and red skittle.
Father: Yes, thank you for coming with me. You are going to go pee pee in the potty.
You are a big boy!
Hudson: A big boy.
Father: Yes, I'm proud of you for using the potty. When you are finished, you will get your Skittles!

Considerations

Hudson's father has developed a well thought out system for rewarding Hudson for steps toward becoming toilet trained. By breaking the toileting behavior into smaller steps (pants check, going pee), he has set up manageable target goals for Hudson. In the scenario above, he times his prompt to go to the toilet well. Hudson has voluntarily stopped spinning and is not engaged in another activity yet. He reminds Hudson of the Skittles reward. He is patient with Hudson's refusal and does not argue or force Hudson to cooperate. At the same time, he is calm and firm with his request that Hudson try to use the toilet. He helps Hudson stay focused on the reward by showing him the Skittles and talking about the colors. He provides a gentle physical prompt to help Hudson start towards the bathroom and then uses enthusiastic labeled praise to highlight this cooperation. Many children on the spectrum rely on consistent routines to help them make sense of their world and to stay regulated. This means that a new routine, like this toileting routine for Hudson, can seem intimidating and scary at first. Hudson's father is making the routine safe by breaking it into steps, labeling and talking about each step, and using praise and incentives to help Hudson practice the steps. As Hudson becomes used to the process, he will need fewer prompts. As Hudson masters and cooperates with the simple steps, his father will be able to increase the complexity of his demand. Eventually Hudson will be able to complete the whole routine with little prompting and without the tangible rewards. Even after phasing out the Skittles, it will be important for Hudson's father to continue with his enthusiastic praise for Hudson's cooperation and toileting accomplishments.

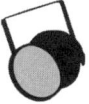

Hudson's father used a combination of a preferred sensory activity (spinning when Hudson cooperated with the dry pants check) and a tangible food reinforcer (Skittles). While using a child's sensory likes or another rewarding activity is an effective ABC way to prompt a child to practice certain behaviors, it can be helpful to add a tangible reward to accomplish a particularly difficult task. For Hudson, the dry pants check was a relatively easier step in the toileting process, whereas peeing in the toilet was quite hard, for he dislikes the feeling of the toilet seat. He needed the extra motivation of the Skittles to cooperate with that step of the process. Remember: the impact of these tangible incentives is much greater when combined with coaching, gestures, praise and parental encouragement.

Using Picture Prompts of Rewards.
For children with limited language, it can be helpful to make picture prompt cards that represent some activities or objects that are reinforcing to the child. For example: pictures of preferred food, object, game, story

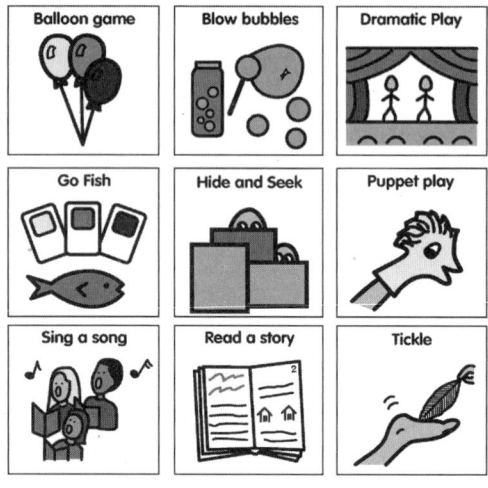

The Picture Communication Symbols ©1981–2010 by Mayer-Johnson LLC. All Rights Reserved Worldwide. Used with permission. Boardmaker™ is a trademark of Mayer-Johnson LLC

book, puppet, or sensory activity. When prompting your child, use pictures to represent both the target behavior and the reward. "When you put on your shoes (show picture of shoes), you can pick grapes or oranges (show grapes and orange cards for child to choose)." Or, parent can pre-choose the reward activity based on knowledge of child's likes: "Teeth first (show picture of tooth brush), then story (picture of book)."

Encouraging Your Children to Praise Themselves and Others

Praising others is an important social skill for children to learn. This is a skill that will help them build positive relationships with other children and adults.

Teaching children to praise others involves two steps. First, you must model how to praise. They will hear your enthusiastic praise to them and to others around you. A few children learn to praise just by modeling the praise they hear, but most children need to be prompted to start giving praise to others. You can prompt your child to praise by giving them the praise words to say such as: "Tell her 'You nice drawing'" or "You can say: 'I like your truck'." It is good to practice this first with a puppet or a doll. It will be easier for your child to focus on giving praise to the puppet or doll than to another child. Once your child is able to repeat your praise words to a puppet, then you can prompt them to praise a sibling or parent. Eventually you can prompt the praise in a play interaction with a peer. For example, you might prompt a child to notice another child's work and compliment them. For example saying, "Look at the castle your friend made. Can you say, 'I like your castle'." If the child follows your prompt, then follow up with praise such as, " That was very friendly. Your friend looks happy." It will likely be a long time before your child can spontaneously give unsolicited praise to someone else. Do not get discouraged. Giving praise or compliments is a skill that also develops slowly and gradually in children with neurotypical development.

For children with less language, you can use a visual prompt to represent praise to someone else. These prompt cards might represent a hug, someone saying thank you, or a thumbs up signal. You can prompt your child to choose one of these cards to give to the person that they want to thank, For example, "You can give the puppet the 'thank you' card to show that you liked that." Or "Do you want to give grandma a hug? You can give her the 'hug' card." If your child understands less receptive language, use fewer words: e.g. "Say 'thank you'?" (showing thank you card) or "Hug Grandma?" (showing hug card).

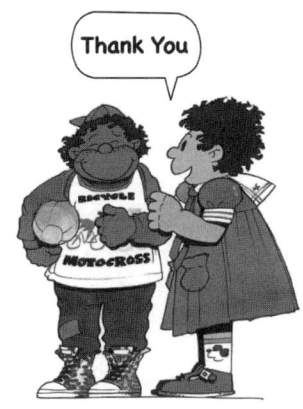

Note: if your child does not like physical contact with others, you would not force them to give a hug to someone else, even a close family member. Instead, you can substitute another friendly greeting such as a wave or knuckle bump or thumbs up.

We also want children to learn to praise themselves, for this can help them persist with a difficult task. For example, the parent or teacher can say, " You look proud of that, give yourself a pat on the back." This focuses on the child's own positive recognition of their work. This is another skill that you could have your child practice with a puppet. Your child and the puppet could take turns saying: "I am good at...." And then patting themselves on their backs. Initially, you will likely need to help your child finish the sentence. They may even want to copy what the puppet says:

Puppet: Let's play a game. Let's say what we are good at. I'll go first. I'm good at jumping. Your turn. What are you good at? I'm good at..."
Child: Jumping!
Puppet: We're both good at jumping! Let's say it together!
Child and Puppet: I'm good at jumping!
Puppet: Give me a high five!

Taking Care of and Rewarding Yourself

By now you have learned a lot of strategies for getting into your child's attention spotlight and building your child's learning into your every day routines. You know how to incorporate concepts such as modeling, imitating, prompting, and coaching into your child-directed play. You have come to understand how your child is incredible and what their strengths and difficulties are. You have learned to identify small goals for yourself and your child, leading to your longer term goal of building your child's social and emotional competence. Parenting is hard work and can be challenging, stressful, and rewarding all at the same time. We hope you have already seen that your effort is worthwhile as your child becomes more engaged and connected with you. These early social and communication interactions will lead to success in years to come.

It takes an immense amount of time and energy to engage your child in the repeated coached learning trials that we have described so far. As you put in the hard work to coach, support, and encourage your child, it is important to "refuel" yourself and your parenting partners. It may be tempting to put aside your own needs and goals as well as those of other family members while you focus on your child with ASD. However, it is very important to consider the needs of your whole family, including yourself. Be sure to take time for your self-care and take steps to be sure you are healthy, both physically and mentally. Here are some tips to taking care of yourself and your family:

- **Take time to focus on your partner and other family members** by listening and communicating about other parts of each other's lives before launching into the subject of your child with ASD. Get a babysitter and plan a date night with your partner or a friend. Build play into your own life with partners, friends, and other family members. These relationships are invaluable supports. Identify a personal goal to be sure this happens.
- **Keep your sense of humor.** Share the funny moments with a friend, partner, or another parent.

- **Schedule time with your other children.** Sometimes siblings of children with ASD can feel left out and lonely and resent all the time spent on their sibling on the autism spectrum. Be sure to set up regular special time with each of your other children and let them know they are special by planning activities that include their "likes".
- **Help siblings and other children understand what ASD is** and why this makes it hard for children with ASD to know how to play with them. Encourage them to play simple games and stay near to coach and support their play interaction. Praise them for their efforts, understanding, and caring. Adjust these discussions of ASD according the age and developmental status of the siblings or friend. Keep it simple for younger preschool children and expand their understanding of ASD as the children get older. Talk openly about any fears or worries siblings may have. Help them voice their feelings, listen, and correct any misperceptions. Reassure them of your love.
- **Be sure to get regular physical exercise, sleep and eat a healthy diet.** This fundamental point about having a healthy lifestyle may get less priority because you are caught up in caring for your child. However, consider this part of your treatment plan for your child with ASD. Build breaks into your daily schedule.
- **Build a strong social network.** One of the most beneficial ways to cope with stress is to build up a strong social network. This can include family and friends who genuinely care about you and whom you can turn to when you need help or support. You might be tempted to avoid being a burden to others; in fact, most people will feel honored that you trust them to share your feelings and problems and to ask for help. Give your family members and friends a chance to be part of this aspect of your life. Share the "How Your Child is Incredible" sheet (Chapter One) with them so they understand how to develop relationships with your child. Parents of children with ASD often find it helpful to talk

with other parents of children with ASD. You can check out the Autism Speaks web site resource guide to find a support group near you. You might want to consider joining a support group with other parents who have children on the autism spectrum.
- **Partner with your child's teacher.** Include teachers in your support network and the team working on behalf of your child. Share with them your child's likes and dislikes and what you find helpful for your child. Ask them for suggestions for things you can do at home that will support their learning at school. Work on your child's behavior plans together. Praise your teachers' helpful efforts and give them support.
- **Give yourself some positive feedback** and think about what you are accomplishing. Coaching your child's social, emotional, and language development is a demanding, time-consuming, and sometimes disappointing process. Avoid belittling or berating yourselves for the inevitable angry, impatient, and frustrated reactions you will have at times or for the seemingly slowness of your child's behavior change. These are normal feelings and thoughts. You can challenge and replace your negative thoughts by staying patient, using positive coping thoughts, deep breathing, forgiving yourself, using positive forecasting for future improvements, and by gaining support from others. It is important that you praise yourself for your successes and take time to reward yourself by doing something that gives you pleasure.

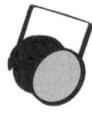

Make a list of some of your own pleasures or rewards such as taking a walk, going to exercise class, having coffee or dinner with a friend, going to yoga, taking in a movie, or having a bubble bath. Taking the time for self-care will refuel the energy it takes to support your child's learning. You are on a different journey from what you expected, but it can take you to unexpected learning and new and rewarding relationships.

Parent Reflections—Using Praise and Rewards

Charlie's Father: *I think Charlie's always worked well with positives. It's hard because he's so impulsive and before he even thinks about it, he's barreling down the wrong path and doing something he should not be doing. But the thing that I am learning to come back to is that if he does 15 things wrong and one thing good, you focus on the one. It's like, find the good and praise it.*

Charlie's Mother: *Yes, and we need to praise him 15 times more to keep the behavior going. With the cat, if we praise every gentle touch, he'll do more gentle touch. When we stop, it's like his impulsive brain takes over, and he squeezes again. But I think that it's getting better. Now, if we get started and praise him at first when he's holding Simba, we can then leave him for a few minutes, and he'll stay gentle. That didn't used to happen. Yes.*

Hudson's Father (about praise): *Praise is tricky with Hudson because he doesn't always look like he hears it. He is engrossed in spinning or whatever activity he's into at the moment. But when I break things up and use the activity to motivate him to practice something, like the breathing, I can feel a small connection when I praise him. Sometimes he smiles spontaneously at me now, and he didn't used to do that.*

Hudson's Father (About incentives): *For toilet training, we need to pull out all the stops, spinning and Skittles and lots of practice. It's a new routine and it's hard for him. In the beginning he really refused to even try. Now, he says "no" but he goes along with it. He likes the Skittles. Without the Skittles, I don't think he'd be willing to sit on the potty. But I can see he's proud when he pees in the toilet. He likes being a big boy.*

To Sum Up...

Once you have learned how to get in your child's attention spotlight, you will be more reinforcing to your child. Your attention, often paired with another incentive, will begin to motivate your child to try new behaviors, learn new skills, and achieve your goals for them. Understanding rewarding antecedents (A) or your child's "likes" and how they can be used to prompt the target behavior you are working on will create learning opportunities for your child. Focusing on rewarding your child's small positive steps with your praise, encouragement, and attention while ignoring or minimizing attention to unwanted behaviors will help those desired behaviors develop and flourish.

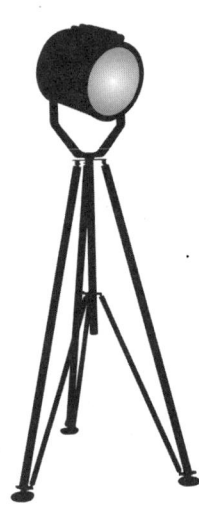

SPOTLIGHTING
Praising and Rewarding Your Child

Praising Your Child
- Prompt your child's attempts to interact with others and praise them for gesturing, talking, sharing, making eye contact, and working together.
- Give labeled and specific praise for target behaviors immediately and consistently.
- Praise with smiles, eye contact, enthusiasm, and gestures. For children with less verbal language combine with a visual praise prompt. Be your child's cheerleader!
- Give pats, hugs, and kisses along with praise.
- Praise your child in front of other people.
- Combine praise with persistence, social, and emotion coaching methods.
- Be sure to get in your child's "attention spotlight" by facing them directly and then praise with lots of smiles, enthusiasm and eye contact.
- Combine praise with a tangible reward for targeted behavior (e.g., hand stamp, sticker, physical activity, crackers).

Tangible Rewards
- Keep your reward program simple.
- Use picture prompt reward cards to help children with less language to choose a reward
- Break down behavior into small steps—be realistic.

- Use spontaneous, inexpensive rewards (stickers, crackers, hand stamp, extra story before bed).
- Get appropriate behavior first, then give reward immediately.
- Gradually replace tangible rewards with your social approval.

 Getting in your child's attention spotlight to praise!

CHAPTER 9

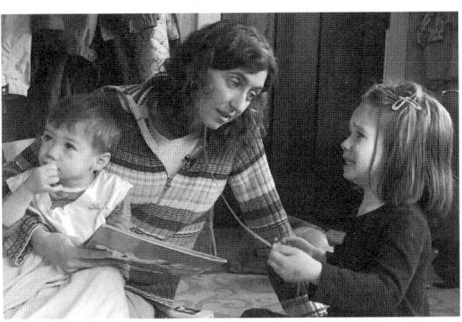

Spotlighting Your Limit Setting and Managing Misbehavior

Introduction
All the coaching and positive attention that you have been working on with your child has likely resulted in your child being more connected to you, more cooperative, and learning exciting new things. But just like any other young child, at times your child on the autism spectrum will be defiant, noncompliant, and will cry, yell, and throw tantrums. This is normal child behavior, not deliberate misbehavior. Children are biologically programmed to explore and test the limits as part of their developmental drive. This exploration stage is thought to help all children develop a sense of independence and eventually self-control. For children with autism, resistance, noncompliance, frustration, or

dysregulation may also occur when they don't understand the adult's verbal instructions or requests. Negative responses may also be a signal of sensory overload or anxiety at a situation that feels out of their control. Overtime, if their noncompliance or dysregulation gets more attention than their compliance or self-regulation, the noncompliance and anxiety will be reinforced and continue.

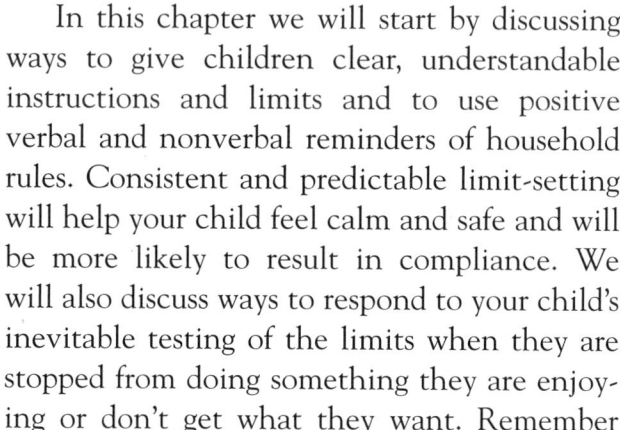

If you are calm and consistent, your child will learn that tantrums and protests don't work to get their way.

In this chapter we will start by discussing ways to give children clear, understandable instructions and limits and to use positive verbal and nonverbal reminders of household rules. Consistent and predictable limit-setting will help your child feel calm and safe and will be more likely to result in compliance. We will also discuss ways to respond to your child's inevitable testing of the limits when they are stopped from doing something they are enjoying or don't get what they want. Remember when your child protests, this is not a personal attack. They are simply expressing their frustrated feelings and testing your rules to see if you are going to be consistent. If you are calm and consistent, your child will learn that tantrums and protests don't work to get their way. On the other hand, if you give in when your child protests, they will probably test harder the next time. When children's feelings are out of control, they need and welcome their parents' ability to stay calm, accept their feelings, and gently follow through and enforce the limit. Children need this predictable parental response to feel safe to do the developmentally appropriate limit-testing that is important to their growth. We will talk about proactive discipline approaches such as distractions, redirections, and ignoring as ways to manage this testing misbehavior.

Positive Reminders

Children on the spectrum will likely need more verbal and nonverbal reminders than neurotypical children because they often do not understand the parental instruction, especially if it involves too much language. In the next scenario notice the way Kalani's mother sets some limits on her son's behavior when he is playing with rocks and water sitting next to his sister. One of her target goals is for her son to be aware of his baby sister and to initiate safe interactions with her. In this case she wants Kalani to learn to let his sister know with his words when he is about to throw a big rock that will splash and perhaps frighten his sister. Think about the approach she takes to remind 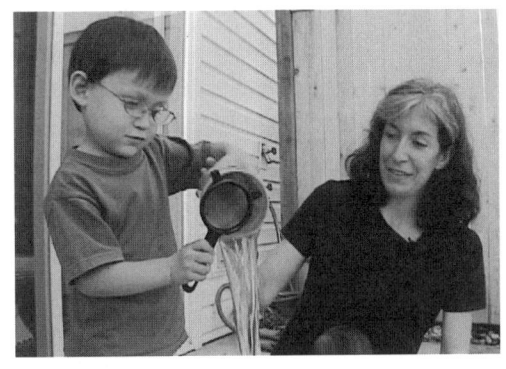 him of her expectations. Mother is sitting with baby Nika in her lap face to face with Kalani and bucket of water between them.

Mother: What are you going to do with your rocks?

Kalani: (no response)

Mother: You found the rock? Are you going to drop it in the water? Oh I think I might move Nika, 'cause there might be a big splash. Okay, now it's safe to throw that big rock.

Kalani: No, I want Nika.

Mother: Throw your rock first, then I will move Nika near you.

Kalani: Throw rock. (throws rock and it splashes. Kalani, Nika, and mom all laugh)

Mother: That was a big splash. Nika thought it was funny too. Let me know if you're going to splash and I'll move Nika.

Kalani: I want to splash.

Mother: Thank you for telling me. I will move Nika. Ok are you ready? Let's go and you can splash. Ready for it go splash?

Kalani: Big rock.

Mother: Big rock, ready splash. Oh, was that a surprise? Those make big splashes, don't they?

Kalani: (Kalani grabs another rock and throws it without warning, splashing mom and Nika. Nika fusses).

Mother: Oh, that was a big rock. Nika got wet. Did you tell Nika: "excuse me Nika, I'm going to make a big splash"?

Kalani: I didn't.

Mother: We don't want to surprise her too much. Kalani, it's a little scary for Nika when she doesn't know it's going to splash. Did you hear her fuss?

Kalani: Big rock. (holding up another rock, but waiting to throw it).

Mother: Thank you for waiting. You can do the big rock. Remember to tell Nika so she knows it's coming. Kalani's getting a big rock. Say "Nika it's going to splash."

Kalani: Nika, it's going to splash.

Mother: Kalani, nice friendly words. You told Nika and she feels safe. You are being a good big brother.

Considerations

This mother patiently teaches Kalani the rules about his rock-throwing game. She coaches him to tell his sister before he throws a big rock. She understands that he needs patience and support to remember to do this. She also knows that she will need to coach him with the words to say to his sister. She praises him when he pauses and waits before throwing a rock, and when he uses his words to warn his sister. When he throws a rock without warning, she points out that this made his sister wet and reminds him what he needs to do next time. She is gently setting a limit and teaching him the positive opposite behavior that she wants. She helps to build Kalani's awareness of his sister's presence in his spotlight by pointing out their shared experience: "Nika thought that was funny too." "You told Nika, and she feels safe." She also points out the link between the splashing and Nika's surprised or scared feelings, so that he can start to understand that his behavior has an impact on others. The mother focuses on supporting the behavior she wants Kalani to do (tell his sister when he is going to throw a big rock and it will splash), and she avoids giving negative "don't" commands.

When your child complies, it is important to spotlight this compliance with a great deal of positive attention and labeled praise.

When your child complies to your requests or instructions, it is important to spotlight this compliance with a great deal of positive attention and labeled praise. For example, this mother praised Kalani for giving a warning before throwing the rock: "thank you for telling me," and for waiting before throwing "thank you for waiting!" She is letting him know that she is pleased that he listened to her coaching.

Sometimes parents overwhelm their child by giving too many instructions at once. This results in the child becoming overwhelmed and may result in the child being noncompliant and frustrated. Most young children can follow one command at a time, particularly if the request is a new behavior or requires the child to exert self-control. This mother focused on one request ("tell before you throw the big rock"), and she restated the rule many times during their play interaction. She used simple phrases and coached Kalani to follow through with her request, giving him the words to say.

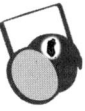

Think about how many directions you are giving your child and the purpose of these instructions. Is every request necessary? Are you giving too many instructions? Are you giving commands at a level that your child understands? Do you give your child time to think about your command or instruction before you repeat it? Do you praise your child's compliance to your requests? Could you remind your child of the command by using a visual prompt of what you expect? For example, a picture of hands-to-self shown to a child who is starting to touch something or someone inappropriately. Or, a picture of putting on shoes when you are asking your child to put on their shoes.

It is helpful to have a few simple household rules as well as some well-established household routines. It is important to teach and practice each of those rules and routines. In the prior scenario, Kalani's mother is teaching him a new rule that is specific to the water play. He is also beginning to learn a more general social rule of letting his sister know when he is going to do something surprising. It will be a long time before Kalani can generalize this specific water rule to the general behavior of being considerate of others, but this rule lays that groundwork.

Think about your own rules and routines. Try to pick 4-5 rules that are important to you. For example: "car seats and seat belts in the car," "gentle and safe hands—no hitting," "food stays in the kitchen or dining room," "no shoes in the house." These rules will be different for different families and are taught, coached, and practiced with your child. Does your child know your household rules? Do you have picture prompts to help cue your child to the rules? You will also have regular routines around daily transitions (getting dressed in the morning, eating meals, getting ready for bed, coming home from school). These are different than household rules, but require similar teaching, coaching, possible picture or object prompts, and repeated practice. When children understand the rules and routines in their households, they feel safer and will be more cooperative.

Transition Warnings

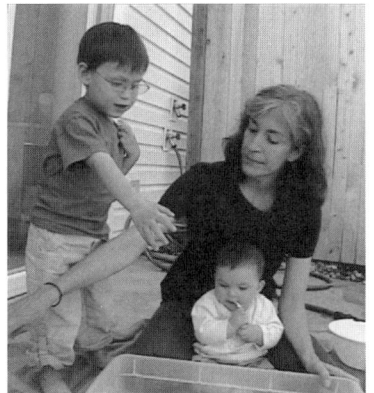

Most children who are engaged in an interesting activity will dysregulate by tantruming, yelling, or crying if the activity is ended abruptly without warning. When possible, it is helpful to prepare your child for a transition—with a warning or reminder of what he will be doing next. In the next scenario notice how Kalani's mother prepares him for ending this fun playtime with rocks and dumping cups of water. Think about what makes her approach effective?

    Kalani: (asks) More splashes.
    Mother: Splashing is fun. It is almost lunch time. Do you want to do two more rock splashes or one more splash?
    Kalani: Two more
    Mother: Okay, two more rock splashes, and then it will be time for lunch. (Kalani throws another rock in the water and his mother continues coaching and praising him).

Mother: That was one splash! What a big splash! Okay Kalani, this is going to be the last splash. Can you tell Nika, "one more splash, Nika."
Kalani: One more splash Nika! (throws rock).
Mother: Good telling, Kalani! That was a good last splash. Now it's all done (uses "all done" sign). It's lunch time. Do you want to hold my hand to go inside or do it by yourself?
Kalani: All by self.
Mother: Thank you for listening and coming! Yes, you can do it all by self.

Considerations

Whenever feasible, it is helpful to give a reminder or warning prior to a command, as this can help for a smoother transition. Kalani's mother realizes that he needs time to make the transition from the fun water play to going inside for lunch. She warns him that it is almost time to stop playing and go inside for lunch. Since Kalani does not understand the concept of time, she marks the transition timing by the number of splashes that he has left, and she gives him a choice of throwing one more rock or two more rocks. When giving a command, it is often helpful to allow children a small amount of control by setting up a controlled choice (two options that are both acceptable to the parent). The mother uses gestures to be sure Kalani understands they will be "all done."

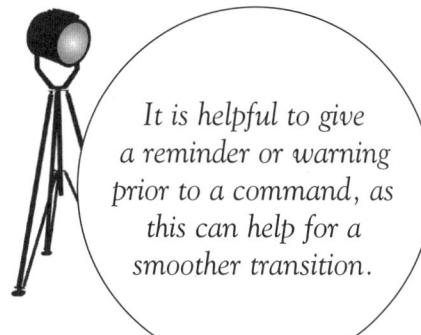

It is helpful to give a reminder or warning prior to a command, as this can help for a smoother transition.

There are many ways to give warnings. For children with limited language or little understanding of time, a timer, music signal, or specified activity can be helpful. For example, "when the timer goes off it will be time to stop playing with the water." Or, "after you put in 3 more cups of water, we will be all done." Or, " when I finish singing this song, we are all done." Always let your child know what will happen next. If the next activity is something your child enjoys, the transition will be easier. For example, "after we are 'all done' with the water, we will go inside, and we have strawberries and cheese for lunch." Even if the next activity is something your child doesn't like, it's still important to keep things predictable by letting them know. "After this book is over, Daddy is going to snug you up in your bed with teddy." Even if the child does not like going to bed, the predictability of knowing what comes next will make the transition easier.

Using picture schedules to help children understand requests, know what is expected and to encourage more independence.
Mini picture schedules: Time is very abstract for all young children, especially those on the autism spectrum. Concrete picture schedules of what happens at certain times of the day can help children know what is being asked, what is happening next, and what to do. Mini picture schedules can be made for the sequence of predictable daily routines and expectations such as how to get ready for bed, morning dressing, and breakfast routines. For example, these pictures show steps for a hand washing routine, placed exactly at the spot where Hudson washes his hands.

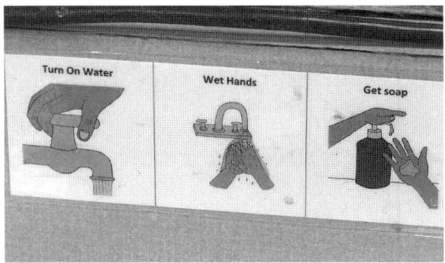 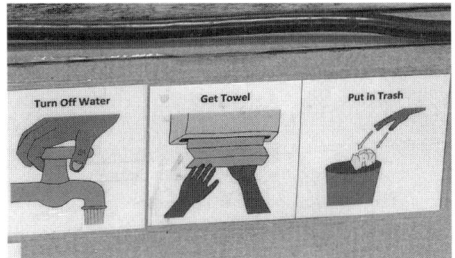

This sequence details of turning on the tap, using the soap dispenser, turning off the tap, and drying hands with a towel. Visual prompts like this can help a child become less dependent on adults, feel more secure, and know what to do on their own. For example, a bedtime routine might include a picture schedule of each activity in the sequence such as: play time, using toilet, taking a bath, brushing teeth, putting on Pjs, and reading a book with the parent. Help your child follow the sequence by pointing to the picture of the current activity and what comes next. For example: "now we are doing play time and then you will sit on the potty." "After the potty, it is bath time. What toy do you want to have in the bath?" Focusing on

Mini picture schedules can be made for the sequence of predictable daily routines.

the positive aspects of the upcoming routine serves to distract the child from his disappointment about stopping the current fun play activity and gives them a visual picture of what will happen next. If your child expresses distress about the transition, you can use emotion coaching to validate that feeling, for example, "I know. You're sad that play time is over. I'm sorry too—that was fun." Ignore excessive protests and calmly focus on what comes next. "We can put the playtime picture away (turn it over). Look at what is next—the potty picture. Do you want to hold hands on the way to the potty or go by yourself?"

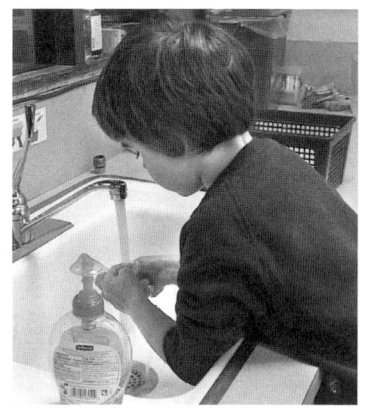

If picture prompts are helpful for your child, you can use a different mini picture schedule for each important routine. These pictures can be line drawings easily found on the internet or actual photographs of your child doing each of the steps in the routine.

The number of pictures in a sequence will depend on the child's communication level. For some it will start with one picture activity such as taking a bath and then proceed, over time, to more pictured activities: first bath, then teeth, and then story... These *"first-then"* picture boards can also be effective for helping children who are resistive to stopping an activity or who find change in a routine difficult. For example, for the child who doesn't want to stop his spinning activity, the parent or teacher can show the stop spinning picture followed by a picture of the next rewarding activity such as picture of reading a book with the parent paired with showing the actual book. For example, the parent can say, *"first stop spinning and then we have our fun reading time."* Eventually, with repetition, just showing the child his favorite book, or the cereal box will help the child understand the sequence or routine for the evening or the morning. Here is an example of a first-then picture program used by a teacher with a child who first had

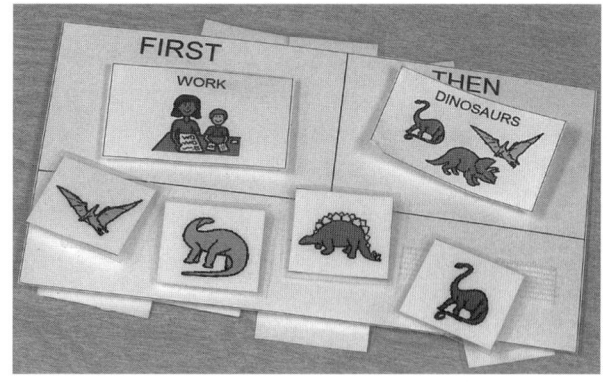

to work on a joint shared work activity for 10 minutes with another child and then he could play with his favorite dinosaur animals alone.

In addition to pictures, parents and teachers can show real objects to signal an upcoming activity such as pajamas to indicate bedtime, a bath toy to indicate bath time, or food or a cup to indicate snack or drink time. Auditory cues may also be helpful such as jingling the car keys to let the child know it's time for a drive to day care, or timer or lights flashing to indicate three minutes to finish. These concrete objects and auditory or visual cues can be especially helpful for a child who is reluctant to transition to a new activity.

Whole day schedules: In addition to using pictures to represent a series of mini schedules in the day, some children find it helpful to have a visual picture schedule for the events of the entire day. For example, first the child goes to Grandma's house (showing picture of Grandma), then having lunch (favorite food item), then watching a video (video), and then being picked up by parent and going home (picture of dad). These concrete picture examples of what happens at certain times of the day helps children understand what is expected. They also can be used as a kind of picture diary for you to later talk about and review what your child has done that day. Some children with ASD can talk about what they are doing in the moment but can't tell you about what happened earlier in the day. These picture diaries help remind your child what they have done and make it easier to tell you without you having to ask questions. If your child is in preschool, you could ask the teacher to send home a brief journal with some pictures of what your child did that day and who they played with. This will help you know what to talk about with your child. Moreover, you could share your picture diary from home with the teacher.

It can also be helpful to use a picture sequence to prepare a child for upcoming and perhaps difficult event such as going to a movie, the babysitter's, grandma's house, or doctor's office, or to prepare for what to do when a visitor comes over. This can be done by showing pictures of the place or activity, and what they will be doing there. Using picture diaries or schedules will help your child to stay calm and to exhibit fewer behavior melt downs during transitions or in new settings because your child understands what will happen next.

Spotlighting Your Limit Setting and Managing Misbehavior 271

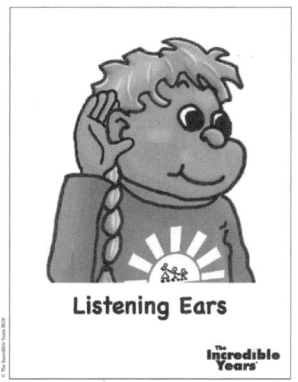
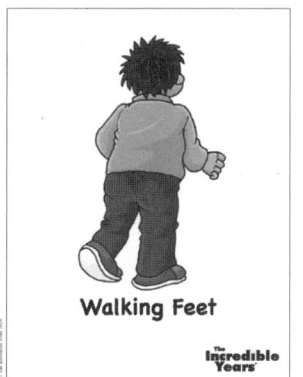
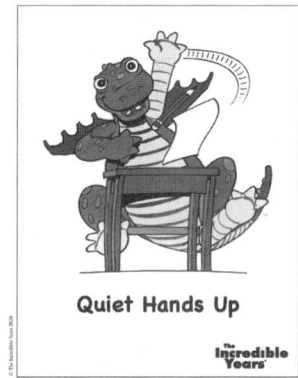

Since schedules and routines may change depending on the day or situation, make your schedule flexible with laminated pictures and Velcro fasteners so you can change the cards when needed. For example, if you get home late and decide there is not time for a bath that evening, you can remove the bath card from the evening routine. If your child is very tuned into the regular schedule, it will be helpful to have them take off the bath card and say: "no bath tonight" so they understand that the schedule is changing.

Household or Classroom Rules: Pictures of household or classroom rules or prompts of expected behavior are very helpful for all children. Some commonly used rules in a preschool classroom are: listening ears, hands to self, waiting, walking feet, and quiet voice. Using the same rules pictures, words, and gestures at home as at school can strengthen

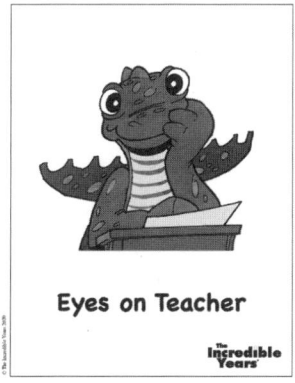
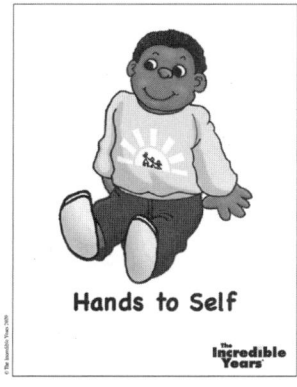
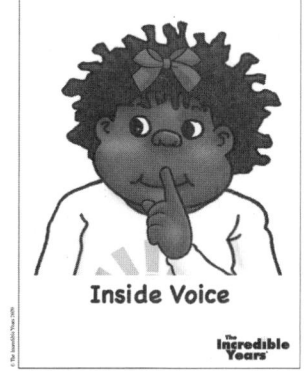

the child's learning of these behavior expectations. It is always best to show pictures of the positive gesture or behavior you want and to model it, rather than show pictures of a negative behavior such as hitting or running inside with a No sign drawn through it.

Establishing predictable daily schedules and routines, offering reminders and warnings for transition changes, and explaining and practicing the important household rules will help your child to learn and cooperate with household and classroom rules. The goal is to reduce unnecessary commands or requests so that your child will learn that your commands/requests are important, and that compliance is expected.

Parents and teachers often need to ask children to do something or stop doing something. These requests or commands are important to help a child function in home and in classrooms. Did you know that commands can be given in ways that make it more or less likely that a child will cooperate? In the next section we will talk about what makes a command effective or ineffective. If you learn to give clear effective commands that are tailored to your child's developmental language level, you will find that your child is much more likely to follow through with what you have asked them to do.

Clear Limit Setting and Follow Through

In the next scenario, Hudson's father is setting a limit regarding the amount of time his son can play on his iPhone. He does this because without some limits, his son can be consumed in this solo interaction for long periods of time. While it might be tempting to place

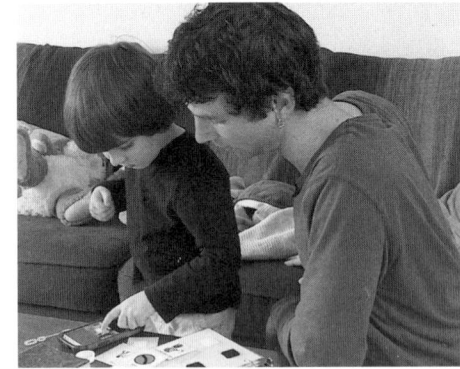

fewer expectations on such a child, this can backfire because it doesn't help Hudson learn alternative social replacement behaviors and may actually reinforce continued use of nonsocial behavior. Notice how the father sets the limit on Hudson's iPhone time and follows through with its enforcement.

Father: (looking at iPhone with Hudson) Okay you can look at the pictures, you can look at the pictures for 2 minutes, I am going to set the timer for that.
Hudson: I'm going to set the timer for that.
Father: Do you want to look at the video? Oh, haven't seen this video yet. What's that? What's Hudson doing? You're riding a…
Hudson: Riding a…(flapping)
Father: What's it called?
Hudson: (flapping) What's it called?
Father: Riding a tricycle, right.
Hudson: Tricycle.
Father: (still looking at iPhone video with Hudson) Peddling all around the play gym that's pretty fun. I'm going to set the timer on the stove since you are using the phone. I'm going to set a timer, and when it goes off, we are going to be all done with the phone okay? Two minutes, okay Hudson?
Father: (looking at iPhone pictures together.) Remember when the timer goes off, the phone is all done. It will go off in one minute now okay? Say, "one minute yes Papa."
Hudson: One minute yes Papa.
Father: You can look at phone pictures for one minute when the timer goes off we are going to be all done. What's that Hudson is eating, ice cream? (looking at pictures on the phone) Wow what are you eating, what kind of ice cream is that? Is that chocolate? There's your potty. You are moving those pictures pretty fast.
Father: Oh, there's the timer… all done. (gets down on Hudson's eye level and makes "all done" sign).
Hudson: Oh no.
Father: Hudson, it's all done. The timer's all done.
Hudson: (runs away with phone) No, no, no.
Father: Hey the timer went off Hudson. Give me the phone please.

Hudson: No, no, no.

Father: (goes over to Hudson.) Give me the phone please, Hudson. Give me the phone please, All done. The timer went off. (takes the phone out of Hudson's hand). Thank you, Hudson. Thank you for giving me the phone. Thank you for cooperating, I really appreciate that.

Considerations

This father sets up a clear limit and instruction about the amount of time that is left for Hudson to use the iPhone by using a kitchen timer. He makes sure Hudson has heard him by prompting him to repeat the transition words, "one minute Papa." Then he engages with Hudson to enjoy the time he has left with the iPhone. When the timer goes off, he gets eye contact with Hudson and gives him a simple and clear "all done" signal. A nonverbal signal is often helpful, especially because children may have a harder time processing language when they are distressed or unhappy. Hudson asserts his independence by running away with the iPhone. The father calmly follows through with his command in a respectful way saying, "Give me the phone please. All done timer went off." He follows through with his command by using a gentle physical prompt of taking the phone out of Hudson's hand. Even though he initiated this action, he still praises Hudson's compliance: "Thank you Hudson. Thank you for giving me the iPhone. Thank you for cooperating, I really appreciate that." He avoids giving Hudson attention for his initial refusal, stays calm and focuses his attention and praise on Hudson's eventual compliance.

Offering two possible choices is strategic because it gives the child some control over what happens next.

When children are upset about ending a fun activity, they may react with protests and noncompliance. It can be helpful to use emotion coaching to recognize their distress: "I know that it's sad when it's time to stop watching movies." It can also be helpful to pair this emotion coaching with a reminder of what options the child does have. For example, the father might offer Hudson a choice of two other preferred play activities by saying, "Now iPhone all done, next playdough or cars?" Offering two possible choices is strategic because it gives the child some control over what happens next, and they may be more likely to be cooperative.

If your child is highly dysregulated, it will not be useful to continue offering choices or coaching statements. Children who are too dysregulated will not be able to process additional input and may become more distressed with continued parental attention. It's also possible that continued parental intervention may inadvertently reinforce the tantrum because the child may believe that there is a chance that the parent will give in if the parent is still engaging in the interaction. Sometimes children need time to work through their frustration before they are able to process the next step. If Hudson had continued to protest loudly, his father would still follow through with gently removing the phone and then allow Hudson's fussing to subside before re-engaging him with a new activity.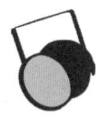

Think about what limits or rules you have regarding your child's activities. For example, how much time does your child have for screen time, spinning, or alone time? Does your child know how much time they can have for preferred activities and when these activities occur during the day? It can be helpful to sequence preferred activities strategically during the day with a preferred activity following an activity that is harder for your child. For example, if your child struggles with getting dressed but loves eating breakfast, then set up the schedule with dressing first, breakfast second. If you would like to have the living room clean at the end of the day, set up 10 minutes of late afternoon family clean up time followed by some screen time for your child while you make dinner. If there are many tasks that are hard for your child, consider allowing shorter, more frequent rewards. For example, you might break up 40 minutes of screen time into four 10 minutes segments that your child can have throughout the day after completing different tasks that are more challenging. If your child relies on visual prompts, make sure that all routines are signaled by picture prompt cards as well as your words.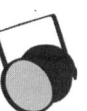

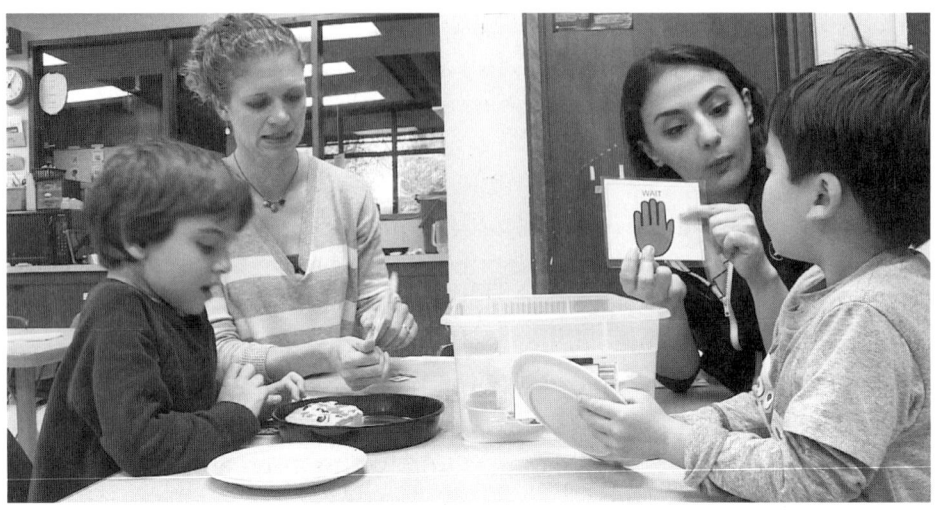

Using Visual Prompt Cards to Help Your Child Understand Your Request/Instruction

For children who are nonverbal and don't understand or follow simple commands, even a two-step picture schedule may be too complex. These children will respond best to limited verbal language (one or two word prompts) and single picture prompts. For example, you might show a picture of a toilet, hand washing, or wearing a mask to indicate the child needs to do one of these things. Again, prior teaching must occur so that the child knows what the picture means before the adult uses the picture alone to prompt the behavior. Command Picture Cards can be put on a key ring to prompt behavior requests such as sit, wait, clean up, quiet, shoes on/off, help, look, all done, walk, and deep breath. Sometimes you might need to physically prompt your child to physically move them through the actions. For example, show the command card, say the command word, and then physically walk them to the sink and put your hands over theirs to wash their hands. Or, put their hands around the hair brush or tooth brush and move them through the brushing movements.

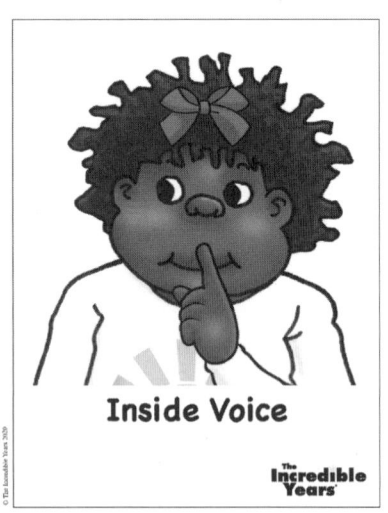

The picture of the stop sign is a useful signal to indicate the child needs to stop what they are doing. The meaning of this visual can be taught by singing a song. Each time the stop sign is held up, the song stops, and when the stop sign goes down, the song starts again.

This is repeated several times so that the child begins to learn the meaning of "stop." The stop sign may be paired with a green "go" sign to provide a visual for starting the activity again. Many other start/stop games can be played using the red stop sign signal while running, chasing, or swinging or spinning and then the green sign to start again. Parents can help children notice real stop signs as they are driving or walking around the community.

Household Jobs

There are many ways your children can participate with you in doing jobs or chores around the house. For example, they can help feed the dog or cat, wash dishes, take laundry from dryer, unload the dishwasher, set the table, help with cooking, and put grocery objects in the cart. Often young children are excited to help with these tasks, and by including your child in these everyday routines, you will continue to encourage cooperation and compliance with requests. Some children will be able to learn to do some of these jobs independently, and other children can work alongside a parent to help out with a small part of the task. For many children helping a parent can be the rewarding antecedent for the target behavior you are working on. Getting to put utensils in the dishwasher, cut up vegetables for soup, or mix the cookies batter can be the rewarding antecedent and the positive consequence for the target behaviors of helping, taking turns, listening, or asking. Use all the same coaching principles for learning new words and social skills as you use during your play times. In these household helping interactions, your child will learn new skills and will feel proud about their contribution to the family.

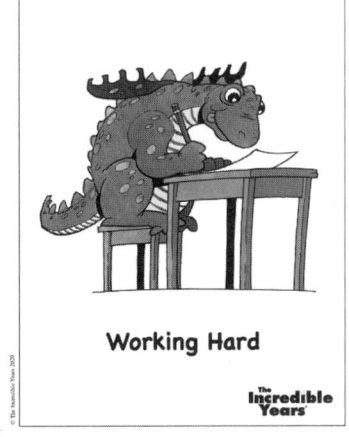

Working Hard

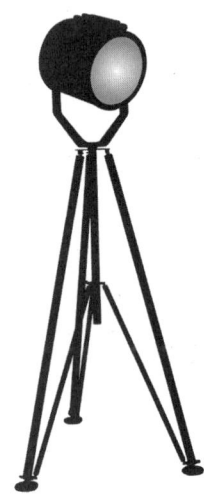

SPOTLIGHTING

Teaching Children to Understand and Follow Commands/Requests

Here are some of key strategies for promoting children's understanding and cooperation with commands and requests:

- Get into your child's attention spotlight before giving a command.
- When possible, give a transition warning about an upcoming behavior or activity change.
- Give a simple request or limit (e.g., "all done, give me phone please"). When possible, include a gesture.
- Use "do" commands or positive requests, "Walk please." "Gentle hands." "Open mouth for brushing." For children with less language understanding, combine word with gesture of action.
- Avoid the use of "no" or "don't" commands and try to focus on what behavior you want, rather than what you don't want. ("Walk please" instead of "Stop running.")
- Use visual command cards for children who are less verbal (e.g., wait, stop sign, sit, toilet, brush teeth, walk etc.).
- Give choices when possible.
- Wait and give your child time to process your request and to respond.
- If your child does not respond, follow through and help scaffold their response with a gesture (point to phone, show washing hands action, or pretend teeth brushing) or prompt child's compliance by whispering a response (say, "all done", while taking the phone away).
- If your child protests, ignore, and when child is calmer, try a redirect or distraction to one of his "likes"(if appropriate).
- If your child is too dysregulated, follow through and then give space for your child to calm down before you re-engage.

- When your child complies with your instruction, give a powerful reward and redirect to another activity ("Thank you, let's go find your favorite book to read").
- Continue child-directed narrated commenting.

Requiring a Response

When you are setting a limit or attempting to distract your child with a different preferred activity, sometimes children, especially those on the autism spectrum, will seem to be ignoring your speech. You may feel you are not making a connection with your child and that your words are not being understood. You might be tempted to move on and make the decision for your child; however, if you don't require a response, your child won't learn the importance of listening or using his speech to get what he wants. It is critical to require a response. In the next scenario watch how the father works hard to get his son's attention and waits for a response. Think about what else he could do.

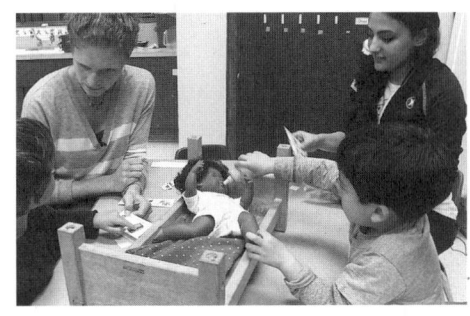

Father: Do you want to have some juice or milk? What do you think? Want some warm milk? Yes or no?

Hudson: (turns away)

Father: Yes, warm milk or no warm milk? (tries to get eye contact) Not sure?

Hudson: (doesn't answer)

Father: What do you think Hudson, warm milk or no warm milk? (tries to get eye contact and child looks away) What would you like? (strokes cheek)

Hudson: (looks away)

Father: (gets out milk picture card and the "no" picture card). Hudson, show me milk or no milk (takes Hudson's finger and points to each card as he labels the options).

Hudon: (still does not reply.)

Father: I think that Hudson wants "no milk" (places Hudson's finger on the "no" card). Can you say: "no milk."

Hudson: No milk.

Father: Thank you for telling me. Do you want juice? (shows picture of juice paired with juice box)

Hudson: (nods head yes)

Father: Yes, please juice (nods head yes)

Hudson: Yes, juice.

Father: Great asking, here is juice.

Considerations

The father does a great job of trying to get Hudson to let him know if he wants some milk or juice to drink. He repeats his request several times, attempting to get eye contact. He remains patient with this process. It might be tempting just to put the juice or milk on the table without requiring his response, but this father's goal is to help Hudson use words to ask for what he wants and to engage in social conversation. Because Hudson continues not to respond, the father tries the picture cards and moves Hudson's finger over each of the cards as he labels what they mean using gestures. He starts first with the milk before moving to juice. In the end, he interprets Hudson's lack of response as a "no" and walks Hudson through the motions of communicating "no milk" by helping Hudson point to the "no" picture and giving him the words to say. Hudson's father is guessing that if Hudson wanted milk, he would be more motivated to communicate, so it is a smart guess to interpret his non-response as a "no." Finally Hudson, repeats the words "no milk" and his father praises his communication. Through his persistence, he is showing his son that it is important to communicate his wishes, both "yes" and "no." Next he moves on to the juice option with the same prompting and gesturing.

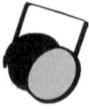

Remember in Chapter Two we talked about how to teach your child to say "no" by starting with the food item or activity your child likes least and reward his "no" response or gesture by putting the object away or turning over the picture prompt. Then offer the more desired food item with the "yes" response or gesture and reward this affirmative response with praise and by giving it to the child.

Waiting for a Response

It is important not to be discouraged or angry when your child doesn't respond to your request. And remember not to resort to just giving them what you think they want. Hudson's father is persistent and calm with his requests even though his son seems to ignore his efforts to engage him. Notice what the father does next and think about what Hudson is learning.

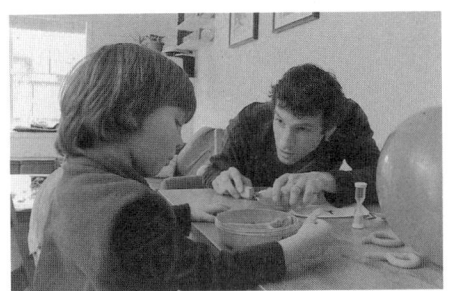

Father: How about I bring over a little snack?
Hudson: (not looking at dad and no response)
Father: Yes for snack or no for snack? Animal crackers and raisins? Yes or no…(tries to get eye contact). What do you think?
Hudson: Yes
Father: Thank you for answering me! You want snack! Do you want animal crackers, raisins, or salami.. what do you think? (brings the snack items to the table).
Hudson: (looking at the snacks, eyes stop on the salami)
Father: (points to salami) Yes salami or no salami, what do you think? Yes salami or no salami, what do you think?
Hudson: Yes salami.
Father: You answered salami! Good telling me, Hudson! Yes salami! Okay, okay dokey, you get a tickle, and I see a smile, I see a little smile. Here is your salami!

Remember not to resort to just giving him what you think he wants.

Considerations

This is a good example showing that initially Hudson didn't seem to be listening or connecting with his father's request. However, when the father shows him the physical objects, names the food items, and asks again for a "yes" or "no," Hudson is able to make a choice. The father continues to try to get eye contact with Hudson when he is asking for a response. He stays patient, recognizing that this is a learning opportunity for Hudson. When he sees Hudson looking at the salami, he does not just hand the snack to him, but coaches him to say "yes, salami." When he finally gets Hudson's response, he is enthusiastic and responds with physical affection by tickling him. Tickling is one of Hudson's favorite sensory activities so doing this adds to the effectiveness of his reinforcement for responding to the question.

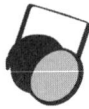

It is easier to coach Hudson to respond "yes, salami" in this scenario than to say "no milk" in the prior scenario. This is because Hudson is motivated by his wish for salami, and his father makes getting the salami contingent on asking for salami. In the prior scenario, since Hudson doesn't want milk, he is not very motivated to say "no." When you are first teaching your child to communicate, it will be easier for them to learn to ask for things that you know that they are motivated to have! However, it is also important they understand how they can say "no" with a gesture or word instead of withdrawing with a nonresponse. It is important to praise your child for saying "no" to indicate that they don't want something.

Using Distractions

All children will protest when asked to stop doing a highly rewarding activity. In Hudson's case, his father limits the use of his favorite activity–spinning—in order to reserve it as a reward for doing other social behaviors. One effective strategy for responding to protests to stopping an enjoyable activity is to distract the child and redirect their attention to another interesting activity. In the next scenario, watch how Hudson's father sets a limit on the amount of spinning activity and tries to redirect his son's protests.

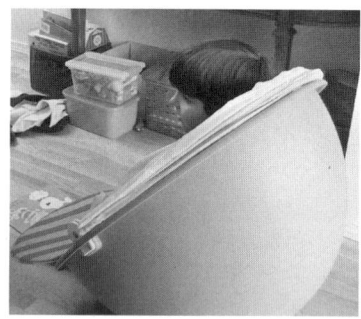

Father: Okay, we'll spin one last time, last time, then we are going to look at the choice board and you can decide what to do next, okay? (*warning of transition*)

Hudson: (protests) No choice board, no choice board.

Father: Whee! Okay all done spinning. Phew I'm all tuckered out.

Hudson: (yells) More spinning. more spinning. I don't want the choice board.

Father: I know it's frustrating to stop spinning. I hear you don't want the choice board.

Hudson: I don't want the choice board.

Father: There are some pretty fun things on here. (*ignores Hudson's protesting and redirects to choice board*)

Hudson: (yells) No, no choice board.

Father: (points to picture on card) We can set up a train track.

Hudson: (not looking) I want to spin some more. (yelling)

Father: We are all done spinning for now. (*repeats limit calmly*)

Father: I'm going to go work on build a track (walks a few feet away from Hudson and pulls out several pieces of track. Puts them together). I'm thinking I'll make a round track for Thomas and Percy. I wonder if I have enough pieces.

Hudson: Spin some more (regular voice, not yelling anymore).

Father: (not looking at Hudson) Hudson is good at making round tracks. I think I need curved pieces. Hudson do you see any curved pieces?

Hudson: (Does not respond verbally but is watching dad and takes a step towards him).

Father: (holds a piece of round track up to Hudson). Do you want to help me put this in?

Hudson: (takes piece and starts to place it on the track).

Father: Thanks for your help! Hey, it looks like your body is feeling calmer.

Considerations

This father does a great job of reminding and warning his child of the limit, telling Hudson that the next spin will be the last one. He tries to prevent Hudson's disappointment about stopping something he loves to do by reminding him of the choice board where he can choose another activity. However, Hudson resists this distraction and asserts his wish to continue spinning. Did you notice that when there is something Hudson wants, his language is more fluid and he is able to communicate a clear want? This suggests that with the snack scene we saw earlier, he was not motivated enough by the milk or snacks to use his words.

Ignore, Redirect, Distract

After setting the initial limit, Hudson's father validates and labels his frustration once, repeats the limit calmly, and then ignores his continued protests. Instead, he diverts his attention to building a train track. This is an activity that Hudson enjoys, although not as much as spinning. Hudson's father does a good job of providing Hudson with opportunities to join in the track building, while also allowing him space to calm down and make the transition to a new activity. When Hudson finally takes a piece of track to help build, his father praises him for helping and labels his calm emotional state.

It is an art to set a limit, ignore protests, and still stay calmly present to help your child transition to a new activity. Above all, it is important for the parent to stay calm, like Hudson's father does. It is understandable for parents to feel frustrated when children tantrum and protest. Unfortunately, when parents show their frustration, children's dysregulation is also likely to escalate. It is also important to know when to disengage from the child's protests. Hudson's father initially labeled his son's feelings about ending the spinning and then calmly reminded him of the limit, but after that, further discussion about the limit or Hudson's frustration would have been counterproductive. Hudson's father engaged him indirectly with the train activity and allowed Hudson to make a transition to calmer behavior before talking to him directly.

Managing Misbehavior

As we just saw, distractions can be a helpful way to support a child who is dysregulated or his having trouble transitioning from one activity to another. However, there are times when a child is too fixated on an idea or too dysregulated to be easily distracted. In these cases, parents' continued efforts to distract a child may be counterproductive. Think about what his happening in this scene with Hudson and his father. What is Hudson learning from his father's continual attempts to distract him? Hudson would like to play with his father's phone, but he has already used his screen time for the day.

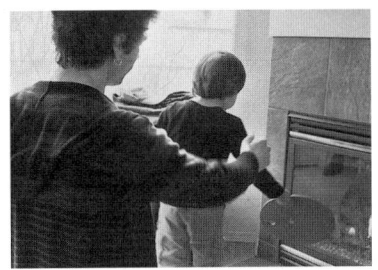

Father: Sorry, no more screen time. Hudson how about if we read one of your library books? (*distraction attempt*)

Hudson: (hits his father)

Father: Hey Hudson, no hitting. We can have a calm body. (*calmly states limit*)

Hudson: (continues to shove father)

Father: We can have a calm body—safe hands. Okay safe hands. (*repeats rule*)

Hudson: (starts shoving and hitting the chair)

Father: I have a different idea Hudson...Do you want to have a little bit of warm milk on my lap? (*Attempts distraction again*)

Hudson: No! (hits chair again)

Father: Say, "I'm mad." (*encourages word use of feeling*)

Hudson: (hits chair again)

Father: Hudson is mad.

Hudson: (hits chair) I want phone. I want phone.

Father: You can take a deep breath, you can take a deep breath, you can practice being calm. (*prompts deep breathing*)

Hudson: No calm! (hits chair again).

Father: When I'm mad, I take a deep breath, (*models taking deep breaths*)

Hudson: (pushes chair over, seems more dysregulated).

Father: I say, I'm going to be okay. I'm going to take deep breaths. (*models positive self-talk and breathing*)

Hudson: No breathing!
Father: You want a hug Hudson? I'll give you a hug. *(attempts to provide support by putting his arms around Hudson to hug him)*
Hudson: *(moves away and rejects hug)*
Father: Say, "no thank you." (calm voice)
Hudson: No!! (yelling)...

Considerations

Hudson's father sets a calm and clear limit and then unsuccessfully tries to redirect Hudson to several different activities (book, warm milk, hug). When he realizes these distractions aren't working, he tries to prompt Hudson to use his words to express his feelings and take deep breaths by saying, "you can take a deep breath and practice being calm." Hudson responds by rejecting these ideas and his behavior escalates to hitting and pushing over the chair. The father responds again with offering a hug and prompting him to say, "no thank you".

This father offers some great distraction strategies and prompts a self-regulation skill of breathing and positive self-talk, saying, "I am going to be okay." It is admirable that he remains calm and supportive during this frustrating interaction. Although his goal is to help Hudson calm down, his continued efforts may be fueling Hudson's tantrum. It is likely that Hudson is too dysregulated to process his father's words and the continued verbal input may be making him more agitated and frustrated. It is also possible that Hudson is holding out hope that he can still have the phone and that he interprets his father's distractions as a negotiation process. Hudson may believe that if he holds out long enough and rejects all his father's ideas, that he will eventually be able to use the phone. In either case, the father's continued attention is serving to reinforce or exacerbate Hudson's protests. After Hudson's father initially tried distraction and emotion coaching, it would have been better to switch to ignoring. He could have turned away, modeled taking some deep breaths, and perhaps started playing with one of Hudson's favorite toys. This would remove the attention that Hudson was getting for his protests and allowed Hudson some time and space to process and move through his anger. Hudson's anger would eventually start to subside and then his father could have reintroduced a distraction.

It is important to know when to stop distracting, prompting, and coaching. Children on the spectrum often need more repetition than neurotypical children, so it is appropriate to calmly repeat a limit, warning, or distraction 2-3 times. Watch for your child's response as you do this. If your child is responsive, begins to calm down, or looks interested in what you are saying or doing, then continuing to engage in this way may help your child regulate.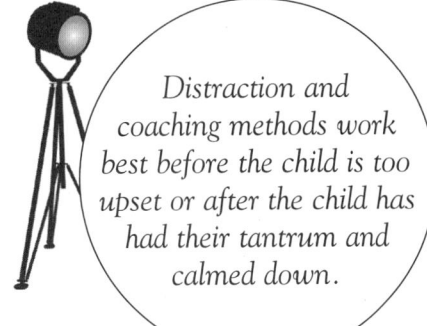

Distraction and coaching methods work best before the child is too upset or after the child has had their tantrum and calmed down.

If, on the other hand, your child gets louder, more agitated, or becomes more aggressive, this is a sign that they are too dysregulated to be able to respond to your distraction or coaching efforts. These distraction and coaching methods work best before the child is too upset or after the child has had their tantrum and calmed down. The problem with continuing to offer further suggestions when the child is dysregulated is that the parental attention is now reinforcing the child's oppositional behavior.

Here are five steps to remember when setting a limit with your child.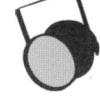

Step #1: Give a clear warning, with lead time, that the activity will soon end; use a timer, bell, gesture or visual prompt to signal the transition. Let your child know what will happen next.

Step #2: Simply state the limit or tell your child that activity is finished with calm voice.

Step #3: Redirect child to the next activity. If possible, give choices (between two activities that child enjoys or of what the child wants to do first if there is a required task); use a picture of possible choices or show actual objects.

Step #4: If defiance continues, ignore and start another activity or task with enthusiasm.

Step #5: Return your attention as soon as your child is calm. Continue to redirect your child's attention to the new activity or task.

Effective Ignoring

Differential Attention: A concept we call *"differential attention"* means that it is important to give attention to and reward behaviors you want to see more of, while not giving attention to and ignoring the undesirable behaviors you want to see less of. Your child will eventually learn there are no benefits to exhibiting misbehavior while there are benefits for positive, prosocial behaviors.

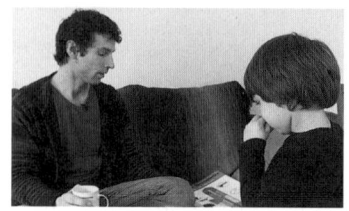

As the scenario with Hudson continues, notice what happens when the father withdraws from the interaction and ignores his son's protests. Think about what makes this approach more effective.

Father: No hug. Okay, guess what? Since you haven't had anything to drink yet, I'm going to make you some warm milk, and you can have it if you want to. (Father walks away into the kitchen to warm up milk and ignores Hudson)

Hudson: (hitting chair)

Father: (not looking at Hudson but at microwave) Almost ready 11, 10, 9… (Hudson stops hitting chair and moves away from it. He is watching his father warm the milk). What do you think? Shall we have it at the kitchen table, or do you want to sit on my lap?

Hudson: Sit on your lap.

Father: Okay, oh you're bringing the arrow back over to the sign…are you going to bring the thermometer with you? You can bring the thermometer over here. Hudson, your body is calm. Thank you.

Considerations

When the father walked away from his son and stopped giving attention to the oppositional behavior, it didn't take long for Hudson to stop hitting the chair and to calm down. This father's ignore strategy was effective because he stayed calm, walked away to do something else, and did not give Hudson any visual or verbal attention. Although he was ignoring Hudson's aggressive behavior, he was on the lookout for a chance to re-engage Hudson in a positive way. As soon as Hudson calmed down a little, his father tried the distraction again. At this point, Hudson seems to understand that the argument for the phone is not going to work and has calmed down enough to accept the distraction. It is interesting that Hudson then brings the Calm Down Thermometer over to his father for discussion.

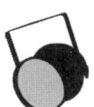

Think about how you respond when your child screams, tantrums, throws things, cries, whines, or ignores your requests. Make an ABC learning plan for giving your attention and rewards for using the positive opposite replacement behaviors such as using a gesture or word to ask for something, taking deep breath to stay calm, or complying to your requests. Try not to provide your child with what they want when they are behaving in inappropriate ways. Instead see if you can prompt your child to use an alternative, appropriate social strategy. Remember, if your child is too dysregulated, you may need to ignore and wait until your child is calmer to reengage, model, prompt, and reward the positive behavior.

Re-engaging and New Learning Opportunities

It is important to remember that after you ignore your child's negative behavior, you should quickly prompt and reinforce your child's positive opposite behavior: that is, the behavior you want to see, as soon as it occurs. As this scenario continues, Hudson brings over the calm down thermometer poster and arrow and they look at some visual picture of feeling faces together. Notice how the father gives his son attention for his calmer emotions and re-engages him into another learning opportunity.

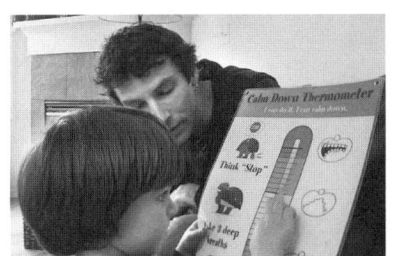

> **Father:** There goes the arrow. Oh, that's when you're mad. You were just a little bit mad a little bit recently. Looks like you're getting calmer. Looks like you are feeling more calm now. You can say, 'I'm feeling okay. I'm feeling better.'

Hudson: I say stop.
Father: Oh stop. Yes, that is what you can do when you feel mad. First you think "stop."
Hudson: (hand flapping)
Father: Stop, take deep breaths. (*models taking deep breaths*) Here you are. What's this?(points to happy face)
Hudson: (hand flapping) Mad.
Father: This one's happy, right. There's a big smile.
Hudson: This one's happy.
Father: This one is mad over here. Grrh. But then happy again. It doesn't take too long. You really like that arrow don't you? That is a cool arrow.
Hudson: He's say mad.
Father: Say mad. Talking about the mad face.
Hudson: He's mad. He's staying mad (has arrow on mad face).
Father: Okay I'll do a pretend mad. Do you want to look at my mad face? Grrh grrh.
Hudson: (arm flaps)
Father: That's pretty funny isn't it... grrh (makes mad face)
Hudson: Talk about this one.
Father: You want me to talk about this one. Can you look at me? What did you say?
Hudson: I want you to do this one?
Father: Can you ask me with your eyes?
Hudson: (looks at him)
Father: Thanks for looking at me. Oh, okay this one is really sad. I'm kind of worried and nervous.
Hudson: Papa. Talk about this one.
Father: You want me to talk about that one? (Tries to get eye contact.)
Hudson: (hand flaps)
Father: What should I say about it? What do you want me to say?
Hudson: Say happy.

Father: Say happy. Okay that's a very happy smiling face—yeah (smiles).

Hudson: (not looking)

Father: Look at my face Hudson, look at me.

Hudson: Say that one, Papa say that one.

Father: Okay but you got to look at me (smiles). Hee hee, oh you are doing it too. Hudson's doing the happy. Can you do a big smile? Show me a big smile. Look at me...let me see your eyes. Okay look at my eyes. Show me your eyes.

Hudson: (Preoccupied with poster but does look at father's eyes.) Papa talk about this one.

Father: Okay well the turtle is thinking stop because he doesn't like to feel mad. He doesn't want to be mad. He wants to be happy again so he says, "first thing I think is stop" and then what is next? What does he do next?

Hudson: Take deep breaths.

Father: That is right this is the word stop. "STOP" spells stop and then take three deep breaths.

Hudson: (moving arrow down)

Father: You can take even more if you want, you can take 10. You can count to 10 and take 10 deep breaths.

Hudson: Papa talk about this one.

Father: Okay we took our deep breaths...swish...and now he is totally happy and cool—he's even acting silly, look he's got a magnifying glass in his mouth

Considerations

This father does a great job of being child-directed and responding to Hudson's interest in the Calm Down thermometer by helping him talk about feelings and practice how to calm down. He makes it funny by showing him an angry face, which Hudson enjoys. Hudson shows his interest by continuing to ask his father to talk about more of the pictures on the chart. Knowing that this is attention grabbing and reinforcing for Hudson, the father uses this as an opportunity to work on helping him practice using eye contact when making a request and teaching emotion language. He is even successful at getting Hudson to tell him what the feeling word is.

Limit Setting & Redirecting

In the next scenario notice how Amelia's mother sets a limit on what ball can be used in the house and redirects her daughter to use the softer ball.

> **Mother:** Would you like to throw it in the bucket?
> **Amelia:** (throws hard ball)
> **Mother:** You know what? This ball is a little hard. How about we do a softer ball? (mother picks up the hard ball and puts it in her pocket).
> **Amelia:** I don't want to do a softer ball.
> **Mother:** I hear that you want the hard ball, but it's not safe. (hands her a softer ball)
> **Amelia:** (throws softer ball)
> **Mother:** Thanks for doing the softer ball so we didn't hit anything or break anything, good thinking.
> **Amelia:** I'm going to throw this... (throws it over shoulder)
> **Mother:** Wow big throw over your shoulder.

Considerations

This mother effectively sets a limit by removing the hard ball and giving her daughter the softer and safer ball. She states the reason for the limit (safety) and then distracts Amelia back to the throwing activity. In all likelihood, the initial protest about which ball to use was likely Amelia's response to wanting to assert independence when a limit was set. Since Amelia's main goal was to throw the ball, once it was clear that the mother was not going to give in or engage in a discussion about which ball, Amelia easily accepted the substitute.

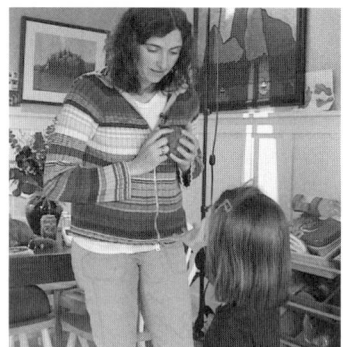

Often, avoiding an argument about the rule or limit and simply offering the alternative will prevent a meltdown.

Ignoring

As the scenario continues notice how the mother effectively uses the concept of "differential attention," that is, holding back briefly on providing what her daughter wants, while prompting and modeling the desired behavior. She ignores the child behaviors she wants to see less of and gives attention to her appropriate behavior. Think about what Amelia is learning.

Mother: (picks up the ball). It's my turn. My turn.
Amelia: (cries) I want it.
Mother: So, you want a turn? How can you ask like a big girl? Do you remember? "May I have a turn please?"
Amelia: Give it right now.
Mother: (bouncing ball in air and ignoring her)
Amelia: (yelling) Give it right now Mama. Give it right now Mama. Give it now Mama.
Mother: (ignoring and bouncing ball)
Amelia: Because Mama, I say give it right now? (Goes to grab it.)
Mother: (whispers) May I have a turn please?
Amelia: May I have a turn please?
Mother: That was such nice asking.
Amelia: Did I say please?
Mother: You did say please. It was so polite. That's a really nice way to ask.
Amelia: I think I just said, "may I"? (throws ball over shoulder)

Considerations: ABC's of Learning

This is a good example of the ABCs of learning. Here the motivating antecedent(A) is the ball, which Amelia wants to have. The mother wants her daughter to learn how to ask for a turn in a polite way. Therefore, she won't give her the ball until she gets the target polite asking behavior (B). She ignores her yelling and prompts the correct behavior by whispering, "May I have a turn please". Once Amelia does ask politely (may I have a turn please) she responds by giving her the ball which is the rewarding consequence (C). Thus Amelia is learning what behaviors will get her what she wants.

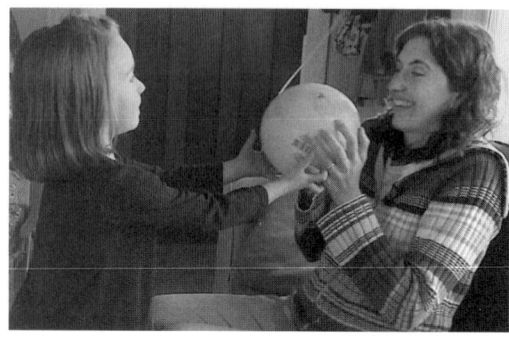

Ignoring and Attending

In the next scenario think about what makes Amelia's mother's ignore strategy particularly effective.

Amelia is getting over-excited with the ball game, and her mother enforces a short running break to calm down which she uses when Amelia is beginning to become dysregulated. Amelia is unhappy about this suggestion.

Mother: Running break.
Amelia: No Mama not a running break.
Mother: Just a short calm-down break.
Amelia: (runs in and hits mother)
Mother: (walks away)
Amelia: What you doing Mama? (comes and touches her arm calmly)
Mother: Playing with the ball. Thanks for calming your body down. That was nice calming your body down so fast (gives her ball).
Amelia: (takes ball from mother and throws it over her shoulder)
Mother: Oh, up in the air (starts to throw ball).

Considerations

Frequently when Amelia begins to get dysregulated, suggesting a running break serves to calm her down. But this time Amelia doesn't like the idea. When Amelia hits, her mother remains calm, patient, and walks away; ignoring this behavior. She gives Amelia no eye contact or verbal contact and has moved her body away. Amelia responds by asking politely what she is doing, and the mother immediately returns her attention, praises her for calming down, and rewards her by giving her the desired ball. It is important to realize that ignores can be very brief and it is important to return attention as soon as the child is behaving appropriately.

Coping with Tantrums

Ignoring is only effective if there is a strong positive relationship between the child and the adult that is strategically ignoring. Ameila's mother has put enthusiasm and time into developing a positive, engaging, and rewarding relationship with her daughter, and this means that Amelia doesn't like it when her mother withdraws her attention.

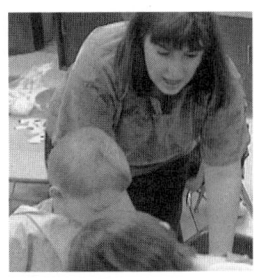

In the next scenario we will see a boy who has no expressive language skills. He is tantruming because his teacher has taken away the bubble wand, explaining it is not safe. He wants it back and tantrums. Notice how the teacher initially tries a distraction and redirection and then realizes she needs to use the ignore strategy.

Bubble table: Hanook is waving a long bubble maker around and it almost hits several other children at the table in the eyes.

Teacher: Stop. Let go, please. Hanook. This one's all gone. You can choose a different one. No, it's too dangerous. Look, you can come and make another choice. *(calmly sets limit and removes bubble wand)*

Hanook: (Fusses, grabs her hand, and tries to take the bubble wand back)

Teacher: You can come and pick a different bubble maker. It's all gone (puts the wand in the hall outside classroom door). It gets in kids' eyes. That's not safe. *(gives reason for the limit)*. Pick another bubble maker? (holds another bubble toy out)

Hudson: (looks towards the table, briefly interested)

Teacher: All right. We okay now? Bubbles need to stay in the table. Do you want to do this? Look, there are lots of other bubble makers in here. *(tries to distract)*

Child: (walks away from teacher to door where bubble wand was put, crying loudly)

Teacher: Oh, Hanook. It's all gone. It's all gone. You can choose doctor, or you can do more bubbles, or you can choose something else. *(tried distract, but Hanook pushes her away and drops to the floor in a tantrum)*

Teacher: (turns away from Hanook and gives attention to other children) Wow, look what Rachel's doing. You're doing a good job Rachel. Look what you're making! Wow! The bubbles look like fun! This is fun. (teacher joins in the bubbles table with the other children and blows some bubbles over in Hanook's direction).

Hanook: (gets up walks towards bubble table. No longer crying.)

Teacher: Oh look, Hanook, look. (holds bubble maker up and Hanook blows a bubble). Oh, Hanook, you're blowing bubbles! Here, Hanook, blow. Whoa, you made lots of bubbles! Good job!

Hanook: (big smile)

Teacher: (excited tone and very positive) Whoa! Oh, Hanook! You made some big bubbles! And Hanook is playing calmly at the bubble table.

Considerations

In this scenario the teacher sets a limit by taking away Hanook's bubble wand explaining it is all gone because it is not safe. She initially tries to distract him with other bubble makers, but he is too upset to listen and starts to escalate, pushing her away. She ignores his tantruming behavior and focuses on the other children. She does not give him eye contact. It is possible to ignore this tantrum, even in a class of other children because Hanook is not lashing out at others. The other children are engrossed in their own play and understand that their teacher is making sure that Hanook is safe. Her positive

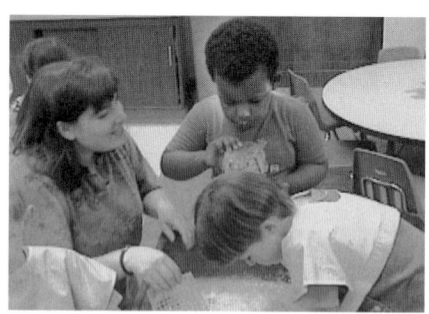

attention to their play reinforces their desire to keep playing and likely helps them ignore Hanook's fussing. Very soon after the teacher begins ignoring Hanook's tantrum, he calms down. At this point, the teacher reintroduces a distraction, blowing some bubbles in his direction to see if he is calm enough to re-engage. As he comes over to the table, she continues to provide opportunities for him to rejoin the play. At the end, she praises his calm body.

What is remarkable about this teacher is her ability to stay calm and patient while waiting for Hanook to self-regulate.

Differential Attention

The next scenario is an example of how Amelia's mother uses differential attention with her puppet to help her daughter learn to be gentle in her interactions. Think about what makes her approach effective.

Amelia:	(grabbed turtle again)
Tiny Turtle:	Oh, that scares me. (turtle sets limit)
Amelia:	(grabs turtle again somewhat aggressively)
Mother:	(takes turtle away and ignores)
Amelia:	Mama don't. Mama don't.
Mother:	(using turtle puppet to talk to Truman) Truman I am a turtle, and I'm scared. Can I come hang out with you? Hi.
Amelia:	Mama don't. Mama can you pass it to me Mama?
Mother:	I think turtle needs you to be gentle. (Truman is looking at turtle.) He's scared when you are rough with him. We need to be gentle with our friends to help them feel safe. He's going in his turtle shell, which means he needs to protect himself to feel better.
Amelia:	(trying to grab turtle)
Mother:	Can you be gentle? Turtle come on out.
Amelia:	(grabs again aggressively)

Mother:	(ignores and talks to Truman) Truman do you want to say hi to the turtle? Oh you are being so gentle.
Truman:	(pats turtle)
Mother:	Truman you are being so gentle.
Amelia:	Can I do that too?
Mother:	Truman was really gentle. I know you can be gentle. You are such a big girl.
Amelia:	Can I do that too?
Mother:	Can you show me how you can be gentle.
Amelia:	I was gentle.
Mother:	Do you want to try again? Show me how you can be gentle.
Amelia:	I want to try again Mama, (gives him a gentle pat)
Tiny Turtle:	Oh thank you for being gentle. I want to be your friend now (kiss each other) because you were gentle with me. Thank you. You are such a good friend when you are gentle. You make me feel safe. That makes me feel so happy.
Mother:	That was nice Amelia, you were so good to him.

Considerations

This mother has been working hard to help Amelia learn to be gentle and friendly with her younger brother and with her peers at school. Through pretend play with the turtle puppet, she can help Amelia learn what turtle feels like when he is poked or treated roughly. She models how turtle goes in his shell to feel safe and calm down. After she prompts Amelia to be gentle and has the turtle tell her he doesn't like to be grabbed, Ameila continues to be rough. At this point, the mother withdraws her attention and praises her brother for being gentle (proximal praise). Clearly Amelia doesn't like it when her mother's turtle attention is given to her brother. Did you notice that the mother needed to withdraw her attention

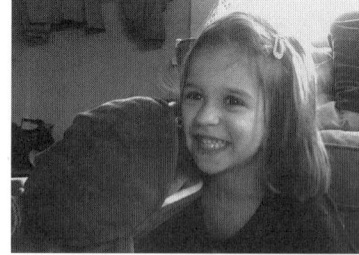

several times before Amelia was ready to be gentle. It's important that the mother gives Amelia multiple chances to try again to be gentle. When Amelia isn't ready, her mother immediately switches back to ignoring without giving more instructions or attention. Amelia finally responds by agreeing to pat the turtle gently. Once she demonstrates gentle behavior, she is rewarded by both the turtle's and mother's positive feedback.

Handling Misbehavior

Now you will see another example of Amelia's mother using the concept of differential attention during her reading times with her daughter. Notice how she ignores Amelia's inappropriate behavior by giving her brother attention and then quickly returns her attention to her daughter when she is calm and speaks politely.

Mother: (stands up)
Amelia: (protests) Here Mama, here.
Mother: Okay one second, my leg fell asleep.
Amelia: (cries)
Mother: Let me just shift. it's okay.
Amelia: You just giving me a…I don't want you to…
Mother: Are you feeling a little sad?
Amelia: (growls angrily, grabs mom's arm)
Mother: (ignores and turns to Truman) Truman do you want to see the book? See the book, see what's in there?
Amelia: Read it Mama.
Mother: It's my turn, it's my turn.(reading dialog from the book)
Amelia: Mama face this way to me, look at me.
Mother: Oh hi you calmed yourself down, that's nice.
Amelia: Read it to me.
Mother: Read it to both of you.
Amelia: Yeah.
Mother: Okay, you've calmed your body down.
Amelia: Why did you not read it to me?
Mother: Do you know why?
Amelia: (grunts angrily)

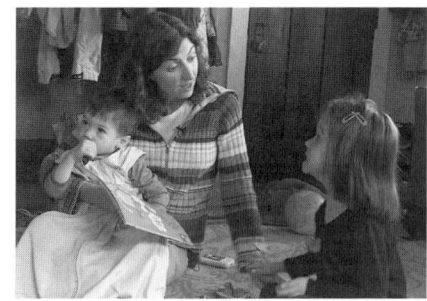

Mother: You got angry, and you were yelling. I can't read when you yell. Did you feel angry? Next time, you can say: "I'm angry."
Amelia: Mama can you read this? Can you say the words?
Mother: Sure, can you say "please?"
Amelia: Mama may I please may I, will you...
Mother: Please.
Amelia: Will you do the words.
Mother: Yeah I will, thank you for asking in such a calm voice.
Amelia: Did I say please?
Mother: You did say please the first time. Thank you for being so calm and being so polite and asking nicely. Oscar and Tilly found a playground.

Ignoring and Taking a Break

In the next scenario we will see that Amelia is upset because the story reading time has ended. The mother uses the ignore technique with her and models some self-calming strategies. Think about why the mother needed to completely remove her attention and ignore her misbehavior.

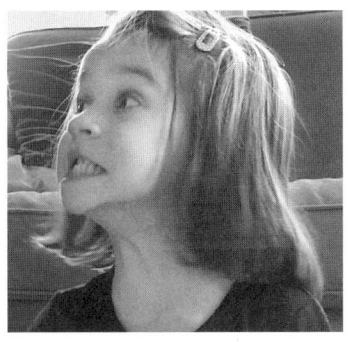

Mother closes the book.
Amelia: (crying) You didn't finish.
Mother: I did finish, honey. I see that you are sad. It's hard when the book is over.
Ameila: (crying)
Mother: Do you need a break to calm down?
Amelia: (screaming) No, no, no, no, you don't, Mama, Mama.
Mother: (turns away to ignore, takes deep breaths)
Amelia: (crying) I want to finish the book Mama...Mama I want to finish it.
Mother: (deep breathing) I can count to three breaths, one......two.......three.......
Amelia: (crying)

Mother: I did finish the book, sweetie. I don't know exactly what you wanted me to finish. Can you tell me?
Amelia: (yells) No (starts hitting her).
Mother: I think you need a break.
Amelia: (screaming) I want you to read this again, Mama I want you to read again.
Mother: (gets up and walks away)
Amelia: (cries and screams) Mama what you doing Mama? Mama What are you doing Mama? (Gets up and follows her to other room) What are you doing Mama? Mama, why did you walk away?
Mother: Are you calmer now? You calmed yourself down.
Amelia: Why did you walk away? Why did you do this?
Mother: You needed a little bit of time honey.
Amelia: Why did you do this?
Mother: You needed a little bit of time sweetie.
Ameila: Why did you do this?
Mother: I told you sweetie.
Amelia: No you didn't.
Mother: You were upset, and I think you needed time to take a break.
Amelia: (yells) No, I didn't, no I didn't…(strikes Mother).
Mother: (walks away)

Considerations

The mother makes the right decision to ignore Amelia's protests and hitting behavior. She tries to prompt her to use one of her self-regulation skills by taking deep breaths, which is a good idea. However, mother does not continue to ignore long enough, and Amelia is able to re-engage her with discussions about why she is walking away. Ameila is still dysregulated and her distress escalates again as her mother tries to explain why she is ignoring. Although it is tempting to explain and answer your child's questions when they are upset, remember that a dysregulated child is not really listening or processing anything that you say. It would have been more effective if Amelia's mother had ignored until Amelia was much calmer and then redirected her to another activity.

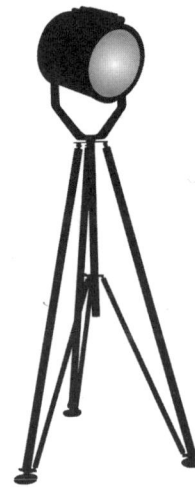

SPOTLIGHTING
Ignoring

- Validate your child's upset feelings (briefly), "I see you are mad." and then ignore if behavior escalates.
- Avoid eye contact and discussion while ignoring.
- Physically move away from your child but stay in the room to assure child is safe.
- Be prepared for testing.
- Be consistent.
- Let your child know once how to get your attention back: "I can listen when you're calm."
- Model using a calm-down strategy without directly engaging with your child: "I'm going to go over here and sit calm. I'm going to take three deep breaths."
- Return your attention as soon as misbehavior stops and your child has calmed down.
- Combine distractions and redirections with ignoring. Use visual prompts of "likes" for possible distractions for what else child can do.
- Choose specific child behaviors to ignore and make sure they are ones you can ignore.
- Limit the number of behaviors to systematically ignore.
- Give more attention to the positive opposite behaviors you want to encourage.

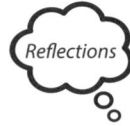

Parent Reflections about Managing Misbehavior

Father: *The idea of differential attention and giving attention to the positives is not something I've always known. The main thing he does is that he'll just start hitting or throwing things and talking about doing things that are dangerous. Like he'll say, "I'm gonna go touch the fireplace." It's been a challenge to just ignore all those things, but I can see that he's usually saying them because he knows they get a reaction. I feel like ignoring has helped quite a bit. In the past we may have thought that we were ignoring these types of behaviors, but gave them some attention, especially if I didn't know for sure whether he was bluffing, but now I figured out* *he's not gonna touch the fire. He knows that that would hurt, so I'm able to just ignore.*

Mother: *Differential attention has really helped our household. The Incredible Years has really helped me solidify that and remind myself to stay in the positive.*

If she's yelling or not asking nicely, I might shift to her brother and describe how he's waiting patiently for a turn and describe what he's doing. And then, usually, quickly, she'll come back and say, you know, "Mama, why are you talking to Truman?" And then I turn to her and say, "Oh your using your big girl words now, that's so great. Thank you!"

Father: *When he has extreme meltdowns, I feel like they're a lot shorter now. Being able to just distract myself with other things helped quite a bit. Even if I'm just pretending to do something else, it definitely helps a lot more than just doing nothing and pretending like I'm ignoring him.*

Mother: *As we learned in The Incredible Years, I try to do it very subtly to not make it a big deal. She knows right away. So I think she knows right away how she's supposed to respond. And sometimes she tries to keep egging me on, like she might yell again and again and see if I'll answer, and then I just wait until I get the nice words, and then immediately shift back.*

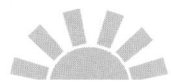

To Sum Up...

Consistency is the essence of ignoring. When your child throws a tantrum, you may be tempted to give in. However, each time you do so, you make the misbehavior worse because you teach your child that she can outlast you. The next time the tantrum will be louder and last longer. Therefore, if you decide to use ignoring, you must be determined to ignore until the misbehavior stops. Effective ignoring is planned, brief, strategic, and paired with giving attention to the "positive opposite" behavior as well as distraction or redirection. Sometimes you are ignoring a part of what your child is doing, while still attending to some other behavior. Above all, ignoring is an active process and requires parents and teachers to remain calm, engaged, and present in the interaction, while not engaging in the child's inappropriate behavior.

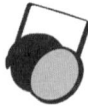

Remember ignoring a child on the spectrum is not likely to be effective unless you have worked hard to be in your child's attention spotlight when they are behaving appropriately and a positive relationship and attachment has been built up between you.

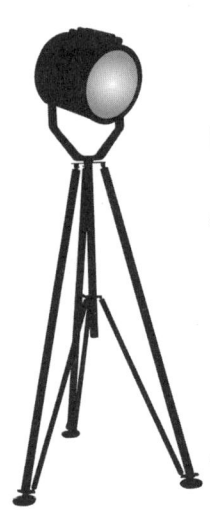

SPOTLIGHTING

Positive Discipline Helps My Child Feel Loved and Secure

- Schedule times daily to engage in interactive child-directed play using prompts and modeling to get your child's attention and spotlight the social behaviors and language you want to encourage; remember you can maximize your child's learning by using these strategies during meals, bedtime routines, and your other care giving routines.
- Use descriptive commenting narrations, pre-academic, persistence, social, and emotional coaching strategies during child-directed play times.
- Use puppets to model appropriate social and emotional behaviors as well as self-regulation skills.
- Use physical sensory routines, praise, and salient rewards to motivate your child's interest in using targeted social and emotional skills and communication.
- Teach your child self-regulation skills using puppets, books, imaginary play, and visual prompts.
- Teach your child how to follow instructions and use reminders, redirections, distractions, visual prompts, and choices to pre-empt misbehavior.

- Withdraw your attention and ignore misbehaviors that are not hurtful to others or to themselves; spotlight your attention on your child just as soon as a positive behavior is used.
- Pace yourself one step at a time.

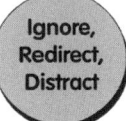

Remember every time a negative behavior is not reinforced and, instead, the positive opposite behavior is rewarded with your attention spotlight and coaching, a productive learning opportunity has occurred. In fact, every interaction with your child is a potential learning opportunity.

CHAPTER 10

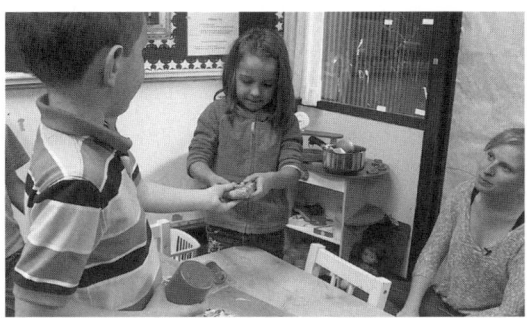

Spotlighting Children's Joint Play with Peers

Introduction
Children on the autism spectrum often show less motivation or ability to play with peers. Sometimes they seem completely unaware of the other children, even when sitting next to them. In other cases, they may desire social interactions but do not know how to initiate or sustain play with another child. They find it difficult to shift their attention from their solitary play to joint play and struggle to take turns, share, help, or respond to other children's ideas or conversation. Play interactions require an understanding of complex social "rules" and norms as well as an ability to engage in reciprocal communication. Many children on the spectrum feel overwhelmed by the

demands of these social situations, and their anxiety, confusion, and frustration can lead to emotional dysregulation, oppositionality, tantrums, aggressive behavior, and a breakdown in the social interaction. As a result, they are often not fun to play with, and so other children may not seek them out. This results in further social isolation and fewer chances for the child on the spectrum to observe and learn from their peers and to practice the skills needed to be successful in social peer interactions.

In the earlier chapters, we focused on the important role that parents and teachers can play in enhancing children's social connections, pretend play, communication skills, social skills, and emotion regulation skills during spotlighted coached play. These one-on-one child-directed interactions with parents and teachers provide a strong base for the next step; widening the child's attention spotlight to include peers and other people. In this chapter we will discuss how to provide small group peer coaching to support children's interactions with other children. We will talk about how to use visual prompts, scaffolded exercises, and adult-child play scripts to help children practice reciprocal interactions and joint play with peers. These scripted scenarios are taken from preschool classroom observations where teachers are

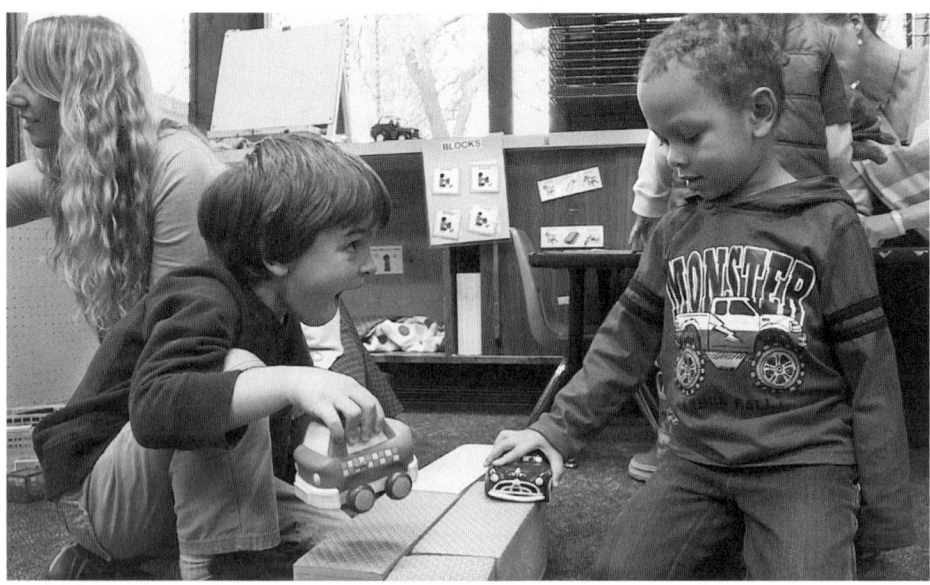

supporting and coaching Amelia, Hudson, and other children on the autism spectrum to learn to socially interact with each other in joint play. Parents can also use these strategies with siblings, during playdates, or when they work in the preschool classroom. Participating in the classroom is beneficial so parents can see how their child interacts with peers and identify possible play mates.

Encouraging Joint Play

In the next scenario, a teacher is playing with Hudson and another child who is also on the autism spectrum. Both children have a toy car and large blocks. Notice the language the teacher uses to help the boys become aware of each other and how she tries to engage them in a joint play activity where she prompts them to decide how to play together.

Teacher: Should we make the blocks longer?
Payton: (shakes head no.)
Teacher: Payton says "no." (*spotlights Paytons' intentional communication for Hudson.*) What do you think, Hudson? Should we make it longer?
Hudson: (nods head yes.)
Payton: (shakes head no.)
Teacher: Yeah? Hudson wants it longer. (*spotlights Hudson's intentional communication*) Okay. Here's the block. Hudson says, "I'm going to make this side longer." (puts block on the end and then both children put cars on road and play together.) Oh! You guys are driving the cars! Uh-oh. Here's a bumpy road. (makes car noises.) What do you think? Where should it go?
Payton: Yeah!
Teacher: Yeah? Bump, bump, bump, bump, bump. (scratches block and makes a scratchy noise.)
Teacher: Payton, where do you think it should go?
Payton: Bumpy side.
Teacher: On the bumpy side? Should it go here, or should it go here? (points)

Payton: Here (points to place).
Teacher: (hands Payton block) Okay. You show me. Good idea.
Payton: (puts block down on his side)
(both children play together each running a car on a block, teacher makes car driving noises.)
Teacher: Ah! Crash! You are playing together and are being so friendly. Nice work.

Considerations

In this scenario the teacher encourages the boys to communicate and make a choice together about how they want to build the road. She spotlights their nonverbal responses of "yes" and "no" to draw the other child's attention to their peer's communication efforts (spotlights their intentional communication). We see that when she repeats the word "bump," Payton responds saying he wants the road to go on the bumpy side. She is child-directed and encourages Payton to choose where to put the block. She gets into the boys' attention spotlights by positioning herself face-to-face with both children, using animated crash and bumpy sound effects, and repeating key words (longer and bump). She enthusiastically labels the friendship skills of being friendly and playing together.

Remember to pause, wait, and give children time to indicate their response with a gesture or word.

This teacher paces her question asking effectively. She spaces out questions with child-directed descriptive commenting in between. When asking questions, it is important to wait and give the child a chance to process the words and respond to the question. If a child doesn't respond immediately, adults often assume that the child didn't hear or didn't understand the question. However, all children take longer than adults to answer questions, and children on the autism spectrum take even longer. Remember to pause, wait, and give children time to indicate their response with a gesture or word. Jumping in too quickly with a second question may actually distract the child and force them to start all over again with the sequence of processing the question and responding.

Unintentional communication is when child does things without realizing their actions, sounds, or words can have an effect on others. Intentional communication on the part of children means the child understands that what they do or say can have an effect on another person. In other words, they communicate with words or gestures on purpose to let someone know something. Teachers and parents can help children hear and focus on the intentional communication of their peers by highlighting their meaning and intentions. For example: the teacher above said: "Hudson wants it longer" when Hudson nodded his head. Payton likely did not notice the head nod but may hear his teacher's words about Hudson's wishes.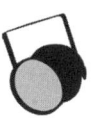

Encouraging Social Peer Communication—Asking and Answering

In the next scenario, children in Amelia's class are having lunch together at a large table. The teacher encourages Amelia and her friend to practice asking and answering questions in a verbal social interaction. Think about what each child is learning and how the teacher supports their social communication. Nica is looking at Amelia's milk box.

Nica: Here (hands back Amelia's milk box).
Amelia: (looking at teacher) That made me feel so happy.
Teacher: Oh, she gave you back your milk box? You could tell her, 'thank you!' (To Nica) That was friendly, Nica. *(prompts child social response)*
Amelia: Yeah.
Nica: I can't see it. Can I see it? Can I see it? (tries to grab Amelia's milk box back to look at pictures on box)
Teacher: (stops Nica from grabbing milk box back.) Oh, you asked a question. You can ask again, and let's wait for Amelia to respond.
Nica: Can I see it?
Amelia: (shakes head no.)
Teacher: Oh, good asking Nica, but she said no. It's hers. *(spotlighting intentional communication)*
Nica: Why?

Teacher: I don't know. You can ask her. (*prompts asking*)
Nica: Why? Amelia, can I have that. I just look at it.
Teacher: Nica, that was friendly asking (*praise for asking*).
Amelia: Because it is from my house.
Teacher: Oh because it is from her house. She doesn't want to drink it, Amelia. She just wants to look at it. (*spotlighting intentional communication*)
Nica: I want to look at it.
Teacher: Good asking. Go ask her again. (*prompts asking*)
Nica: Can I look at it?
Amelia: (Shakes head no.)
Teacher: Amelia says "no." Nica, that was such friendly asking. You waited and listened for her answer and asked again. I am proud of you for staying patient. (*labeled praise for friendly asking*)

Considerations

This teacher sets up an effective communication practice to encourage Nica to ask Amelia for what she wants rather than just taking Amelia's milk box. She helps Nica to learn to repeat her request despite being told no. Then she helps Amelia explain to her friend why she is not sharing. The teacher respects Amelia's decision not to share. Then she showers her positive attention spotlight on Nica for her ability to verbally ask for what she wanted, to wait for Amelia's reply, and to stay patient when Amelia still didn't want to share. The teacher turned this potential conflict into a powerful communication learning opportunity for both children.

Encouraging Social Peer Communication—Listening

In the next scenario the children continue having their lunch together. Notice how the teacher uses descriptive commenting and questions to encourage social communication sharing. Think about why the teacher makes sure Amelia has heard the other child's response. Think about what she is helping Amelia learn?

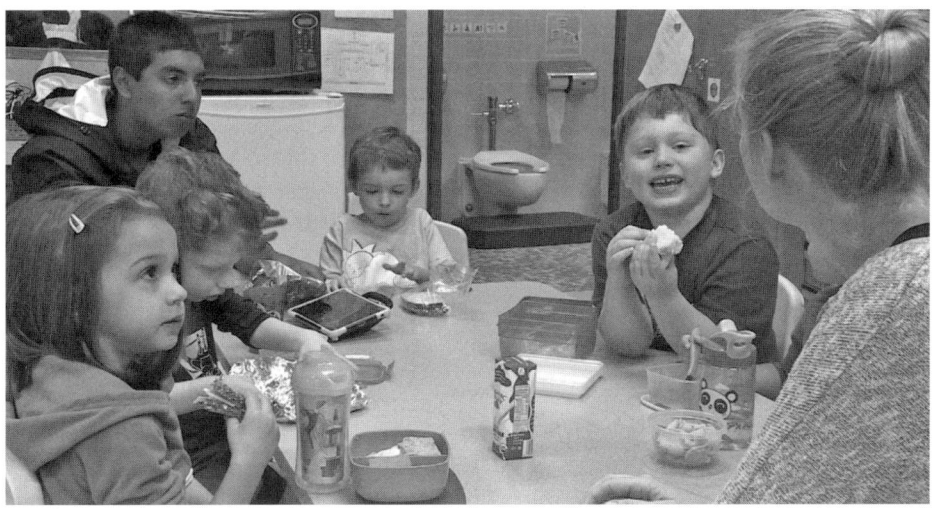

Teacher: Look at the table. Joe, Atlas, Nathan, and Amelia all have sandwiches. Four out of five kids have sandwiches.

Teacher: What is on your sandwich, Amelia?

Amelia: Um, my sandwich has…my sandwich is turkey and cheese.

Teacher: Nice answering Amelia. Hey, Joe, what's on your sandwich?

Joe: Hmm, cheese and meat.

Teacher: What kind of meat?

Joe: Ham.

Teacher: Ham. Hey Amelia, did you hear that? (*spotlighting intentional communication*) Joe has ham and cheese and you have turkey and cheese. You are both being friendly; telling what is in your sandwich. I wonder what the difference is between turkey and ham? Does anyone know?

Considerations

The teacher tries to structure the lunch time to make sure the children interact and communicate with each other. She models how to initiate social communication by asking Amelia and Joe what kind of sandwiches they are each eating. Eventually, with this modeling, the children will learn they can start a conversation with each other by asking a question. The teacher also repeats Joe's responses to make sure Amelia is aware of and understands what he has said to her. She praises them for talking together and prompts possible extension of their communication by asking them if they know what is the same and different in their sandwiches.

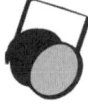

Think about how you can spotlight intentional communication for your children at mealtimes; that is, helping your child to be aware of what someone else at the table is doing or saying. Prompt your child and their siblings to ask questions of each other and share their likes and dislikes. If your child is an only child, then model this information communication between your child, yourself, and any other adults. Help your child on the spectrum to understand what someone else has said by spotlighting intentional communication.

Teacher-Directed Practices—
Asking and Sharing

Teacher child-directed descriptive commenting and social coaching supports children's ability to develop positive relationships with peers. It works because the teacher is modeling and prompting peer social interactions and because it shows the children that the teacher is interested in their development of friendships. For children on the autism spectrum, teachers work to get into their student's attention spotlight to scaffold short teacher-directed ABC practices between children based on the children's "likes". This is similar to the ABC one-on-one scenarios discussed in the earlier chapters only expanded to several children.

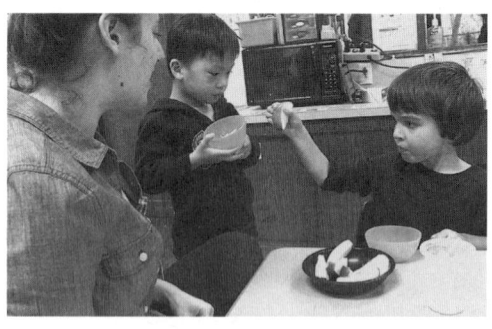

In the next scenario you will see a teacher setting up language practices at snack time. These children, who all have some language delays, are practicing how to ask for and tell each other what they want. Notice how the teacher scaffolds these learning experiences and think about how you might set up similar practices in your setting.

Teacher: Hudson, what would you like? Would you like apples, animal crackers or cheese? (points to each one in 3 bowls.)
Hudson: Crackers.
Teacher: (points at John) John is in charge of the crackers. So, Hudson you can go tap him on the shoulder. Go tap him on the shoulder (gives Hudson empty bowl) and ask for some animal crackers. That's a good choice.
Hudson: (gets up from table.)
John: I want some more apple.
Teacher: More apple? Well guess what? Hudson's going to ask you a question first, then you can ask Hudson for apple. Here comes Hudson to ask you a question, John.
John: I want some apples (starts to give a cracker to Hudson).
Teacher: John, wait for Hudson to ask. Hudson, say: "crackers please."
Hudson: Crackers please.
Teacher: Nice asking Hudson! And now John is sharing the crackers with you!
John: (puts crackers in Hudson's bowl and Hudson goes back to his seat)
Teacher: Good sharing, John.
Teacher: Okay, now John, you can go ask Hudson for some apples.
John: (goes over to Hudson's chair.)
Teacher: Nice listening John.
John: (taps Hudson on shoulder.) I want apples.
Hudson: (gives John apples.)
Teacher: Good asking John and nice sharing Hudson. You guys are doing such a good job being friendly and sharing with each other.
Teacher: (prompts Hudson to ask another child at the table for water)
Hudson: (taps Cazé on shoulder.)

Teacher: Hey Cazé, I think Hudson has a question for you. *(spotlight intentional communication)*

Cazé: I think a big bee. I think a big bee. (lost in own world)

Teacher: Hudson you can say "water please." *(prompts asking)*

Cazé: I think a big bee. (still not focused on Hudson)

Teacher: Hey, Cazé, listen. Hudson's trying to ask you something. *(spotlight intentional communication)*

Teacher: (to Hudson) What do you say? Water please.

Hudson: (mumbles softly and hard to know what he said) Water please.

Teacher: Good asking Hudson. Here comes Cazé being a big helper.

Cazé: (pours water into Hudson's glass.)

Hudson: (hands flapping.)

Teacher: Nice job asking Hudson.

Teacher: Wow Cazé, you're so good at pouring water. That's a good friend.

Teacher: Wow, Hudson, you got a lot of water. You look happy that your friend shared.

Considerations

The teacher has strategically set up this ABC practice learning opportunity by using the boys' food likes as motivators (A) for them to learn to ask for what they want and to share. She lets Hudson know he can ask by tapping John on the shoulder and saying, "crackers please" (B). She keeps the request simple and achievable to assure success. Then John has an opportunity to repeat this asking practice which was first modeled by Hudson. Each child is rewarded for verbal asking by getting the desired food item (C). Furthermore, the teacher praises them for their friendly social behaviors of helping and sharing. Next the teacher sets up another practice opportunity for Hudson. She coaches Hudson to ask: "water please" and makes sure that his peer, Cazé, understands his request. Hudson's hand flapping seems to indicate that he is pleased to have a

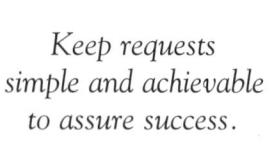

Keep requests simple and achievable to assure success.

friend help him with the water. He has learned that using his words to ask results in him getting what he wants. The teacher labels Hudson's feelings, facilitating his understanding that his verbal asking behavior is connected with getting what he wants and to his feeling happy.

Parents can facilitate similar interactions between siblings or with a peer by setting up a snack practice with two desirable snacks. Each child can be put in charge of one snack item and the parent can support the children to ask for snacks and share with each other.

Using Visual Prompts to Enhance Lunch Time Language

In the next scenario, the teacher of younger children (2-3 years) uses both visual pictures of a snack menu and concrete objects of foods to help a group of 6 children indicate their snack choice verbally or nonverbally. Notice how this teacher uses the visual prompts and her language differently for children who are at diverse stages of communication.

Teacher: Let's take a look at our menu. Let's see what we have. (shows picture of snack food menu.) Hmm. First thing on our menu is cereal. There's the cereal. (shows bowl of cereal and points to picture of bowl of cereal on card.)

Jessica: I want cereal.

Teacher: Great talking Jessica! It's crunchy. I will give you some cereal in just a minute! And then next we have raspberries. Raspberries that are sweet and juicy, and cheese. Yeah. (shows bowls and pictures of cheese and raspberries .)

Teacher: Okay I'm going to give everybody a little bowl. I'll start with a little bit of cereal for everybody.

Jessica: I want a bowl.

Teacher: Jessica asked for a bowl. Ian, can you give this to Jessica, please? That'll be Jessica's bowl. *(prompting Ian to help)*.

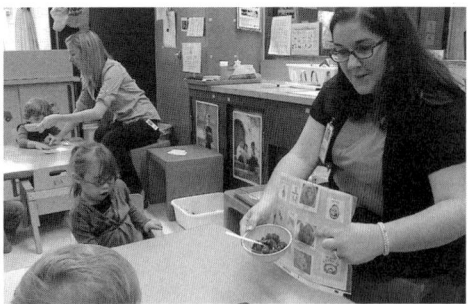

Ian: (passes bowl to Jessica)
Teacher: Good helping, Ian.
Teacher: Okay Vivian, and what would you like? Berries or cheese? (offers choice)
Vivian: (points to picture of berries)
Teacher: Buh, buh, buh. Berries. Vivian pointed to berries. I'm going to give you a few berries and a fork so you can poke them if you want. Pretty cool. Okay, Ian, what would you like?
Ian: Berries.
Teacher: Ian is talking too! Berries. I want berries. One, two, three, scoop. *(uses the one-up rule: "I want berries")*
Forest: I want milk in this. (child models teacher's "I want" language)
Teacher: You want some milk in yours? Forest, I can get you some milk in your cereal. Sure thing. Can you pass me your bowl please? And I'll put in more cereal with the milk. Crunchy cereal. And here comes some cold milk. (more words for Forest who has good receptive language)
Forest: I, I want spoon.
Teacher: A spoon please. I thought you might want a spoon. That's a great idea, Forest. Okay. Do you want milk in your cereal, Ian? You're helping out your friend there.
Vivian: (Vivian points to picture of berries.)
Teacher: Berries. Sure thing (teacher gives her a small amount of berries and then Vivian points again at cheese)
Teacher: Oh, cheese, too? More berries and more cheese. (Vivian points to all 3 pictures.) Good pointing! Okay, here's more berries. Ready? You can give them a poke.

Considerations:

The teacher's language is simple, slow, repetitive, descriptive, and responsive to each child's receptive language understanding and expressive language.

Scenario Continues.

Ian: Milk.
Teacher: Milk, okay. Cup of milk for Ian. Jessica, do you want something to drink?
Jessica: Cup.
Teacher: A cup of milk?
Jessica: (nods head yes.)
Teacher: A blue cup?
Jessica: Sure.
Teacher: Here comes a blue cup. Vivian I see you pointing to some food over there. Is there something you'd like? I've got more water and cereal. Which one? (shows her water and bowl of cereal.)
Vivian: (points to cereal)
Teacher: Cereal. I want cereal. I want cereal. (points to menu picture as she says words.) I want cereal. (models words for Vivian) There's the cereal Vivian. Cereal. Alright. It's pretty yummy, huh? I hear you crunching on your cereal.

Considerations

This teacher effectively adjusts her language according to each child's stage of communication. Vivian is able to point to indicate what she wants but is only making a few audible sounds and is using no words. For Vivian, the teacher relies on the visual cue cards and simple one-word descriptors. Ian is making one-word requests ("berries"), so his teacher uses the one-up rule to repeat his request in a simple sentence: "I want berries." Jessica and Forrest are already using simple sentences, so the teacher repeats their sentences back and adds additional descriptive information. "The cereal is crunchy" or "Here is some cold milk." For Forrest, who has the most language, the teacher also adds additional questions, "Can you pass me your bowl please?"

Using Snack Talk Cards to Promote Social Communication

Preschoolers benefit from teachers modeling and providing structured scaffolding to help them learn to talk with peers about common interests. Children with autism need even more support in this area and can

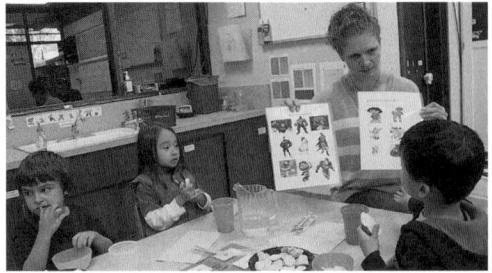
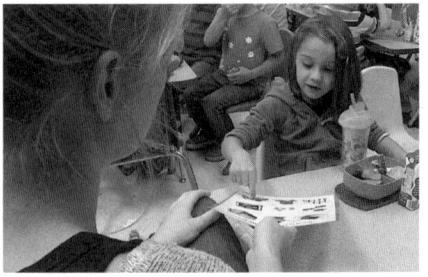

benefit from visual prompts to structure these discussions. In the next scenario, notice how the teacher uses "snack talk" visual cue cards to give these preschool children ideas for what to talk about during snack time.

Teacher: (holding snack talk card of pictures of favorite toys such as balls, crayons, cards, Legos, playdough, etc.) This talk card says, "What is your favorite toy?" (points to words on card).

Teacher: I'm looking at the card. My favorite toy is playdough. (*Teacher models and points to playdough on picture as well as naming it. Then she hands card to Amelia.*)

Amelia: I'm looking at it. My favorite toy is playing this with Truman. (points to picture of stuffed animals.)

Teacher: Playing stuffed animals with Truman?

Amelia: Yeah.

Teacher: (to all children at table) So Amelia said her favorite toy is playing stuffed animals with Truman. (*spotlighting Amelia's communication to her peers*) Amelia, ask your friend. (*prompts verbal interaction with boy.*)

Teacher: You can ask Nathan next. You hold the card so Nathan can see.

Amelia: (looking at Nathan) What is your favorite— Nathan...?

Teacher: Good asking, Amelia!

Nathan: (points to a picture.)

Teacher: Ooh, what did he say?

Amelia: Marble maze.

Teacher: Cool. Okay So, Amelia you can pass the card to Nathan? Nathan, you can ask Atlas. (*hand over hand: physically moves Amelia's hand to help her pass card to Nathan.*)

Teacher: He's right there. (points to Atlas.)

Nathan: (looks at pictures and points at marble maze.)

Teacher: Yes, Nathan, you like the marble maze. Can you show the card to Atlas and ask what do you like? (*prompts words to say*)

Teacher: (helps Nathan move the card to Atlas (*physical prompt*) You are showing it to Atlas.

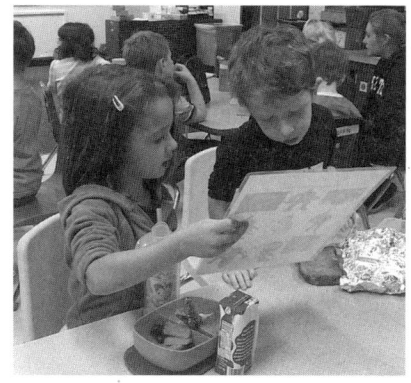

Considerations

The snack talk cards show how pictures can help children talk about their favorite play activity or character. These cards provide a simple way to prompt them to share and communicate their likes to others. Children with different language levels can use the cards in different ways. Amelia has good language skills but is hesitant to initiate with others. The card gives her ideas of what to say, and the act of handing the card to another child and asking Nathan for his preference provides her with a structured way to interact with a peer. Nathan is not using words to communicate, but he is able to point to show that he likes the marble maze, letting Amelia know his preferences. He also has trouble following the teacher's verbal prompt to show the card to Atlas, so the teacher helps him connect her words with the physical action by physically helping him move the card over to Atlas. As children discover each other's likes and dis-

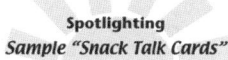

Who is your favorite character?

Dina Dinosaur	Elsa	Buzz Lightyear
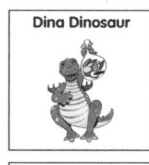	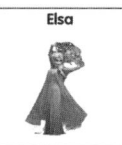	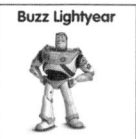
Tiny Turtle	**Dora the Explorer**	**Minions**
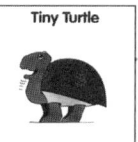	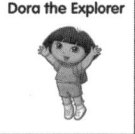	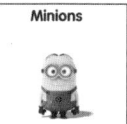
Mickie and Minnie Mouse	**Wally & Molly**	**Spongebob Squarepants**
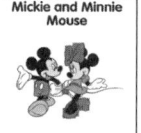	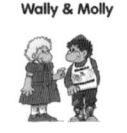	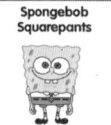

likes, they get to know each other as individuals and begin to develop friendships.

Using Dramatic Play to Prompt Verbal Social Interactions
Getting Joint Play Started

Dramatic play around a theme such as pretending to cook dinner, taking care of a baby, building something together, or playing a fishing game can be a great way to encourage and coach children's social interactions with peers. Pretend play does not come naturally to children on the autism spectrum because it is linked with language skills and giving attention to others, but both can be improved by coaching experiences with neurotypical peers who do readily engage in pretend play. In these interactions,

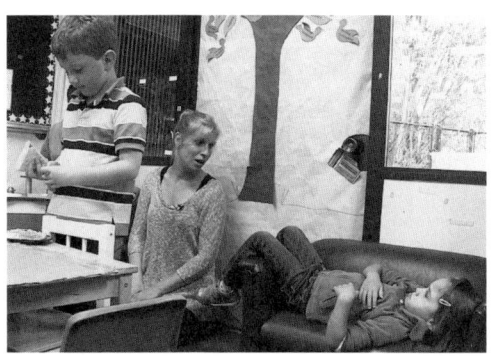

socially adept children can model friendship skills for their peers on the autism spectrum. However, because children on the spectrum often have difficulty knowing how to respond to these social skills, it is important for the interactions to be supported by teachers who can model, prompt, and scaffold a shared joint play experience.

In the next scenario sequence, you will see a teacher working with Amelia, who has good expressive and receptive language but rarely initiates verbal interactions with other children. Without a teacher to provide social coaching with her peers, she usually ends up playing alone. In this play experience in the pretend play kitchen area, the teacher deliberately pairs Amelia with two boys who are very social and comfortable with imaginary play. Notice how the teacher starts by making sure Amelia will be involved in this drama play activity.

    Amelia: I'm going to lay in my bed. (lies on couch away from boys)

    Teacher: You're going to lay in your bed. You better tell Atticus so he knows. Maybe he could make you some food. *(prompts peer interactions)*

    Amelia: (mumbles) Atticus, I'm going to lay in my bed.

Teacher: (whispers) He can't hear you.
Amelia: (mumbles) Atticus, I'm going to lay in my bed.
Teacher: He can't hear you. You might have to go get his attention.
Amelia: (yells) Atticus, I'm laying in my bed. Make me some food.
Atticus: I can make you food. I can cook bacon.
Teacher: I like how you got Atticus's attention by being super loud. He's a good friend! He's going to make you bacon. Oh, you look cozy in your bed. Hey, Theo. Amelia might need something in her bed. What do you think she might need?*(prompts 2nd boy's involvement)*
Theo: A pillow?
Teacher: That's a good idea. Amelia, Theo will get you a pillow *(spotlighting Theo's communication for Amelia)*
Amelia: I don't need anything. I don't need anything.
Teacher: Tell your friends. *(prompting Amelia's communication to peers)*
Amelia: Friends, I don't need anything. I'm good.
Teacher: She looks like she's good. Amelia, it's good that you're talking to your friends. Atticus, what is your plan? *(spotlights intentional communication to let boys know of Amelia's response and praises her communication efforts)*
Atticus: I'm making her some bacon.
Teacher: (looking at Amelia) How do you feel about that?
Amelia: (whispers) Yeah, good.
Teacher: Atticus, Amelia said she said she feels good about bacon. I love bacon. I'll help. I'll get some plates down. *(spotlighting Amelia's intentional communication to Atticus)*

Considerations

This teacher prompts and encourages Amelia's verbal communication and social exchange with the boys by prompting her to communicate and praising her for speaking up. She also finds a way to encourage the boys to include Amelia in their play, even though she is lying on the couch slightly apart from them. The teacher makes sure that the boys hear her requests and feelings about their cooking plan so that there can be shared joint play with her intentional communication. She encourages the cooking plan by saying she wants to help and models how to help in joint play. She has strategically picked two boys for this play who will model social skills and will be willing to include Amelia in their play.

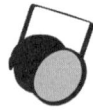 **Setting Up Playdates**

Parents can facilitate similar interactions between siblings or can invite another child over for a coached play date time. It is helpful to choose a friendly and flexible playmate who has good social skills. Children who are slightly older than your child may be more forgiving and responsive to this kind of coached play interaction and may be more likely to include and accommodate your child in their play. On the other hand, a younger child may be more agreeable to less complicated play interactions and more accepting if your child does not immediately respond in the way that they expect. A younger child may also be happier to engage in some parallel play, with parental social coaching to make joint connections. Teachers are a good source of suggestions for which children from your child's school peer group would make good play companions. It will be important to provide lots of praise and attention to both children and to spotlight intentional communication to help your child be aware of the other child's activities, requests or ideas.

It is helpful to choose a friendly and flexible playmate who has good social skills.

Set up these play dates with a defined and consistent structure such as lunch or snack, then some unstructured, unpressured play (e.g., video, playground, or park outing) so children can get acquainted. This can be followed by more structured play with your social coaching. Using a picture schedule of what will happen in the play date will let the children know the expectations. Be sure to schedule at a time when your child is not too tired. To start, it is good to limit the time of the overall playdate and keep these more structured playtimes short. A playdate that lasts 30-45 minutes may be enough to start with. For some children on the spectrum, playing with another child for even 5-10 minutes is emotionally tiring at first. Provide toys such as Legos, marble towers, doll houses, cars, or blocks that promote interaction. If possible, provide duplicates of your child's favorite toys so that imitation can occur. If the play mate is neurotypical, you can help them understand your child and his likes. For example, saying, "Hudson has trouble understanding and talking sometimes. You can help him by using simple words and showing him what to do. He may not look like he wants to play but keep trying." Or, "you can tell him when it is your turn and when it is his turn. I am sure you will be a good friend." You can ask the play mate what some of their likes are, what songs they can sing, or particular books they like to read about. Where there are similar interests, try to provide these books and objects to encourage the children to share their passions by playing, talking, reading, or singing together. Finally, help your child and their friend know how to indicate they are finished playing together and how to say good bye. Try to end the play time before your child becomes tired and overwhelmed. In the beginning, your presence to coach and model play will be critical. Over time, when the routine and activities have been established, you can begin to fade out and enjoy seeing more independent play.

Prompting and Scaffolding Joint Play

Next, notice how the teacher encourages Amelia to participate more actively with the boys.

Theo: Hurry, Atticus. Bacon very hot.
Atticus: It is. (to Theo) Put it right up here.
Theo: (puts pan on stove top.)
Atticus: Now we click the timer.
Theo: To ten.
Teacher: That's a good idea, count to ten. Alright, Amelia. After they make you bacon, we're going to join them at the kitchen, and we're going to make something. What are you going to make? *(prepping Amelia for a transition to more interactive play)*
Amelia: Um, pancakes.
Teacher: That is an excellent idea. So after you get the bacon, you can go to the kitchen and join the boys and make some…

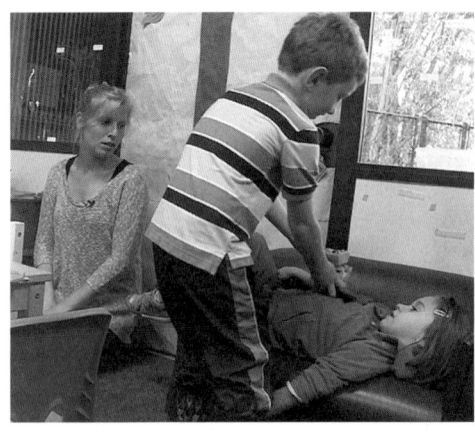

Amelia: Pancakes.
Teacher: Pancakes! Real nice.
Theo: Four, five, six, seven, eight, nine, ten. Ready. (dumps bacon on plate.)
Atticus: (takes plate to Amelia.) One plate full of bacon.
Theo: And here's the bacon.
Amelia: Thank you.
Teacher: Nice friendly words.
Amelia: (hands back plate) I'm all done with my egg.
Theo: She's all done with her egg. I'm putting it in the trash.
Teacher: Are you done with your bacon?
Amelia: After the boys come, after Theo and Atticus come.
Teacher: Come where?
Amelia: Come to me.
Teacher: You can ask them to come to you. (*prompts request*)
Amelia: Come to me. I'm done with it.
Atticus: (comes over and takes plate) I'll throw this in the trash can. Here's the trash.
Teacher: Alright, nice talking, so, Amelia, remember your plan. You finished the bacon. You were going to go to the kitchen. What were you going to do?
Amelia: Make pancakes.
Teacher: You're right. I can't wait to taste it.
Theo: I'm making applesauce.
Teacher: Did you hear that, Amelia? Theo said he's making applesauce. (*intentional communication to be sure Amelia heard Theo*)
Atticus: He's making applesauce, but I don't know how to make it. (walks away.)
Theo: You just mash up some apples.
Amelia: This is in the oven. I'm going to put all the food in the oven and make applesauce.

> **Teacher:** Good idea. Theo, did you hear that? Amelia said she's going to put all the food in the oven and make applesauce. Was that similar to your plan? *(intentional communication to promote joint play)*
> **Theo:** (nods yes).
> **Atticus:** No.
> **Teacher:** So Amelia and Theo are working together on apple sauce. (to Atticus) What's your plan?
> **Atticus:** Making pizza.
> **Teacher:** Awesome. Applesauce and pizza. You are a cooking team. That sounds delicious. *(intentional communication to promote team work)*

Considerations

The teacher coaches Amelia to join in the cooking. She gives her a transition warning (after the bacon comes, then you'll cook) and gives her a choice about what she is going to make, prompting more language and decision making. The teacher continues to draw the boys' attention to Amelia and to prompt Amelia to talk with them. Once Amelia is up from the couch and is with the boys, she gives up her pancake idea and, with the teacher's help, makes a plan to make applesauce with Theo. The teacher praises their ideas and teamwork. Without this teacher scaffolding, Amelia would likely be playing alone while the boys pretended to cook together. However, this teacher's coaching efforts have encouraged Amelia to bring the two boys into her attention spotlight to foster some joint play that she can enjoy.

Promoting Verbal Expression of Ideas

As the cooking drama scenario continues, notice how the teacher continues to help Atticus and Amelia to communicate and compromise as they both try to cook in the same oven.

> **Amelia:** (putting things in the oven.)
> **Atticus:** I'm having trouble, there's lots of food (wants to put his pizza in the oven, but Amelia's food is in the way).

Teacher: (to Atticus) Talk to Amelia. See if you guys can compromise. Come up with a plan. *(prompts Atticus to interact with Amelia)*

Atticus: I'm putting this right down here. (puts pan on one side in the oven)

Teacher: That's a good plan. Amelia, Atticus put his things on one side so there is room for your food too. *(spotlighting intentional communication for Amelia)*

Teacher: (to Atticus) You could ask Amelia if she needs some help with her cooking, since yours are in the oven. *(prompting more interaction with Amelia)*

Amelia: (ignoring other children and continuing to put food in oven.) Pizza and cheese, and more carrots.

Atticus: (puts another pizza in oven.)

Amelia: (yells) No, I don't want pizza in here.

Teacher: Amelia, can you tell Atticus in a friendly voice? *(prompts friendly interaction)*

Amelia: (to Atticus) No thank you. No thank you, you can move that.

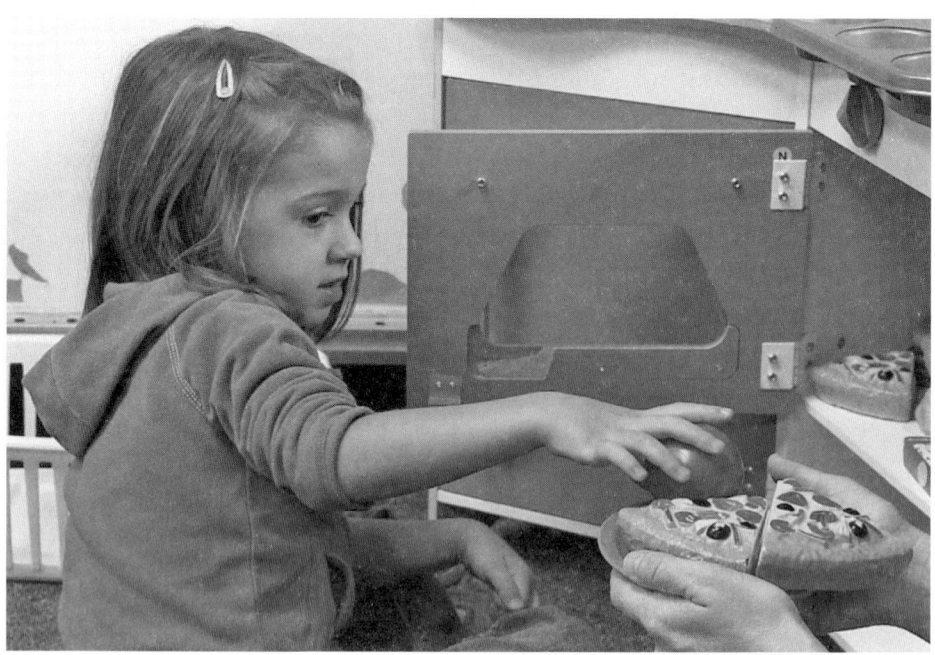

Teacher: That was a friendly way to ask.

Theo: (has been watching the interaction and steps in to help). I'll take the pizza, Amelia. I'll take the pizza to cook in the pan. (takes pizza and puts it in his frying pan.)

Amelia: Okay.

Teacher: Theo that is good helping your friends! Good problem solving Theo. Let's check to see if that's okay with Atticus. Amelia, can you ask Atticus if it's okay to cook the pizza in the frying pan? (*prompts and models communication*)

Amelia: Atticus is that okay?

Atticus: Okay, we can cook in the pan.

Teacher: Amelia I like the way you used your words to check with Atticus, And then Atticus agreed with you. He's being flexible. You guys are all working together like a team. You are being friendly and helping each other.

Considerations

When Amelia seems to be ignoring what the boys are doing, the teacher narrates their actions to spotlight their play. She prompts the boys to initiate communication with Amelia to try to get her more involved in the joint play and to problem solve the issue of oven space. When Amelia protests Atticus's attempt to put the pizza in the oven, the teacher coaches her to use friendly words to ask. She supports the children to come to a compromise. These boys are quite accommodating to Amelia's wishes and cooperate with her demands. The teacher asks Amelia to check with Atticus to see if he is okay with the plan to cook his pizza in the frying pan. This gives her practice in thinking about the feelings of others. The teacher ends by praising all the children for working like a team and being friendly.

This joint interactive play expands Amelia's spotlight to include sharing her attention with the boys. This scenario illustrates the rationale for setting up these practice coaching sessions with peers who are flexible and friendly. If Amelia were playing with another child who had difficulty compromising or who was stronger willed, it would be more difficult to coach them to a positive resolution. For a child with fewer social skills than Amelia, you would start with one other prosocial child to reduce the complexity of the interaction. If your child is not ready to play with another child, then you can coach them in a play interaction with yourself or with a puppet, as described in earlier chapters.

> *If your child is not ready to play with another child, then you can coach them in a play interaction with yourself or with a puppet*

Modeling and Spotlighting Intentional Communication to Promote Sharing

Now the teacher has successfully helped Amelia express her words and feelings. Next notice how she models, prompts, praises, and spotlights intentional commenting to help Amelia learn to share and interact more in joint play with the two boys.

Amelia: Applesauce is done.
Teacher: Awesome. (Theo hands teacher some pizza.) Thank you. You should ask the rest of your friends if they want some pizza. (*prompting Theo to share.*)
Theo: Do you want some pizza, Atticus? (Theo shares pizza.)
Atticus: Yes.
Amelia: Here's some applesauce. (Amelia shares with teacher.)
Teacher: Thanks for sharing with me. Is it hot? (*modeling how to praise*)
Amelia: It's a little bit warm.
Teacher: Okay. You can put it on my pizza. (Amelia puts applesauce on teacher's plate.) Thank you.
Teacher: Would you like a piece of my pizza? (*models sharing.*)
Amelia: I'm good.
Teacher: So, no thank you? (*prompts manners*)
Amelia: No, thank you.

Teacher: Nice words (pretends to eat applesauce). This is delicious applesauce. *(models praise.)*

Theo: Are you done with your pizza?

Teacher: I, I didn't even take a bite yet. But can I share some of Amelia's applesauce with you? *(models sharing.)*

Theo: (takes applesauce and pretends to eat it.)

Teacher: Oh, how does it taste? *(prompts Theo to praise.)*

Theo: Good.

Teacher: Oh, Amelia. Theo said the apple sauce tastes good. Can you see if Atticus wants some applesauce? *(prompts sharing)*

Amelia: Here's some more applesauce for you. (Amelia shares with Atticus.)

Atticus: Thank you (takes applesauce).

Teacher: That's great sharing with Atticus. Let's see if he likes it. Atticus, what do you think about the applesauce?

Atticus: It's good applesauce. Do you want pizza (offers to teacher and Amelia).

Teacher: Amelia, Atticus likes your applesauce. Let's try the pizza and tell him if it's good. *(intentional communication and prompting further response)*

Amelia: It's good pizza Theo.

Considerations

In this scene, the teacher is working to help Amelia be more connected and responsive to the boys. She participates in the play, modeling accepting pizza from Theo and complimenting him for it. Have you noticed that most of Amelia's unprompted initiations are with her teacher, not with her peers? This is common for children on the spectrum who may perceive adults as safer and more predictable. The teacher accepts Amelia's offer of applesauce and compliments her for it. Next, she transfers Amelia's attention to her peers by prompting her to share with Atticus. Finally, she prompts the children to compliment each other on their cooking. By participating in the play, the teacher becomes a powerful social model for Amelia, expands Amelia's attention spotlight to be aware of the boys, prompts social interactions, and makes her feel safe to try out social interactions with the boys.

Now notice how the teacher continues to spotlight intentional communication to help Amelia be aware of the boys' feelings and responses. Think about what she is helping Amelia learn next.

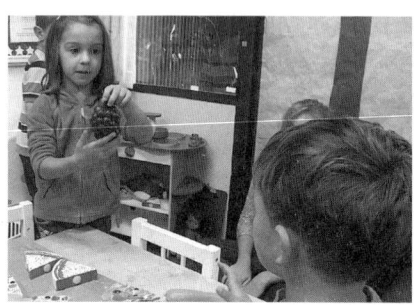

Scenario continues.

Amelia: Are you all done with this?
Teacher: I am, thank you.
Amelia: Okay.
Atticus: I love carrot applesauce.
Teacher: I heard Atticus say, "I love carrot applesauce." (*spotlight intentional communication*)
Amelia: I'm going to have grape applesauce (holds grapes).
Teacher: You can ask Theo or Atticus. (*prompts communication with boys*)
Amelia: Theo, here's grape applesauce for you.
Theo: No, thank you.
Teacher: Oh, he said "no thank you." What about Atticus? (*prompts sharing request.*)
Amelia: (offers grape applesauce to teacher.)
Teacher: I'm full. I already had some applesauce and some carrot apple-sauce. But Atticus hasn't had any. (*prompts sharing again*)
Amelia: Theo, do you want applesauce?
Teacher: Oh, I heard Theo already say "no, thank you." (*intentional communication to help Amelia understand*)
Amelia: Atticus, would you like some grape applesauce?
Atticus: Yes.
Teacher: Ah, so friendly. You shared your grape applesauce. Atticus was excited to try it. (*promotes connection between social skill and friends' feelings*)

Considerations

In this scenario Amelia is making progress with her efforts to widen her spotlight and to initiate interactions with her peers. With some prompting from her teacher, she offers them applesauce. The teacher helps to make sure that Amelia stays focused on the boy's response by spotlighting their intentional communication ("Theo said, no thank you," "I heard Atticus say he loves applesauce.") When Amelia directs her communication to the teacher, the teacher encourages her to talk with the boys directly, saying: "No, thank you, but you can ask Theo or Atticus." When Amelia shares with Atticus, the teacher highlights his positive response. Thus she connected Amelia's social sharing with Atticus's feelings.

Promoting Peer Communication

This teacher has strategically choreographed dramatic play to skillfully model appropriate social skills for all the children. She has tailored her coaching to help Amelia, who is less socially skilled than the boys, to understand what they may be feeling, wanting, or not wanting. This strategy of letting Amelia know what someone else is feeling or wanting is sometimes called prompting *intentional communication*. Next, think about how the teacher continues to help Amelia sustain her initiation of verbal interactions beyond asking a single question.

Amelia: Theo, do you want—Theo, Theo, Theo, Theo, Theo, Theo, Theo, Theo do you want that applesauce?

Theo: Sure.

Teacher: You can ask Theo how it tasted. I wonder if it was crunchy.*(prompts and models asking)*

Amelia: Theo is it crunchy?

Theo: It was mushy.

Teacher: He said it was mushy. *(spotlighting intentional communication)* You must have tried a different kind of applesauce.

Amelia: Atticus, would you like vinegar?

Atticus: I will want that on my apple.

Amelia: (sprays vinegar on apple.)

Atticus: Thank you.
Amelia: Atticus, Atticus. Would you like carrot applesauce?
Atticus: Yes.
Amelia: And you have, you have to put it in there when you're done, okay? Thank you.
Amelia: Theo, would you like orange applesauce?
Atticus: I do.
Amelia: Theo, Theo would you like orange in applesauce?
Theo: (shaking cheese on pizza) No thank you.
Amelia: Okay... (accepts no and starts to walk away).
Theo: Yes, yes.
Amelia: (smiles and looks at teacher.)
Teacher: Nice sharing, you are offering applesauce to your friends. They're excited to try your applesauce creation. You are being friendly.

Considerations

In this scenario, we see that Amelia is enjoying offering applesauce to the boys. She is now doing this without prompting and is starting to listen to their responses. When Theo at first says "no" Amelia accepts his response and says "okay." Amelia is pleased when he changes his mind and the teacher praises Amelia for this nice sharing with friends and celebrates that they are excited to try this creation.

Prompting Peer Sharing and Praising

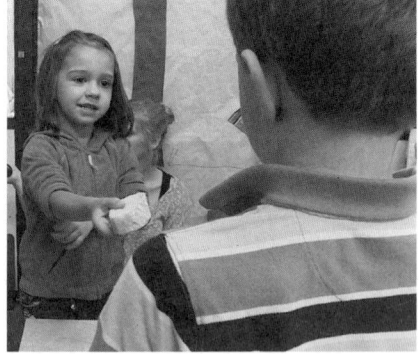

The teacher has been using dramatic play to help Amelia learn to initiate verbal interactions and cooperate in joint play and to help her see the connection between her offers to share and the resulting feelings of the boys and their developing friendship. Next think about how the teacher helps Amelia learn how to ask for what she wants and to learn to praise Theo's cooking.

Amelia: I would like ketchup on my pizza.
Teacher: You should tell Theo, maybe he'll let you try some.
Amelia: Theo, let me have ketchup on my pizza.
Theo: (hands her pizza) Here you go.
Teacher: Taste it.
Amelia: That made me feel happy.
Teacher: Ah. That's awesome, you feel happy he shared with you.
Teacher: Is it good?
Amelia: It's, it's, it's yucky and good.
Teacher: Oh, you should tell Theo it's good, he's the chef.
Amelia: Theo, it's yucky and good.
Theo: Do you like it?
Teacher: Tell him what the good part is.
Amelia: The ketchup is good.

Considerations

Here we see that Amelia understands the connection between Theo's sharing his pizza and her happy feelings. This indicates she is enjoying sharing her attention spotlight with the boys. Then the teacher prompts Amelia to use another social skill (giving a compliment) by cuing her to tell Theo what she likes about the pizza.

Think about how you could set up drama experiences with your child and a friend or a sibling. Amelia is very verbal and, with coaching and support, she seems to respond well to being with 2 children. Seeing the boys model social skills with each other is a good learning experience for her. However, for children like Hudson or Kalani it would be best to start this joint play time with just one other child. Playing with two children could be too complex and overwhelming for children with more limited language or play skills.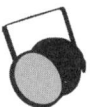

Coaching, Listening, Asking & Sharing

In the next scenario notice how the teacher has set up a small group playdough activity for Amelia and the two boys. Notice how she and prompts, coaches, and models their social skills. Think about what Amelia is learning in this coached peer joint play.

Teacher: Alright, Amelia, I'm going to give you all the playdough. So if anyone wants any playdough, they can ask their friend Amelia.
Atticus: Amelia, can I have some playdough?
Teacher: Atticus asked you nicely!
Amelia: Sure.
Teacher: That was nice. You listened to your friend Atticus, and you shared some of your playdough. Amelia, may I have some playdough? *(models asking)*
Teacher: (Amelia hands her playdough.) Thank you. I just need a little bit.
Atticus: You can ask too of me, you ask too for me. (holds out his toys to the teacher).
Teacher: Can I have that red turtle toy?
Atticus: Yeah.
Teacher: Thank you Atticus. You shared with me.
Theo: Could I, could I have some playdough, Amelia?
Amelia: Sure.
Theo: Thank you.
Teacher: That was really friendly. Our friend Theo asked, and Amelia listened and then shared some playdough.

Considerations

The teacher strategically gives Amelia all the playdough. This provides an opportunity for her to learn to listen to the boys' requests and to share with them. The teacher also participates in the interactions, modeling

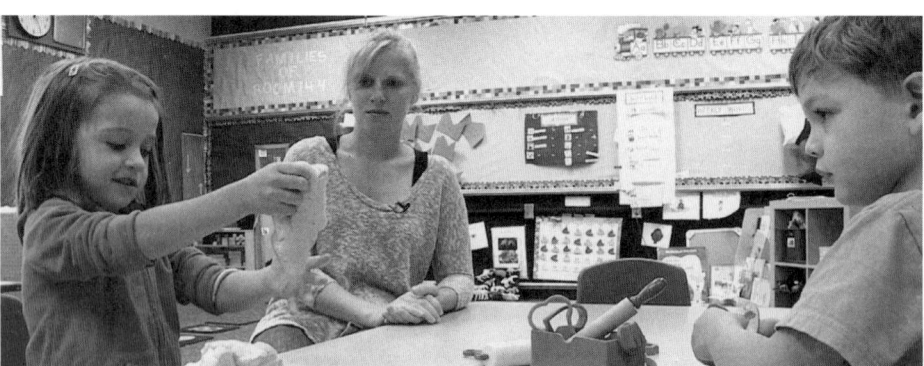

polite asking by asking Amelia for playdough and Atticus for a turtle toy. She praises all the children for listening, sharing, and saying thank you.

Coaching Waiting for a Turn

As this playdough play continues, the teacher continues to model and prompt the desired social behaviors and uses praise that labels the specific social behavior she is proud of. In this activity there are only two rollers for the three children. Notice how the teacher helps the children learn to wait their turn. Amelia and Atticus are using playdough rollers and Theo would like one.

Theo: Can I have a roller, Atticus?

Atticus: You can have it in one minute.

Teacher: Theo that was nice asking and now you are doing good waiting.

Theo: Could I have that roller, Amelia?

Amelia: In one minute.

Teacher: Nice asking again, Theo. If you look over by the sink, there's a green timer with one minute on it. You can go grab that. (Theo gets timer and puts on table)

Atticus: You want this roller, or her roller? I got a shape roller. I got one like these.

Teacher: Yep, Theo so there's a shape roller for you, I heard Atticus suggest using that.

Theo: I don't want a shape roller.

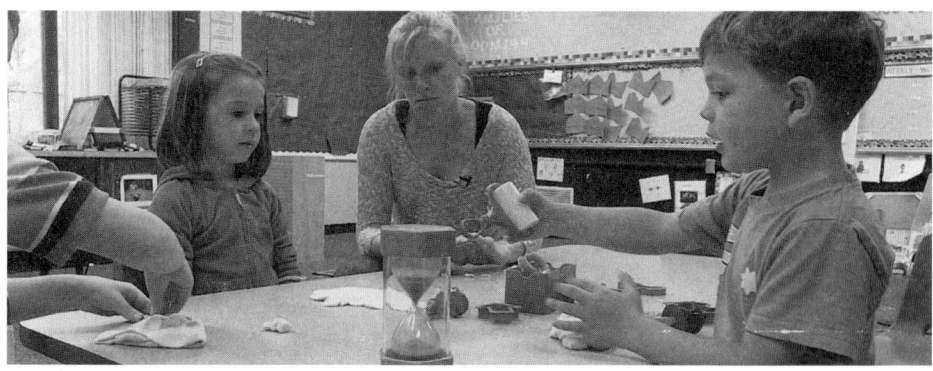

Teacher: Okay, Atticus he doesn't want a shape roller. Nice idea. Theo is going to wait for the other roller. (one minute passes while sand goes through time).
Atticus: The sand is done.
Teacher: That's right. Now it's Theo's turn for the roller. Theo, which roller did you want?
Theo: I want the blue roller.
Teacher: Okay, can you ask Amelia politely for a turn with the roller.
Theo: Amelia, can I have the roller please.
Amelia: In one minute.
Teacher: Theo already waited one minute. Can you share now? Then you can use the time to wait for your turn.
Amelia: (shares her roller and takes the timer).
Teacher: That was good sharing, Amelia. You can have another turn soon.

Considerations

In this scenario the teacher has set up the activity so that there are not enough rollers, and the children need to learn how to share with each other. The teacher gives attention to and praises their polite asking and waiting their turn. The teacher also uses a sand timer to help the children understand how long one-minute is. From this coaching the children learn that they can say 'no' politely and that their friend will be supported to wait with the teacher's attention and praise.

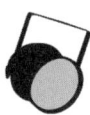

Think about how you could set up a peer play activity with one child to promote your child's practice of sharing, asking, and waiting with another child. Plan to have less drawing or cutting or cooking materials than the number of children so they are motivated to wait, ask, share, and take turns.

Promoting Cooperative Play

So far the children are working independently at the table, each on their own activity. This is an important first step in interactive shared play. Next think about how the teacher tries to encourage some cooperative play with a joint activity.

Amelia: Maybe Theo will make a big road.
Teacher: Alright, it sounds like you want Theo to make a big road. I wonder what Theo wants.
Theo: Maybe we could use all our playdough to make a big road.
Teacher: You guys could get started on that now. You should talk to Amelia, and see if she likes that plan.
Theo: Do you like that plan, Amelia?
Amelia: Yeah.
Teacher: So, you just told Amelia that you wanted to make a big road, and she agreed. So, what is your plan?
Theo: Atticus, do you want to make a big road?
Atticus: Yes, yes.
Theo: So, you got to make flat like a road.
Atticus: I'm making some lines for the road.
Teacher: You are all working together. Amelia's pushing it down with her knuckles to make a flat road.

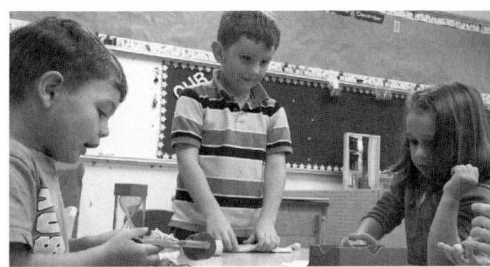 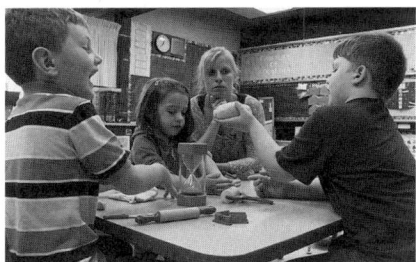

A new boy takes Atticus' place in the play. Notice how the teacher handles the situation when the new boy wants to do something different.

Atticus leaves table and a new boy, Joe, joins in
Theo: Let's make the road super big.
Teacher: Theo has an excellent idea.
Theo: Make a big road.
Teacher: So Theo, Joe doesn't know your plan. Can you tell him what you are doing?
Theo: We can make a big road.

Joe: No, no, not that. A low vampire castle.
Amelia: I'm, I'm, I'm almost done with making it flat.
Teacher: (whispers to Amelia.) Wait a second. Did you hear what Joe just said?
Amelia: What?
Teacher: Ask him. (prompts asking)
Amelia: What did you want?
Joe: I want to build a low vampire castle.
Teacher: He wants to make a vampire castle. (intentional communication) Ameila what was your plan?
Amelia: My plan was making a castle at the end of the road.
Teacher: Joe, did you hear that? You and Amelia have the same plan on making a castle.
Theo: You make a castle with Joe. I will make the road.
Teacher: (to Amelia) So Joe is making a vampire castle. What kind of castle are you making?
Amelia: Um, a mountain castle.
Teacher: Oooo, that sounds exciting.
Joe: And…
Teacher: I bet vampires live on mountain castles.
Joe: (pats Theo's arm) Um, excuse me. But, I mean, do you want to help me make a low vampire castle? Hmm?
Theo: Hmm. I want to make my own one.
Teacher: (to Joe) Theo doesn't want to do that now, but Amelia might want to help you. (intentional communication and prompt)
Joe: You want to help me make one?
Teacher: Oh, Amelia didn't hear you. Try asking again.
Joe: Amelia, do you want to help me build a low vampire castle?
Amelia: Sure.
Teacher: Awesome you are a team. You guys can combine your playdough. So Joe, what's your first step to make this castle?

Considerations

The teacher promotes cooperative play by getting the children to talk about their plans with each other. She makes sure they listen to each other and understand each other's suggestions. As Joe and Amelia decide on making a vampire mountain castle together, she praises their teamwork. If Amelia had less verbal language, the teacher could praise their work together with a thumbs-up gesture and perhaps show them a team work visual prompt as she says, "great teamwork".

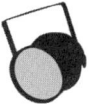

Remember that cooperative play is a developmental process. At first, children will engage in parallel play where each is involved in their own ideas and imaginary world. At this stage, joint play is playing near another child, sharing space, and some resources, without noticing or engaging with each other. As children develop, this parallel play will shift to being able to take an interest in a peer, ask a question, share, and wait for a turn, but each child may still be primarily interested in their own play plan. Finally, children will learn to work together on a shared goal or to engage together in the same imaginary world.

Promoting Cooperative Play

The teacher has successfully helped two of the children to continue to work cooperatively on a joint activity. The third child, Theo, continues with his independent play idea. Negotiating a joint activity and sustaining their attention with several peers is challenging for most children this age. It is even more difficult for children on the spectrum to navigate social interactions with more than one child at a time. Notice next how the teacher continues to help them cooperate in a joint play plan. Think about when you might support independent play and when to encourage cooperative play.

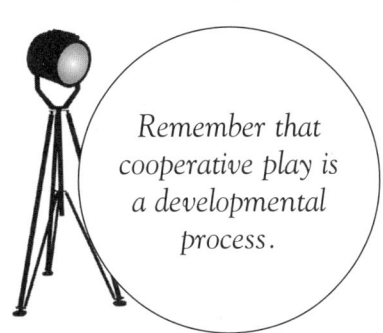

Remember that cooperative play is a developmental process.

    Amelia: No, don't do that. (Joe was moving her flattened playdough)
    Joe: No, I'm just helping you.

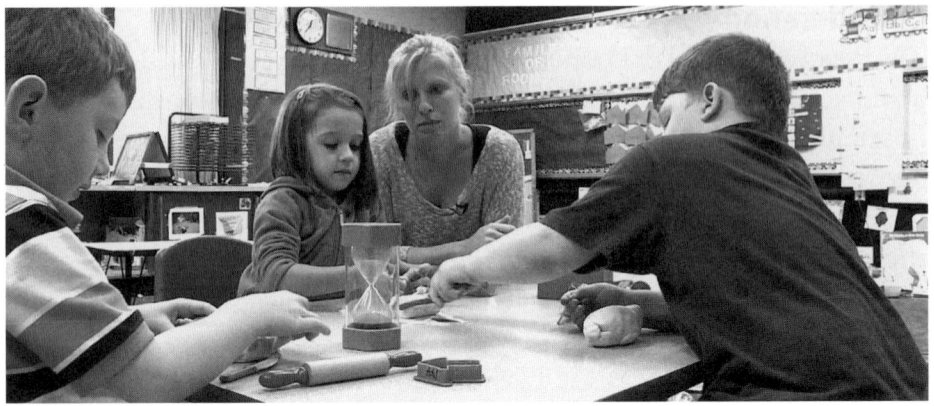

Teacher: Um-hmm. Because you guys agreed to make the vampire castle together. So Joe said he's going to help you make the floor, by flattening it out.
Teacher: (to Amelia) What is your plan with the floor?
Amelia: Um, putting it together.
Teacher: So, Amelia is putting it back together and Joe is flattening.
Joe: (rolling the playdough.)
Teacher: Theo is making a pretty good turtle nest over there, or a cave. (includes Theo even though he is not working on the castle with Amelia and Joe)
Amelia: Um, I'm, I'm finishing on my castle.
Teacher: (gives her a thumbs up signal.)
Joe: Wait it's our castle (rolls playdough more).
Amelia: No, Joe.
Teacher: Amelia and Joe, I see you both helping with the castle!
Joe: I'm just helping you making the floors.
Teacher: Okay, so the floors are done. What's the next step?
Joe: The next step is…
Theo: Build the castle.
Joe: Ahh, that was what I was going to say. Next we have to build the low vampire castle.
Teacher: Now Theo is helping too!

Considerations

This teacher is able to use social coaching to help these three children learn about the cooperative skills involved in a joint play project. She encourages them to describe their plan, help each other, and learn to accept a friend saying no to a request. At this age, negotiating social interactions to work together on a single activity is hard work because it requires a high level of shared problem solving and will be difficult for most children. This teacher gives the children brief opportunities to try this out while also supporting their independent creativity. For Amelia, who is the only child with autism, the teacher coaches her to notice what the other boys are doing or suggesting and support her own independent ideas. The fact that they are all sitting together and making a vampire castle is definitely a shared joint activity, allowing for some independence.

Using Picture Play Scripts to Promote Shared Joint Play

Every child on the autism spectrum is unique, with a different set of developmental delays and challenges. We have seen that Amelia has language skills and can be coached to communicate socially with her peers. However, Hudson has far less language, is less interested in social interactions and is more interested in exploring nonsocial objects by himself. As is common for many children on the spectrum, his play is often repetitive and non-imaginative. One of the goals for Hudson is to expand the variety of his play activities as well as to help him initiate a social interaction with a peer. Earlier in this chapter, we saw a teacher using child-directed narrated coached play with Hudson and one other boy while they were driving their cars on block roads.

In the next scenario this same teacher uses some picture play card sequences to help Hudson and his friend learn new ways to play with the blocks, other than driving cars. These scripts break down the multi-step play sequences into simple steps that show them exactly what to do.

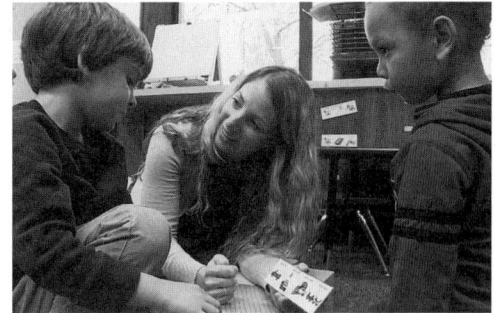

Notice how the teacher uses the picture play script cards to help facilitate the interactive shared play and think about how you could use this idea with your child.

Teacher: Hey, you guys. What do you think we should do next? Payton, what do you think we should do next? (shows them picture cards of four options with cars and points to each one.) We drove our car. We could have a race. We could make a tunnel. Or, we could make them crash. What do you think, mister?

Payton: Um... (points to race on picture card).

Teacher: Oh, Payton says race. Hudson, what do you think? Should we race? Look. *(intentional communication)*

Payton: I won!

Teacher: What? We didn't say go. Do you want to race or do you want to drive? (leans over to get eye contact with Hudson.)

Hudson: (looks at pictures and points.) Drive.

Teacher: Oh, Hudson says, I want to drive. All right. We'll drive, and then we'll race. (makes driving noises.) Come drive with us Payton! (makes driving noises.) Come on over. We're going to drive, and then we're going to have a race. (makes driving noises.) I'm going to get a race ready. Yeah. What do you think? Are you ready to race? Alright. First we drove. Now it's time to race. (shows the card again.) Okay. Ready Hudson? I made a racetrack.

Hudson: (moves away ignoring them and playing alone with his car.)

Teacher: Check it out, bud. (taps Hudson on his back.) We'll start our cars here, and what shall we say? One, two, three, go?

Hudson: (still with back to teacher playing with his own car.)

Teacher: Ready Hudson? Come on over. (he turns around to watch) Okay, this is Payton's, and this is Hudson's. (points to ramps.) Let me set it up. Okay, ready? You want to count? Say one, two, three go? Okay. Do you want to count, Payton?

Payton: Yeah.

Teacher: Okay, all right.

Payton: One, two, three, go! (both children send cars down on slide.)

Teacher: Go! nice one! You are friends having fun together.

Considerations

This teacher is incredibly enthusiastic, using lots of gestures and sound effects. She points to the pictures on the visual sequence prompt to get them to make a decision about whether to race, drive, go through tunnel, or crash. The picture prompt gives the boys ideas for what they can do. The boys have different ideas so she incorporates both wishes into the play sequence: "first we'll drive (Hudson) then we'll race (Payton)." She works hard to keep Hudson involved in a joint play activity with

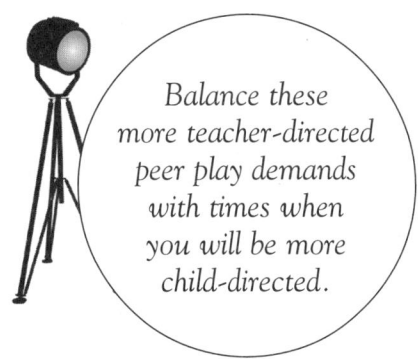

Balance these more teacher-directed peer play demands with times when you will be more child-directed.

Payton as he easily withdraws into solitary play. She makes the race seem exciting and accessible by building two ramps and setting up the cars for the race. This makes it easier for Hudson to shift from driving to racing, and he and Payton and race cars together down the ramp. This is a big accomplishment for Hudson. This kind of coaching is quite teacher-directed. This teacher asks for each boy's choice about what to play, but then she structures the play and prompts them to participate, even when they both revert to their own solitary play. In this case, the teacher has made the choice that it is important to push these two boys into each other's attention spotlight for this brief joint-social interaction. Without her coaching, they would not try this activity and would not experience the fun of racing together. She will balance these demands to play together with times when she goes back to more child-directed coaching so that each child can experience her attention without the demands to engage in the joint social interaction.

Using Picture Play Scripts to Promote Social Confidence

Next notice how the teacher uses the picture scripts to encourage Hudson to try to play in a different way with the blocks. Notice how the predictability of these visuals seems to give Hudson more confidence in his play because he knows exactly what comes next.

Considerations

For children like Hudson, the visual picture play scripts helps them think of other ways to play and shows them exactly what to do. The predictability of the simple steps often helps a child to feel more confident about what he might do next. Earlier, we saw one of Hudson's difficulties is that he plays the same way repetitively. The goal is to encourage him to learn some new play behaviors. In this scenario, Hudson learns three different things he can do with the cars and the blocks. The teacher is still child-directed in that Hudson is given the choice of which play idea he wants to do.

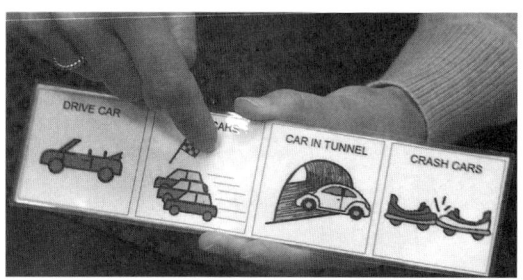

Encouraging Social Interactions with Picture Activity Scripts

Notice how the teacher uses social coaching and a play activity visual script to encourage Hudson's and Payton's social interactions with playdough. Think about what makes her approach effective in this scenario.

Teacher: (coaches Hudson to show playdough script to Payton) Hudson, show Payton what you're doing. Let's show him. Let's show him the picture. (Takes Hudson's hand in her own with the picture and shows it to Payton. With Hudson's other hand she pats Payton on shoulder.) (*physical prompt*) You can say, "Hey, Payton." Tap him again.
Payton: What?
Teacher: Do you want to make a snowman?
Payton: No.

Teacher: Oh, he said "no." Should we ask him what he wants to make?

Payton: I'm done. I'm done. (cutting his playdough)

Teacher: Are you going to cut it up?

Payton: This goes here.

Teacher: Oh, he's cutting it up. Let's do what he's doing. We'll use this tool. (hands Hudson a tool.) Let's cut it up.

Hudson: (starts cutting.)

Teacher: Yeah, you guys are both cutting. Well, you like a rolly cutter and Payton's got a cutter too. Cut, cut, cut. Cut, cut, cut. Nice you guys. Cut, cut, cut. Nice cutting, Hudson.

Teacher: Oh, it's sharp. Cut, cut, cut. Hey, Payton, your friend doing? (points to Hudson.) Check in, Mr. P. Look. What's Hudson doing? He's cutting. He was doing what you're doing. Look. You have one, too. (Payton looks and holds up his cutter) Yeah. Now you both have those rolly cutters. Cut, cut, cut. Check it out, Hudson. Payton has one, too. It's little. You have a big one. You are both working together. (*intentional communication to promote children's awareness of each other*)

Considerations

The teacher (using a physical prompt) takes Hudson's arm to pat Payton on the shoulder to get his attention. She encourages Hudson to watch what Payton is doing when cutting up the playdough. She gives Hudson a similar tool so he can imitate what Payton is doing.

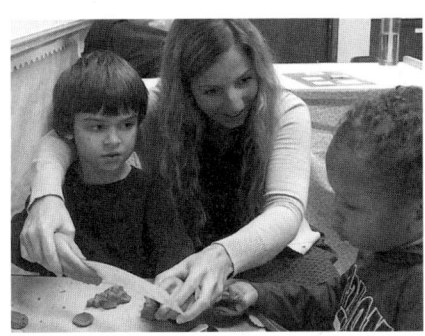

She repeats the words cut, cut, cut and reinforces Hudson's cutting so she can help him understand what the word cut means. She helps each boy be aware of what the other boy is doing. They are learning new ideas for playing with playdough and also how to let another child into their attention spotlights.

Social Coaching on the Playground

Without teacher social coaching and support, Hudson withdraws from play or stands alone away from his peers, flapping his arms. For outside play, teachers also use social coaching to help him engage in the communication steps needed to initiate a play interaction. In the next scenario notice how the teacher uses the sequenced picture cards on the playground to help Hudson make a choice for what play activity he is interested in.

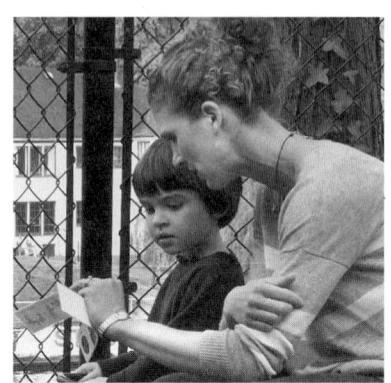

Hudson and Cazé are playing near each other. Each has a ball.

Teacher: (to Hudson) Ready? You've got the ball. You can ask Cazé to play? You can say, "Throw it." (Hudson kicks the ball). Go for it. (kicks ball back to him.) There you go, nice.

Hudson: (hits ball then walks away.)

Teacher: (to Cazé) Ah oh, Cazé, do you want to do one more, or are you all done with the ball? All done?

Cazé: (nods head he is done)

Teacher: Hey, Hudson. Cazé's all done. Do you want to do more ball, or do you want to make a different choice? (shows him the card with playground choices.)

Hudson: Choice.

Teacher: (pointing to card) Which one, which one do you want to do? Race bikes, throw ball, or play in sand?

Hudson: (nods head with ride bikes)

Teacher: Okay, ride bikes, we need to, get a friend. We're going to race bikes with a friend. Who do you want to invite?

Nolan: Hi, who came here?

Teacher: Let's see. Hudson, Nolan's right here. Say, "Nolan, let's ride bikes."

Hudson: (to Nolan) "Let's ride bikes."
Teacher: Good asking. Where's the bike? Let's go find the bikes. We're going to go find the bikes. Nolan found a bike. There you go. Hudson's going to find a bike.
Hudson: (gets a bike and starts riding.)
Teacher: Good job asking your friend Nolan to ride bikes.

Considerations

The teacher has been effective in using pictures to help Hudson chose his preferred playground activities (balls and bikes). She coaches Hudson to notice another child who is also playing with a ball and then helps him initiate a request for another child to ride bikes with him. She gives Hudson the actual words to ask Nolan to play bikes. When Hudson copies her words, she praises him for asking. Think about how you could use visual prompts and social coaching when your child or student is at a playground with other children.

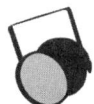

Because Hudson's social anxiety is significant, it might be helpful for the teacher to offer a reinforcer (such as stickers or hand stamps) for his small steps at initiating an interaction with a peer. It is possible that riding the car is not motivating enough for him to ask a friend to play. Remember that when he was practicing toileting behavior at home, his father used Skittles to reinforce the step that was hardest for Hudson (sitting on the toilet).

Social Coaching–Asking to Play

Hudson and Nolan and ride their bicycles around the playground but don't interact. Nonetheless Hudson has initiated an interaction and made a play choice. These are big steps for him. They stop riding bikes, and Hudson again seems at a loss for what to do. In the next scenario notice how the teacher coaches and supports Hudson to try a different outside play activity.

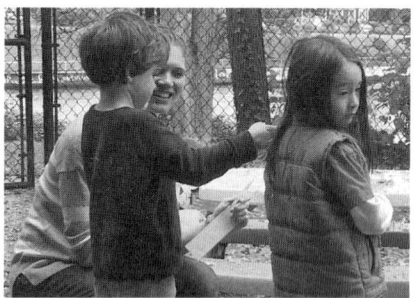

Teacher: Hey, Hudson. Check it out, friend. We already rode bikes. What do you want to do next? Do you want to play catch, or do you want to do teeter-totter? (shows pictures)

Hudson: (points to picture of playing catch.)

Teacher: Playing catch? Cool! Check it out. Here's what we need to do. Hey, Hudson. Check it out. First is, 'Get ball.'

Hudson: (looks around for a ball and finds one.)

Teacher: Oh, okay. Good deal! We got the ball. Next is, hey, Hudson, check it out. (shows picture card again.) Next says, 'Ask a friend to play.' Who should we invite to play? Do you want to ask Nolan or Cazé?

Hudson: (looks around unable to make a decision and then withdraws, going to face into corner of fence.)

Teacher: (shows him picture card again.) Okay. Check it out Let's ask Cazé. You can show him. You can say, "Cazé let's play." Your turn

Hudson: (flapping arms and looking up at sky.)

Teacher: (they arrive next to Cazé) Here... You can say, "let's play." Go up to Cazé. Tap him on the shoulder. (models tapping Cazé on shoulder.)

Hudson: (taps boy on shoulder.)

Teacher: There you go. Nice. Hey Cazé. Hudson's trying to say, "Let's play catch." (shows him the card.)

Cazé: Ok.

Teacher: Great! Cazé and Hudson are going to play catch together.

Considerations

The teacher helps Hudson make a decision about what to do next using picture cards of possible activities. He chooses to play ball so she coaches him with the picture sequence of getting the ball and asking a friend to play. Finding someone to play with is hard for Hudson, and the teacher provides coaching and a physical prompt to help him tap Cazé on the shoulder and show the ball picture. While Hudson is capable of using words to ask, he is likely so overwhelmed by the social situation that he is not able to make the verbal request. The teacher supports him by speaking the words for him, while she helps him make the gestures. In the end, his request is successful, and Cazé agrees to play.

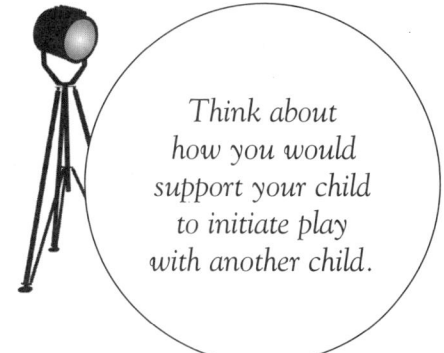

Think about how you would support your child to initiate play with another child.

Hudson's learning could also be broken down into smaller steps with more reinforcement at each success. For example the teacher could use more labelled praise and small rewards (e.g., hand stamps, fish crackers) for making a choice of activity, for trying and moving closer to another child (e.g. Cazé), for saying, "my turn," and for tapping Cazé on shoulder. The teacher's requests could also be simplified with fewer words.

Based on what we have learned here in the prior scenarios, think about how you would support your child to initiate play with another child. Based on your child's social and language developmental levels, you may use picture prompts, physical prompts, gestures, or verbal prompts and coaching to help your child make a request or suggestion to another child.

This coaching for Hudson is complex and potentially fraught with anxiety, especially if the other children, who are also on the autism spectrum, don't comply to his requests or model social skills for him to learn from. Ideally when Hudson is coached to ask for something, the other child will agree so that he is immediately reinforced for asking. In the real world this will not always happen. Sometimes children's requests will be met with a negative response from the other child. When this happens, adults can

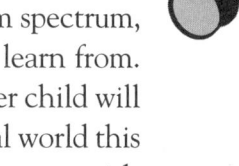

continue to support both children. First, praise the child who asked by saying "Hudson, you asked very politely." Then acknowledge the other child's feelings or response: "Sounds like Cazé doesn't want to play." Then provide a coping strategy or alternative response to the first child: "You're staying calm and can make another choice." Or, "I can play ball with you." Or, "Let's find another friend." This sequence helps children learn to try again when a first request doesn't work.

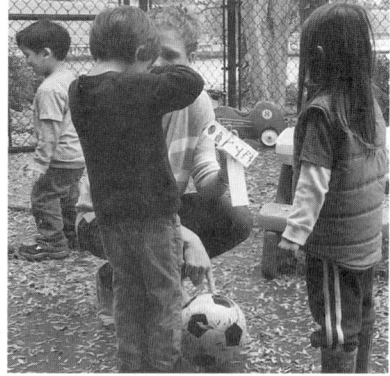

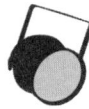 Remember you can use some of your other social skills visual prompts during these play times to remind the child to use social skills such as waiting, asking, saying sorry, trading, and taking turns. (See also Chapter Four)

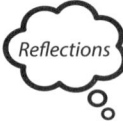
Teacher Reflections about Hudson
In addition to supporting language, we also use a lot of visual supports to help build social engagement. Playing catch back and forth between two peers is something that a lot of our friends start with. It is very basic turn taking social interactions. We have a play schedule that shows first get a friend, then get a ball, then throw the ball, catch the ball, and repeat. It is a foundational skill for more complex turn taking skills. And it also targets how to initiate an interaction; meaning, how do you invite a friend to play?

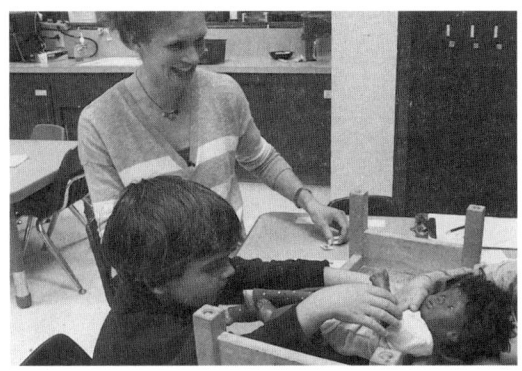

In the classroom for students with autism, the sociodramatic play is something everyone is working on. So it is a skill we want to be sure all students want to engage in because so much learning happens through play. We have some play sets around feeding a baby, rocking a baby, kissing a baby, making pizza, setting table, and putting the blanket on the baby. The way we teach it is to use the visual support that shows the individual steps and sometimes we model it, so it is a big, important goal for all of my students.

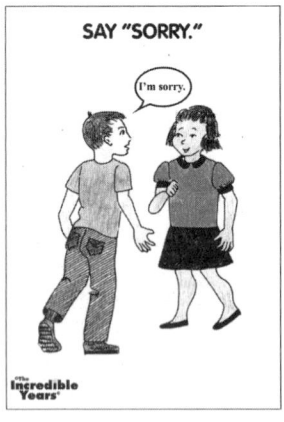
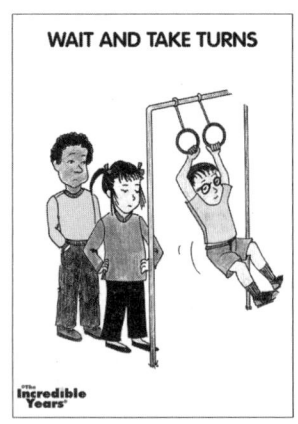
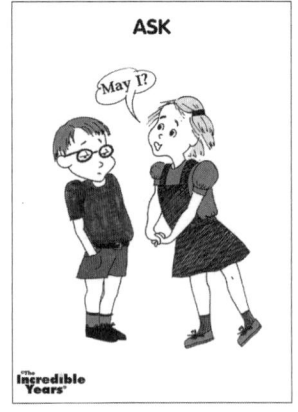

Another teacher: *I've also structured some of our play scripts to include a peer so the first step is to get a friend, get a puzzle, put the pieces together. One of Hudson's goals for this year is allowing children in his space. He is not one to go over and start building on someone else's structure or tolerate someone in close proximity to him. I think he gets nervous about unpredictable behavior. Keeping things safe and structured and limiting kids to one or two other peers is a good place to start.*

Teacher Reflections about Amelia

In dramatic play, one of Amelia's goals is to participate in cooperative play with her friends. So coming up with a common theme and then working on that together and working with a small group of kids. 1-2 other students. In dramatic play we were working on how she wanted to maintain her idea of taking a nap while the other boys wanted to cook or make a restaurant. So to initiate those cooperative interactions, at first it was for the boys to bring Amelia food and the boys lead that play. Then we worked on getting her to join in and play with or near the boys.

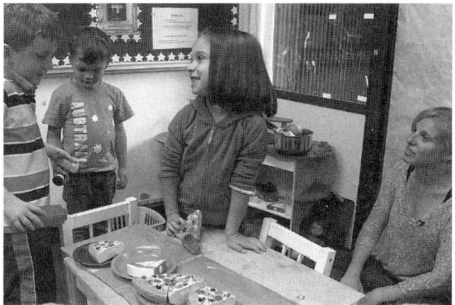

When we were playing with playdough, my goal for them was to notice what their friends were doing and try to build on that. So, throughout the play interactions, I provided support and prompts. For example, "Amelia look at what your friends are doing. He's doing this, and he's doing that". Then they could work together or at least acknowledge they were doing a similar activity differently. We want them to be able to have some boundaries and to say that they want to play or not play. One boy said, 'no I don't want to build a castle' and that was okay. He stayed at the table. He was still with his friends, but they weren't just having the same idea. So they were still participating together.

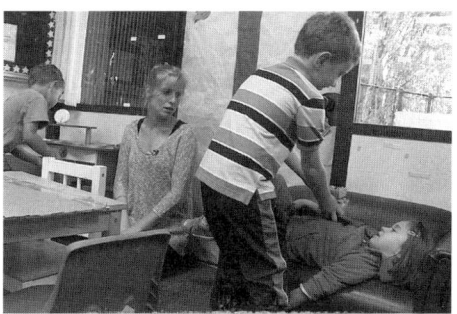

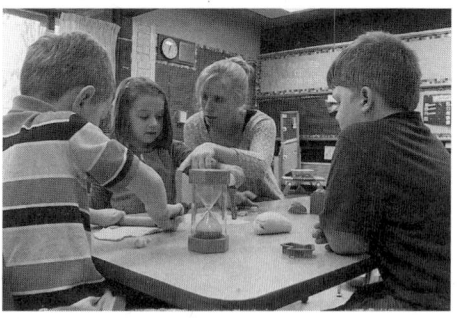

Turn taking is such a huge peer interaction. And one way we do it is to use a timer. It is a really clear visual for kids to know they will eventually get a turn with something they want and in return they will also have to give something up. We use a little green sand timer and it's one minute and so the kids have learned over the course of the year that if they want a turn and the other child is not willing to relinquish their toy right away, they can go get a sand timer and flip it over.

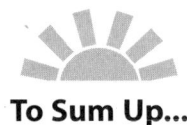

To Sum Up...

In these last scenarios during drama, a playdough joint play, and on the playground, we can see how complex it is for teachers to use social coaching in a developmentally appropriate way with groups of children each at a different social development stage. In the case of Hudson, one-on-one play with the teacher would begin the process of expanding his attention spotlight to include one other person. As Hudson finds this child-directed coached play enjoyable, then the teacher can begin by incorporating one other child into joint play. Preferably this would be a child who is compliant, interested in Hudson, and has some social skills that can be modeled for Hudson. Having the sequenced picture play cards will help a child like Hudson know some things he can do in the play and increase his confidence. Once children like Hudson learn to enjoy these peer interactions with one child, then another child may be added to the mix. However, it is important to pace this learning slowly and carefully for we don't want Hudson to develop further anxiety and frustration about peer play.

Amelia is ready to be coached and supported with 2 other children. She learns from the teacher and peers' modeling and is receptive to the teacher's intentional communication, prompts and scaffolding of her attempts to interact with the other children.

In all these peer interactions, the learning will only happen if the adult (parent or teacher) is there to model, prompt, scaffold, and praise the social interactions and to help the child be aware of the other children's requests, suggestions, and other friendship skills. While one-on-one child directed play is about building the relationship between the teacher or parent and the child, peer coaching is about strengthening the connections between the children with each other. When the child on the spectrum has become comfortable with another child in his spotlight, he can then begin to learn from the peer modeling and social interaction experiences.

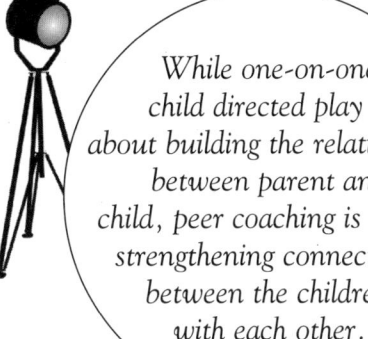

While one-on-one child directed play is about building the relationship between parent and child, peer coaching is about strengthening connections between the children with each other.

SPOTLIGHTING

Coaching Children's Social Peer Interactions: Model, Prompt, Coach, Imitate, Reward, & Use Intentional Communication

- Model social skills such as asking to play, offering to share, waiting, taking turns, asking for help, using gestures, making eye contact, apologizing, and praising.
- Prompt child to ask to initiate interaction, play, share, or take a turn; Let it go if child doesn't respond to prompt.
- Model the actual words and nonverbal gestures for the child to say and copy (e.g., "my turn" and patting chest to indicate your turn.)
- Imitate, coach, and praise child's friendly behaviors when they occur (e.g., initiating interactions, sharing, helping, taking turns, waiting, being polite, apologizing, giving compliments, pointing/gesturing, patting shoulder, or eye contact).
- Carefully select peers who will complement the social goals for the child on the spectrum (consider the peer's temperament, skill level, and developmental age)
- Occasionally prompt child to notice what another child is doing or to help him understand what another child has said. (Spotlighting Intentional Communication).

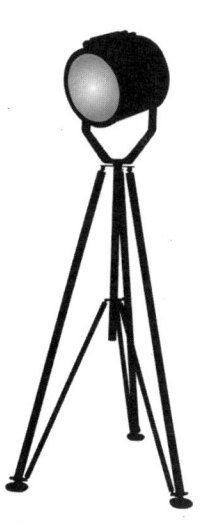

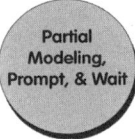
Partial Modeling, Prompt, & Wait

- Help a child understand sharing or helping makes other children feel happy, so the child can see the connection between their social behavior and the other's feelings.
- Help child accept a peer's refusal to share by reinforcing their waiting and patience and by distracting them with other interesting activities.
- Keep peer play interactions short at first. Notice cues that children are becoming tired and try to stop while the play is still going well.
- Use visual prompts, sequenced play scripts, and gestures to promote practice of targeted social behaviors for children with limited language.
- Encourage pretend or drama play with puppets or action figures to model social skills such as asking to play, offering to help, taking a turn, and sharing.
- Give more attention to positive social behaviors than to inappropriate behaviors.

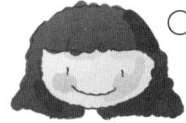

"Your friend is looking for a red block, can you help him?" (Prompt.)

"That's so friendly. You are sharing your cars and waiting your turn. Your friend looks happy." (Connect social behavior to feeling.)

"You are both helping each other like a team." (Show helping visual card.)

"You waited and asked first if you could use that. Your friend listened to you and shared." (Connect behaviors to positive outcome.)

"You both worked together to make that tower. That was great cooperation." (Enthusiastic praise.)

SERIES SUMMARY

Caring for a child on the autism spectrum is stressful and challenging at times. Parents have also told us that once they learn how to get into their child's attention spotlight, strategically respond to their behavior, and see their child start to make progress, they feel rewarded and fulfilled by their efforts and the new journey. Remember, it is important also to consider the needs of your family and, especially, to take care of yourself. Take time to give and get emotional support from your partner, other family members, friends, and your child's preschool teacher. Share with others some of the techniques that work with your child so that their learning opportunities will increase. Give child-directed special time and attention to your other children as well and help them understand why their sibling with autism sometimes doesn't play or talk with them. Give them some suggestions for how to play with their sibling. Many parents also find it helpful to be in a parent group to share joys and sorrows and ideas with other parents in a supportive and collaborative way. Remember that you are the expert in your child and know their likes and dislikes and how they learn best.

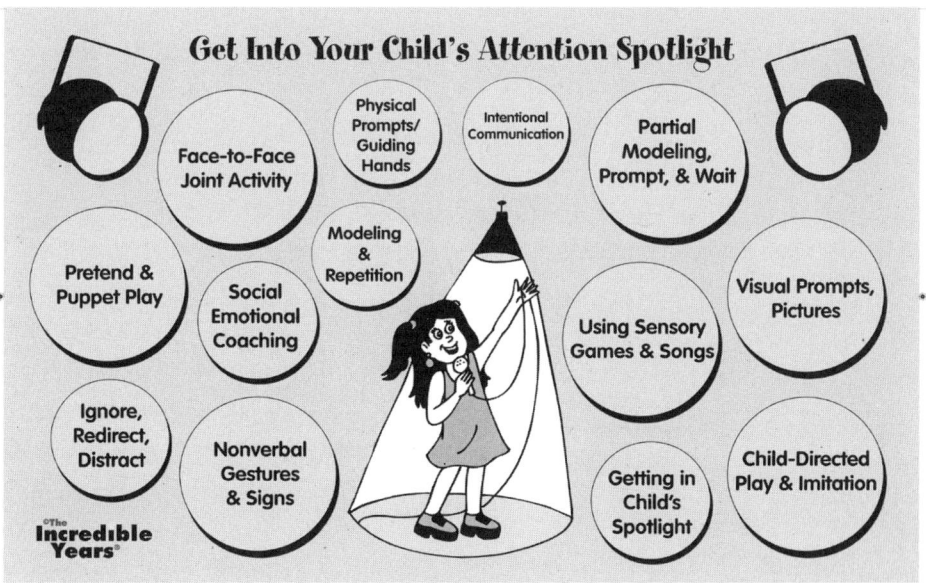

APPENDIX

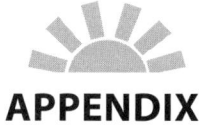

Incredible Years® Parent Strategies Questionnaire for Children with Autism (2-5 years)

Parent/Caregiver (name): _____

Parents learn extensively from self-reflection regarding their interactions with their children and the strategies that are working or not working. From these reflections you can determine personal goals for making changes in your approaches to bring about positive learning for your child. Use this checklist to think about your strengths and to assess areas you might want to work on for future goals.

Promoting Social, Emotional, Language and Academic Development in Children with Autism In this section we would like to get your idea of how confident you are in using the following strategies.	Very Unconfident	Somewhat Unconfident	Neutral	Confident	Very Confident
1. Simplifying and tailoring your language according to your child's individual language development?					
2. Identifying the specific ABCs: antecedents (A) that will motivate and prompt your child's target behaviors or words (B) and rewarding its occurrence with positive consequences (C).					
3. Being able to get in your child's attention spotlight to engage him or her in social and emotional learning opportunities?					
4. Being able to ignore and redirect your child's unwanted behaviors, giving your attention back when she or he behaves in the targeted way?					
5. Helping your child regulate his or her emotions?					
6. Using puppets and pretend play to teach your child social and emotional skills and to enhance communication?					
7. Using your child's sensory likes and dislikes such as auditory, tactile, visual, smell, taste/oral, proprioception (body space/balance/need for movement or stillness) to enhance his or her learning opportunities?					
8. Adapting teaching and materials to use your child's most effective learning mode (visual, auditory, motoric, sensory/tactile)?					
9. Managing your child's challenging behavior and following through with behavior plans and goals?					
10. Working with your child's classroom/early childhood teachers?					
11. Setting up structured play dates to help your child practice specific social skills?					
12. Developing and using visual supports (e.g., choice boards, command cards) to enhance your child's social, emotional and language learning?					

continued on next page

A. Specific Teaching Techniques to Enhance Language Development

In this section we'd like to get your idea of how often you use the following strategies to promote your child's language learning.

	Rarely/Never	Sometimes	Half the Time	Often	Very Often
1. Participate in child-directed, narrated play to increase interactive involvement and joint attention from my child.					
2. Use enthusiastic voice tone, songs, imitation, modeling, simple language, repetition and commenting using the "one up rule" to increase my child's verbal communications.					
3. Use descriptive academic coaching language to promote language skills (e.g., colors, shapes, positions, names of objects).					
4. Use visual prompts, gestures, preferred objects, books, and sensory likes, to strengthen language communication and joint interaction.					
5. Use verbal prompts, partial prompts, and pauses to wait for my child to look, gesture, or respond verbally before continuing.					
6. Use puppets to model and engage children in social communication.					

B. Specific Teaching Techniques to Enhance Social Development

In this section we'd like to get your idea of how often you use the following strategies to promote your child's social learning.

	Rarely/Never	Sometimes	Half the Time	Often	Very Often
1. Use social coaching to model, prompt practice, label, and praise social behaviors such as sharing, waiting, eye contact, helping, listening, asking, turn taking, and initiating an interaction.					
2. Use puppets to model, prompt, label, and practice social behaviors.					
3. Praise and reward my child for using appropriate social friendship skills.					
4. Identify specific social behavior goals for my child according to his/her play stage.					
5. Use books, games, and visual pictures to prompt, signal, and practice targeted social behaviors with my child.					
6. Use sensory social routines to enhance my child's arousal for learning.					
7. Comment on and praise prosocial peer models to increase my child's focus on appropriate social behavior					
8. Use intentional communication to help my child be aware of other children and their needs, interactions and to promote their joint attention and empathy during play activities.					
9. Set up peer playdates to promote my child's interactions with others and provide social coaching during these interactions.					

C. Specific Teaching Techniques to Enhance Emotional Development and Self-regulation

In this section we'd like to get your idea of how often you use the following strategies to promote your child's emotional development.

	Rarely/Never	Sometimes	Half the Time	Often	Very Often
1. Use emotion coaching to model, prompt, and label emotion language in my child.					
2. Model emotion language through words and facial expressions for my child.					
3. Use persistence coaching language to encourage my child's continuous effort to do a task. (e.g., "that's hard, but you keep trying!")					
4. Use pictures cards and photographs that portray people in various feeling states to teach my child emotion vocabulary and prompt his or her to use these visuals to express emotions.					

continued on next page

C. Specific Teaching Techniques to Enhance Emotional Development and Self-regulation *(continued)* In this section we'd like to get your idea of how often you use the following strategies to promote your child's emotional development.	Rarely/Never	Sometimes	Half the Time	Often	Very Often
5. Help my child understand how others feel through modeling, acknowledgement, mirroring back, labeling feelings, voice tone, and intentional communication.					
6. Recognize early cues of emotional dysregulation in my child and prompt his or her use of calm down strategies.					
7. Focus more of my attention on positive emotions than on negative emotions.					
8. When coaching negative emotions, also coach appropriate coping strategies (e.g., you are feeling mad but you are taking three deep breaths to calm your body down).					
9. Use story books to teach my child emotion words and promote empathy and guided practice.					
10. Use puppets that share their feelings to prompt my child's emotional language, social responses and empathy for others.					
11. Use visual self-regulation cards such as calm down thermometer, breathing, or turtle picture with my child.					

D. Specific Teaching to Enhance Behavior Management Strategies In this section we'd like to get your idea of how often you use the following strategies to promote your child's positive behaviors and decrease their inappropriate behaviors.	Rarely/Never	Sometimes	Half the Time	Often	Very Often
1. Give my child choices when possible.					
2. Use visual prompts, verbal and nonverbal signals and/or command cards to remind my child of our household rules, schedule, and appropriate behavior.					
3. Prepare my child for transitions with a predictable and visual routine.					
4. Give face-to-face praise paired with smiles, eye contact, enthusiastic tone of voice, and sensory likes to reward desired behavior.					
5. Reward self-regulation, joint attention, and responses to instructions with child's sensory likes.					
6. Wait for my child's response when asking a question about his or her wants.					
7. Use visual cues, gestures, and simple words to distract and redirect when my child is angry or frustrated.					
8. Ignore misbehavior that is not dangerous to my child or another child.					
9. Help other siblings or peers to understand my child's misbehavior and to respond to it with understanding and without reinforcing its occurrence.					
10. Set up problem solving scenarios with puppets to practice appropriate social responses to situations that are difficult for my child. (e.g., ask a friend to play, going to a birthday party)					

E. Strategies for Working with Teachers and School	Never	1–2 Times a Year	Once a Month	Once a Week	Daily
1. Use a system for regular school communication about my child (face-to-face communication, texts, notes, calls, meetings).					
2. Ask my child's teacher to tell me about how I can help support my child's school learning goals at home.					
3. Set up opportunities for to participate in classroom activities.					

continued on next page

E. Strategies for Working with Teachers and School *(continued)*	Never	1–2 Times a Year	Once a Month	Once a Week	Daily
4. Partner with teachers to provide ideas, materials, and support for classroom activities.					
5. Share with teachers my awareness of my child's sensory likes and dislikes and how these can be used to help motivate my child's learning.					
6. Share with teachers the ABC of behavior change in my child.					
7. Collaborate with teachers on a home-school behavior plan and share goals for my child.					
8. Becoming more aware of local opportunities to attend parent groups specifically for parents of children with autism.					

F. Planning and Support	Never	1–2 Times a Year	Once a Month	Once a Week	Daily
1. Review my progress in achieving the goals for my child and myself.					
2. Collaborate with other parents for solutions and support.					
3. Read the *Incredible Years Parent Book*.					
4. Manage my stress level utilizing positive cognitive strategies and gaining support from friends, family and teachers when needed.					

Appendix 363

Sample "How I am Incredible!" form for Hudson

My support people: Hudson.. 3 years old 9 months Family.. father primary caregiver; mother works full time; no other siblings	My Language Level *(e.g., no spoken language, visual language, 1-2 words, echolalic, good language)*: Limited eye contact Points to visual Sometimes echo's what is said Nods agreement –responds to verbal partial prompts for food & preferred toys Does not talk to peers and withdraws from their verbal overtures
My Play Level *(e.g., play alone, anxious or withdrawn, want to initiate play with others but don't know how, initiate but inappropriate)*: Some functional solo play – cars Play repetitive with no variation Doesn't seem interested and/or is anxious with peers Supported with play scripts reluctantly Reciprocal play with one child can be encouraged with social coaching, prompts & imitation (2 peers is too much stimulation and he withdraws)	My Sensory Likes *(e.g., trucks, swinging, music, water play, bananas)*: Enjoys spinning, being swung in a blanket Loves small skittles and will work for them Avoids social interaction Flaps when excited Withdraws in certain social situations - pulls clothing over head and is anxious
My Sensory Dislikes *(e.g., loud noises, certain smells)*: Doesn't like loud noises Upset when routine changes or his asked to stop spinning	My Parent's Goals for Me: *(e.g., make a friend, more words, follow directions)*:

©The Incredible Years®

Sample "How I am Incredible!" form for Amelia

My support people:

AMELIA'S FAMILY
~ 2 parents, younger toddler sibling, supportive parents

My Language Level *(e.g., no spoken language, visual language, 1-2 words, echolalic, good language):*

Responds to greetings from parents
Speaks in 3-4 word sentences when prompted at centre. Does not initiate verbal exchanges with other children and does not respond to their overtures
No emotion language

My Play Level *(e.g., play alone, anxious or withdrawn, want to initiate play with others but don't know how, initiate but inappropriate):*

Some parallel play
Needs adult support to model and prompt co-operative play with 1-2 peers or sibling
Limited self directed social interaction with peers
Interested in peers

My Sensory Likes *(e.g., trucks, swinging, music, water play, bananas):*

Likes play dough, reading books, games, puppets, running and jumping
Likes long, thin plant leaf which is with her constantly and she spins it
Joins mat times, sits with others in classroom
Does not like fine motor activities (some delays)

My Sensory Dislikes *(e.g., loud noises, certain smells):*

does not like fine motor activities

My Parent's Goals for Me: *(e.g., make a friend, more words, follow directions):*

©*The Incredible Years*®

REFERENCES

The Incredible Years (IY) parenting programs are a set of developmentally designed interventions (birth to 12 years) focused on strengthening parent-child interactions and improving parenting skills in order to prevent or reduce children's behavior problems and to promote their social, emotional, and academic competence. The effectiveness of the Toddler and Basic Preschool parent programs first developed in 1980 have been widely researched in multiple randomized control group trials, showing improvement in terms of parent stress levels, depression, and parental coping, as well as in children's social and self-regulatory behaviors and reducing their behavior difficulties.

Menting, A. T .A., Orobio de Castro, B., and Matthys, W. 2013. Clinical Psychology Review. See web site link for this meta-analysis review of 50 parent studies for Incredible Years Programs. https://www.incredibleyears.com/article/effectiveness-of-the-incredible-years-parent-training-to-modify-disruptive-and-prosocial-child-behavior-a-meta-analytic-review/

First Study with Children on the Autism Spectrum

One of the first studies carried out with parents of young children on the autism spectrum was conducted using the original IY Basic preschool parenting program designed for neurotypical children (Dababnah & Parish, 2016). The results showed promising outcomes but indicated the need for more specificity and video examples related to autism symptoms.

Dababnah S, Parish SL. Incredible Years Program Tailored to Parents of Preschoolers With Autism: Pilot Results. *Research on Social Work Practice*. 2016;26(4):372-385. doi:10.1177/1049731514558004 https://www.incredibleyears.com/article/incredible-years-program-tailored-to-parents-of-preschoolers-with-autism-pilot-results/

Webster-Stratton, C., Dababnah, S., & Olson, E. (2018). The Incredible Years Group-Based Parenting Program for Young Children with Autism Spectrum Disorder. In M. Siller and Morgan, L. (Eds.),

Handbook of Parent Coaching Interventions for Very Young Children with Autism (pp.261-283). Switzerland: Springer. https://www.incredibleyears.com/article/the-incredible-years-group-based-parenting-program-for-young-children-with-autism-spectrum-disorder-2/

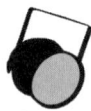
Subsequently two IY autism programs were specifically developed to target the needs and concerns of parents, child care workers, and preschool teachers of children ages 2-5 years on the autism spectrum or with language delays. The research regarding these recently developed programs is in the beginning stages. In New Zealand, the University of Canterbury published a report (2021) evaluating both of these programs with two cohorts of parents and teachers pre- and post-training and at follow-up. Both parents and teachers consistently reported that children's self-regulation, imagination, and social and emotion skills had "improved" or "greatly improved" post-participation in the program. The impact on the program parent participants wellbeing and coping skills was considered "very good". The results for the teacher program showed increased teacher confidence and frequency of use of the strategies learned as well as optimism about their future use of social and emotion coaching strategies with these children.

This New Zealand report and presentation may be found on the IY web site authored by Associate Professor Laurie McLay, Dr. Cara Swit, Professor Neville Blampied, Dr. Anne-Maire McIlroy and Dr. Dean Sutherland, University of Canterbury. https://www.incredibleyears.com/download/administrators/implementations/Ministry-of-Education-IYA-2021-evaluation-presentation-final-draft.pdf

Currently another study is being conducted in Spain in a program called FIRST STEPS. The protocol for the Spanish study published (2021) can be found on our web site by the authors Fátima Valencia, Elena Urbiola, Marina Romero-González , Inmaculada Navas, María Elías, Alexandra Garriz, Almudena Ramírez and Laia Villalta.

Valencia, F., Urbiola, E., Romero-González, M., Navas, I., Elías, M., Garriz, A., Ramírez, A., and Villalta, L. (2021). Protocol for a randomized pilot study (FIRST STEPS): implementation of the Incredible Years-ASLD® program in Spanish children with autism and preterm children with communication and/or socialization difficulties. *Trials 22*, 291.https://doi.org/10.1186/s13063-021-05229-1 https://www.incredibleyears.com/article/protocol-for-a-randomized-pilot-study-first-steps-implementation-of-the-incredible-years-asld-program-in-spanish-children-with-autism-and-preterm-children-with-communication-and-or-socializat/

A third study is being conducted at the University of Wales. See web site for this published research protocol. https://www.incredibleyears.com/article/the-incredible-years-autism-spectrum-and-language-delays-parent-program-a-pragmatic-feasibility-randomized-controlled-trial/

Williams ME, Hastings RP, Hutchings J. The Incredible Years Autism Spectrum and Language Delays Parent Program: A pragmatic, feasibility randomized controlled trial. *Autism Research.* 2020;13(6):1011–22.

Other reports can be found on our web site. These include:

McAleese, M., & Nesbitt, A. (2018). *The Incredible Years® Autism Spectrum and Language Delays (IY-ASLD) Programme for Parents delivered for Northern Health and Social Care Trust (NHSCT).* Northern Health and Social Care Trust, Northern Ireland. https://www.incredibleyears.com/article/the-incredible-years-autism-spectrum-and-language-delays-iy-asld-programme-for-parents-delivered-for-northern-health-and-social-care-trust-nhsct/

Evans, S. & Crumpton, J. (2017). Incredible Years® Autism Spectrum Parent Programme: Pilot Study, Powys, 2015-2017. Powys Teaching Health Board. https://www.incredibleyears.com/article/incredible-years-autism-spectrum-parent-programme-pilot-study-powys-2015-2017/

Dababnah, S., Olson, E.M., & Huntington, S. (2017). Tailoring an Evidence-Based Practice to Parents Raising Preschoolers with Autism: Pilot Trial of The Incredible Years. Presented at

International Meeting for Autism Research https://www.incredibleyears.com/article/tailoring-an-evidence-based-practice-to-parents-raising-preschoolers-with-autism-pilot-trial-of-the-incredible-years/

Muschietti-Piana, V.E. (2019). *Changes in Parental Self-Efficacy Following "Autism Spectrum Disorder & Language Delay Incredible Years®" Parenting Program* (Unpublished dissertation). Middlesex, London. https://www.incredibleyears.com/article/changes-in-parental-self-efficacy-following-autism-spectrum-disorder-language-delay-incredible-years-parenting-program/

You can continue to check the IY web site for new studies emerging from evaluation of these IY autism parent and preschool teacher intervention programs.

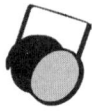

There is a wealth of impressive autism research and evaluation of different interventions using the ABA model, Pivotal Response Training (PRT) (e.g., Koegel, Schreibmann) and the Early Start Denver Model (ESDM) (e.g., Rogers, Dawson, Stern). Many of these programs are described in the following book, which also includes the Webster-Stratton, Dababnah, & Olson (2018) chapter referenced above on the Incredible Years autism programs.

Siller, M. and Morgan, L. (Eds.), Handbook of Parent-Implemented Interventions for Very Young Children with Autism (2018) Switzerland: Springer International Publishing.